Foundational Issues in Human Brain Mapping

Foundational Issues in Human Brain Mapping

edited by Stephen José Hanson and Martin Bunzl

A Bradford Book
The MIT Press
Cambridge, Massachusetts
London, England

MIT Press books may be purchased at special quantity discounts for business or sales promotional use. For information, please email special_sales@mitpress.mit.edu or write to Special Sales Department, The MIT Press, 55 Hayward Street, Cambridge, MA 02142.

This book was set in Stone Serif and Stone Sans on 3B2 by Asco Typesetters, Hong Kong. Printed and bound in the United States of America.

Library of Congress Cataloging-in-Publication Data

Foundational issues in human brain mapping / edited by Stephen José Hanson and Martin Bunzl.
   p. ; cm.
"A Bradford Book."
Includes bibliographical references and index.
ISBN 978-0-262-01402-1 (hardcover : alk. paper)—ISBN 978-0-262-51394-4 (pbk. : alk. paper)
1. Brain mapping. 2. Brain—Magnetic resonance imaging. I. Hanson, Stephen José. II. Bunzl, Martin.
[DNLM: 1. Brain Mapping. 2. Brain—physiology. 3. Data Interpretation, Statistical. 4. Magnetic Resonance Imaging. 5. Research Design. WL 335 F771 2010]
QP385.F68   2010
612.8'2—dc22   2009036078

10 9 8 7 6 5 4 3 2 1

Contents

Acknowledgments

We gratefully recognize the support of the Office of the Vice President for Academic Affairs at Rutgers and the McDonnell Foundation in providing funds for the meeting that led to this volume, the unflagging patience and enthusiasm of our editor Tom Stone, the valiant and the precise work of Helen Colby in wrangling our contributions into presentable shape.

Introduction

This is a watershed moment in the field of neuroimaging. At least three emerging trends have been slowly reframing the field for the last five years. Each one of these trends intersects with a foundational issue in human brain mapping, affecting the measurement or methodological or theoretical nature of the overall field. First are methodological problems that have arisen concerning nonindependence of samples—in effect the lack of cross-validation procedures applied in the field, especially in social neuroscience (SN). This has caused a systematic reevaluation of scores of SN studies reporting correlational results literally "too good to be true," because they weren't. This type of methodological problem, at first glance, may appear arbitrary and due to an oversight of some sort; however, it actually relates to a larger set of methodological issues that are at the very foundation of the neuroimaging enterprise itself. The overall scale of the typical neuroimaging dataset, the intrinsic noise level, and its intrinsic multivariate nature have all been an enormous challenge in the field.

To compound these issues, statisticians early in the enterprise advised those developing new tools (e.g., statistical parametric mapping or SPM) to take a conservative approach to statistical analysis, estimation, and design in neuroimaging. Unfortunately, this led researchers to apply the general linear model (GLM) to single voxels and to engage in Neyman-Pearson hypothesis testing. But for what hypothesis? Apparently, that each voxel was significantly different from its level in a "minimally different" condition, the so-called Donders paradigm. Unfortunately, this approach suffers from the lack of cross-validation, which promotes the painting of voxels as "active," "engaged," or otherwise "on" when they actually may be false alarms. More disturbingly, in that brain mapping's *sin qua non* is to localize function, many voxels that should be mapped would simply not be mapped.

The second trend is, in fact, a direct response to the foundational nature of the neuroimaging data itself. New methods have begun to appear in the human brain mapping field that directly assess the voxel covariation in that they classify conditional on the multivariate patterns of voxels. At a micro-level, these new methods attempt to exploit the obvious neural level of interactions that are contiguous within areas of the brain. These methods are based on statistical learning theories that have been developed and applied for more than a decade in the neural information processing field for many kinds of problems and applications. They are standardly cross-validated, nonlinear, multivariate, and regularized. In effect, they can provide valid and reliable estimates of cortical diagnosticity and reveal maps of the stimulus waveform resulting in new visualizations of cortical structure and similarity. This trend is likely to cause significant changes in human brain mapping as new questions and answers often result from the second generation of scientific methods that supplant and revisit the foundational questions that ignited the field in the first place.

The intersection between the first trend and this second one leads to new concerns about localization and modularity. Is there a "face area," a "place area," and so on? Or are these well known results in the brain mapping literature a result of a methodological artifact promoted by features of the standard methods? These newer multivariate classifier methods raise many important questions about the original framing of the brain mapping problem and the nature of the brain response at the spatial level functional magnetic resonance imaging (fMRI) affords us. Wherever these new methods lead us, the human brain mapping field is evolving and is beginning to search for new metaphors, measurement, and data structures.

There is a third trend that follows in the footsteps of the second, which relies on new methods from computer science and machine learning, and focuses on a new data structure—*the graph*. Recent trends have focused on the relationship between regions of interest and their interactivity. The brain is, of course, composed of sets of distinct and overlapping networks somehow creating cognitive and perceptual processing. In the past ten years, interest has accumulated concerning the identification of various brain networks. One of the more commonly encountered networks is the so-called mirror system, which appears to have some functional relationship to the nature of perception action coupling. Other "social" networks seemingly have been identified, including "mentalizing" and "face recognition" as well as "self" or "intrinsic" networks.

All this is well and good, except for the fact that data structures more complex than a single region of interest (ROI) or node require search, since even simple networks of four nodes or more have greater than 59,065 possible alternative graph hypotheses. This kind of localization is therefore not possible without some sophisticated search methods. Unfortunately, graph search must be predicated on node localization, which, as we just discussed, is under some revision in terms of methods and tools. Graph search also depends on time series extraction, which with the blood oxygen level–dependent (BOLD) signal, provides some time resolution challenges that may allow extraction only to greater than 100 ms, making simpler perceptual processing out of reach with fMRI and proper graph search. Nonetheless, it does open the door to many of the mid-size networks that many cognitive and social neuroscientists find plausible.

Consequently, this shift toward graphs from nodes requires yet another reframing of the field, which focuses on processes over localization. Graph methods in neuro-imaging have been primarily confirmatory and created the illusion that graph structure itself was easily extracted from a few statistically significant blobs that had some modal relationship to atlas-based brain areas. Clearly, whatever methods emerge for graph estimates, they will have to require search and cross-validation, as well as confirmation across experiments that attempt to predict graph modulation, edge variation, and specific graph structure.

These trends in the field seemed urgent enough to discuss and examine in a workshop that brought together neuroimagers with a unique sounding board consisting of a group of philosophers. We developed an agenda based on these trends and invited leading neuroimagers and philosophers sophisticated in cognitive science and cognitive neuroscience. This created an exciting workshop the two of us organized in the late spring of 2007 in New Brunswick, New Jersey. Because of its special nature and the lack of connection between participants, this workshop certainly had the potential of falling into the usual set of fossilized positions, with little or no interaction between the various participants. More of a concern was the lack of familiarity many neuroimagers might have had with methodologies or arguments resulting from philosophers examining the same research. In fact, the venue and participants exceeded our expectations concerning the level of discussion, debate, and interaction between philosophers and neuroimagers. More interesting, debates focused on central issues neuroimagers had resolved or put to rest and not reexamined over many years. Often, a well placed query from a philosopher, looking for clarification, sparked heated debates between neuroimagers. This volume represents an attempt by the workshop organizers to capture some of the liveliness of these debates with a subset of the meeting participants along with other contributors whose work seemed relevant and important to the overall themes of the book.

What follows is organized around a set of specific foci that cross-cut the emerging themes discussed in this Introduction. Throughout the meeting there was clearly a level of controversy that we have attempted to reflect by inviting specific commentaries and conversations concerning the various pieces by different authors.

The first section (Location and Representation) intersects with emerging trends that involve both localization (trend 2) and statistical measurement (trend 1). In this section, we revisit the idea of localizers and the implications for brain localization more generally (Kanwisher, Friston). This section also includes a contribution concerning trend 2, specifically in which multivariate pattern analysis as an alternative to the standard methods is framed and formally proposed (Haxby) and further discussed in the context of high-resolution methods (Grill-Spector in Section III: Design and the Signal). The section ends with an informal discussion that attempts to replicate the tenor of our meeting and provides a larger perspective on the nature of localization and the tacit assumptions of neuroimagers about how modularity of function and localization in the brain are related (Bunzl, Hanson, Poldrack).

In the next section (Inference and New Data Structures), intersections occur with both trend 1 and trend 3, with a contribution about the controversies concerning correlations of fMRI data and social attributions (Vul, Kanwisher). A focus of the chapter is on the nonindependence or lack of cross-validation that has plagued the social neuroscience field more specifically. A dissenting comment by Poldrack follows as well as a riposte by Vul and Kanwisher, which we hope provide some degree of resolution of these claims and counterclaims. The next contribution (Mole and Klein) discusses what inferences can be drawn from neuroimaging data and lays out the importance of the "consistency fallacy." Harman further clarifies this discussion and adds inference worries regarding the use of neuroimaging data. This section concludes with a chapter that offers a framework for a new neuroimaging data structure, the graph, which, according to the authors (Hanson and Glymour) has been misappropriated without proper methods of estimation or search.

The third section (Design and the Signal) addresses the underlying signal properties of BOLD and the design issues related to inference. The problems that ensue when simple statistical questions are posed cut across trends 2 and 3. The standard inferential design approach in neuroimaging is rife with assumptions of factorial independence of processes and underlying neural signal that are unlikely to be true (Poldrack), and much of the resting state properties of BOLD appear to be systematic, with some intrinsic activity state that is typically more activated during "rest" conditions (Biswal). All of this is further compounded by individual differences in anatomy and functional response (Poline).

The final section (Underdetermination of Theory by Data) ties together all the trends in more philosophical treatments of the nature of what we are trying to measure. Contributors here have asked foundational questions about the nature of the representations neuroimaging presents (Roskies) as well as just what inferences we are entitled to make from them (Loosemore and Harley; Bechtel and Richardson). The section closes with a wide-ranging discussion (Coltheart) of many of the papers in this volume, posing the key question of just what brain imaging is for.

This volume documents the many challenges the field of neuroimaging faces, but it is noteworthy that it is the very researchers in the field who have helped develop and popularize the standard human brain mapping framework that have been among the most ardent critics of this same framework. As the field evolves, we think it is essential to continue to revisit foundational questions. In this sense, we offer this volume as the opening round of what we hope will be an ongoing and lively debate framing the foundations of human brain mapping.

I   Location and Representation

1 A Critique of Functional Localizers

Karl J. Friston, Pia Rotshtein, Joy J. Geng, Philipp Sterzer, and Rik N. Henson

The use of functional localizers to constrain the analysis of functional magnetic resonance imaging (fMRI) data is becoming popular in neuroimaging. This approach entails a separate experiment to localize areas in the brain that serve to guide, constrain, or interpret results from a main experiment. The need and motivation for functional localizers are often not stated explicitly and sometimes unclear. Nevertheless, several colleagues have encountered reviewers who thought that omitting a functional localizer did not conform to good or standard practice. The purpose of this commentary is to provide a reference for people who do not want to use functional localizers and have to defend themselves against the contrary attitudes of reviewers (see appendix 1.A for some verbatim comments).

The term *functional localizer* is generally used in the context of stereotactic neurosurgery or radiosurgical treatment planning. It refers to a functional (e.g., fMRI) experiment that is used to disclose eloquent cortex (e.g. Liu et al. 2000). The word *functional* distinguishes this localization from the anatomic information in structural MRI or computed tomographic (CT) scans. The human brain mapping community has adopted this term to refer to an auxiliary fMRI experiment that constrains the analysis or interpretation of a main fMRI experiment. Although every fMRI study is a study of functional localization in the human brain, we will take functional localizer to mean a separate scanning session that has been divorced from the functional experiment proper.

Our aim is to frame some issues that may be useful when motivating and critiquing the use of localizers (or not using them). Specifically, we focus on four issues:

- Functional regions of interest (fROI), such as the fusiform face area (FFA), the lateral occipital complex (LOC), or visual word form area (VWFA), are often viewed as useful vehicles to characterize functional anatomy. Although fROIs are sufficient to establish functional selectivity, they preclude inferences about functional specialization. This is because functional specialization entails anatomical specificity (i.e., the specialized region exhibits more functional selectivity than another region). This anatomical specificity cannot be addressed with a single fROI.

• The validity of fROI constructs depends on their context sensitivity. For example, the VWFA may process words in one context, but not another. Equivalently, the voxels comprising the FFA may change when processing one facial attribute relative to another. Unless an fROI is context-invariant, it may not provide the most appropriate constraint with which to analyze responses in a different context. Indeed, the introduction of factorial designs to neuroimaging was driven by context-sensitive specialization implied by interactions between factors, and the empirical failure of pure insertion (Friston et al. 1996). This leads to the next point.

• Separate localizer designs often represent missed opportunities, in relation to factorial designs. Eliciting main effects in the localizer and main experiments separately precludes tests for interactions (i.e., differences in activation between the localizer and main sessions). Localizer designs could be regarded as a slightly retrograde development in experimental design, in that inferences about effects in the main experiment usually rest on simple subtraction and pure insertion. Clearly, many designs cannot be made factorial. However, when they can, there are compelling reasons to use factorial designs. Our main point here is "people who like localizers should like factorials even more." (Jon Driver, personal communication).

• The practice of averaging responses over voxels in an fROI has clear advantages in simplifying analyses. However, averaging entails some strong assumptions about responses that practitioners may not have considered. Some of these assumptions are untenable (e.g., homogeneity across the fROI), and historically have led to the development of voxel-based analysis (i.e., statistical parametric mapping or SPM). In this sense, fROI represents another retrograde development.

• An advantage of fROI averages is that they summarize subject-specific responses without assuming anatomical homology over subjects. However, there may be more sensitive and principled approaches to the problem of functional–anatomical variability.

Several other issues, which are not the subject of this critique, include the following:

• The labeling of regional responses using anatomic or functional information from another study. This study could be a localizer, a retinotopic mapping study, or indeed someone else's study of a related effect. We are concerned only with functional localizers that are used to constrain analysis, not the post hoc use of localizing information to label the results of an analysis.

• The use of functional (as opposed to anatomical) constraints to characterize regional responses. This is an important component of many analyses, particularly in the context of factorial designs. Functional constraints per se are essential for hypothesis-led and powerful inference. Our focus is on the use of fROI averages to summarize regional responses, not on their useful role in constraining searches to regional responses within the fROI.

• The principled use of localizers in designs that require separate sessions or are not inherently factorial. This commentary is organized as follows: First, we review the functional localizer approach to fMRI data analysis, its motivation, and its relation to conventional multifactorial experimental designs. We then deconstruct two recent experiments reported in the literature, which used functional localizers, to reprise the main points of the first section. The first is an example of functional localizers in the study of object-defining properties. The second uses functional localizers to characterize evoked responses associated with attentional shifts.

Theoretical Issues

Functional Localizers and fROI

Functional localizers can be thought of as the splitting of a study into two parts. One part (the localizer) involves the comparison of two or more conditions (e.g., pictures of faces versus pictures of houses) to isolate a functionally specialized region (e.g., the fusiform face area; Kanwisher et al., 1997). The other part constitutes the main experiment and usually involves comparing further conditions that have not been explored previously (e.g., pictures of dogs that are named at either the basic level—"Dog"— or subordinate level—"Dalmatian"). These are used to establish the functional selectivity of the fROI. The results of the functional localizer (i.e., the fROI) are used to constrain, anatomically, the search for effects in the main experiment. When the conditions in the functional localizer and the main experiment share a factor, there is an implicit factorial design, in which the localizer can be considered as a level in an extra factor (localizer versus main). See figure 1.1 for two examples.

Functional localizers raise two issues. First, why include an extra factor in the experimental design and, second, why perform it separately? The following section addresses these two questions.

Why Use Functional Localizers?

Attribution Versus Constraints Functional localizers assume there is some effect that has an important role in interpreting or constraining the analysis of the effects in the main experiment. One common use of localizers is to inform the labeling of region-specific effects identified in a separate analysis of the main experiment (e.g., retinotopic mapping). Here, the results of the localizer are used to either a priori constrain the analysis of the main experiment to a subset of voxels according to some cortical parcellation scheme (e.g., retinotopy) or post hoc to assign labels to regional effects of the main experiment (e.g., V2). The usefulness of such constraints depends on their anatomic and physiological validity. The use of functional localizers is common in studies of early visual processing, because the fine-grained retinotopic organization of early

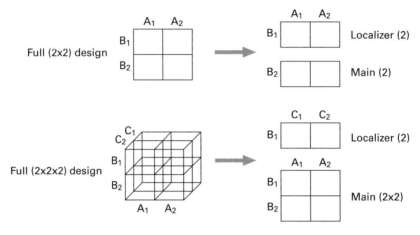

Dissembling full designs to create functional localizers

and the implicit loss of cells

Figure 1.1
A schematic showing the relationship between functional localizers and their multifactorial
parents.

visual areas is well established and largely cue-invariant. This calls for a characterization of structure–function relationships on an appropriate spatial scale.

This critique is not concerned with the use of localizers that inform the analysis, attribution, or interpretation post hoc. It is concerned with the use of localizers as constraints on the analysis per se. These constraints may or may not be valid. Such
constraints appear to operate in several ways. First, the inclusion of the localizer enables one to constrain the search for significant effects of the main factors by looking
only in areas activated by the localizer. Here, the objective is to increase the sensitivity of searches for regionally specific effects in the main experiment (by reducing the
problem of multiple statistical comparisons). Second, one can assess the effects of
the main factors on the average response of the areas activated by the localizer. The
latter is a special case of constrained inference that is not concerned with where
effects are expressed (the localizing fROI prescribes this). The question here is what
effects the main factors have on the average response. We will deal with these two
cases in turn.

Functionally Constrained Searches   If the localizer is chosen carefully, it can provide a
tremendous increase in sensitivity because it reduces the multiple comparisons problem entailed by searching over large volumes of brain. The anatomical constraints
functional localizers afford usually take the form of regions of interest. These are de-

fined operationally by reliable effects in the localizer. The search for significant effects in the main experiment can then be constrained to voxels showing maximal responses within the fROI (ideally using a Bonferroni correction for the number of such maxima). Alternatively, a random field correction, as implemented in SPM, is applied to all voxels within the fROI. This is known as a small volume correction (SVC) (see Worsley et al. 1996). Constrained searches would be preferred if one wanted to search for functionally heterogeneous responses within an fROI. For example, only part of the V5 complex, defined by visual motion, may be engaged during the perception of apparent motion.

Constrained searches of this sort are standard practice in conventional fMRI analyses that do not use functional localizers. Perhaps the most common examples are searches for differences among event types in event-related designs limited to regions that respond to all events relative to the interevent baseline. This constrained search relies on the fact that differences among event-related responses are orthogonal to their average (i.e., do not bias the inference). In balanced factorial designs, the main effects and interactions are, by design, orthogonal. This means that one can take the maxima, or fROI, of one effect and constrain the search for the other effects to the ensuing voxels. For example, two effects might define plasticity in the motor system: a main effect of movement (motor-related responses) and a movement-by-time interaction (learning-related changes in those responses). The search for interactions can be restricted to maxima exhibiting a main effect of movement to infer motor plasticity. This example highlights an important point, namely, main effects usually constrain the search for interactions. This is because finding a significant interaction between factors A and B in the presence of a main effect of A entitles one to say that responses to A, in A-selective regions, depend on B. We will see in the following text that these interactions are usually precluded in localizer designs.

This well-established approach to constrained statistical searches does not rely on a separate localizer. The key thing to appreciate is that contrast testing for a particular effect can be used as a localizer for the remaining (orthogonal) effects. In this sense, any factorial fMRI study has as many functional localizers, embedded within it, as there are orthogonal contrasts. A typical two-by-two design has three orthogonal contrasts. The natural conclusion is that all fMRI experiments are simply collections of functional localizers. This is quite sensible given that human brain mapping is about functional localization. In short, the use of localizing contrasts to provide constraints on the search for orthogonal effects has a long history (e.g., Friston et al. 1996), is principled, and rests an explicit or implicit (localizer) factorial design that may or may not be balanced.

Note that this approach assumes a modular functional architecture. For example, basing functional constraints on faces versus houses assumes that all face-related processes occur only within regions that show a stronger response to faces compared to houses. More generally, one should be aware that constraining the search for interaction to regions showing main effects will miss crossover interactions. For example, a region that activates in one context but deactivates in another will exhibit no main effect and will be missed in a contained search. All constraints should be used in an informed and careful fashion. Next, we discuss approaches that do not constrain the search for functionally selective responses but examine the functional selectivity of the fROI itself.

Functional ROI   The second reason one might want to use a localizer is to restrict the analysis to the responses of the fROI itself (i.e., responses averaged over voxels within the fROI). In this case, there is only one statistical inference and no need to adjust the P value. The motivation goes beyond simply increasing sensitivity, because the nature of the response variable is changed qualitatively, from a collection of regional responses at each voxel to a summary of their collective response, that is, average. In this context, responses elsewhere in the brain are not of interest; the researcher has reduced functional anatomy to a single brain region, defined operationally by the functional localizer. This is perfectly tenable, with the qualification that inferences relate to, and only to, some ad hoc fROI.

This approach has the advantage of being focussed, providing for uncomplicated accounts of responses within a prespecified fROI. However, fROIs could be regarded as colloquial in the sense that they are not derived from any formal functional ontology. The point here is that an ad hoc fROI cannot participate in structure–function ontologies unless it has some structurally invariant functional properties. In short, a useful fROI should comprise the same voxels in different contexts. There are many examples of functionally segregated regions that do this. For instance, all the anatomical and physiological evidence suggests that V5 is specialized for motion processing. Similarly, the anatomical profile of selectivity in V1 units is largely context-invariant (e.g., ocular dominance columns). However, even in V1, extra-classical receptive field effects and attentional modulation confer context sensitivity at some level of analysis. This context sensitivity is assessed with interactions in factorial experiments. The simple and logical critique of fROI, defined by localizers, is that the context sensitivity of their anatomy cannot be assessed because localizer designs preclude the assessment of interactions. This means that localizers are unable to establish the structural invariance properties of the fROI they are designed to study.

Functional Selectivity Versus Functional Specialization   A more fundamental problem with fROIs is that they preclude any inferences about functional specialization in the brain. There is a subtle but important distinction between functional selectivity and functional specialization. Functional selectivity is defined operationally by demonstrating functional responses in a single unit or area that are selective or specific to some stimulus or task attribute (i.e., orientation of a visually presented bar or category of an object). Functional selectivity implies specificity in terms of what elicits a neuronal response. In contrast, functional specialization is not an operational definition; it is an inference that a particular unit or brain area specializes in some function or computation. This inference rests on an anatomical specificity in terms of where functionally selective responses are expressed. For example, V5 or MT expresses functionally selective responses to motion and is functionally specialized for motion because motion-selective responses are restricted largely to this area. In short, functional selectivity implies responses that are specific to a domain of function or stimulus-space. Conversely, the specificity in functional specialization refers to structural or anatomical space.

The distinction between functional selectivity and specialization has important implications for fROIs; fROIs are entirely sufficient to establish functional selectivity because one can examine their responses in a large number of contexts. However, they cannot be used to infer functional specialization because they are blind to responses elsewhere in the brain. Put simply, for every face-related process, there may be another area that expresses a more selective response than the FFA. The only way one would know this would be to employ a conventional SPM analysis. A simple example may help to clarify this point.

Imagine a study of implicit face recognition using an incidental same-different judgment task. The design has two factors; face versus nonface and familiar versus unfamiliar. A conventional analysis reveals a main effect of faces in the FFA and a main effect of familiarity higher in the ventral stream. Critically, the interaction between faces and familiarity elicits the greatest response in a face-recognition area (FRA). One might then infer that the FRA was specialized for facial recognition and that the implicit recognition of faces involved a set of areas that included the FFA and FRA, specialized for presemantic processing and recognition, respectively.

Functional ROI analyses afford a much more limited inference. The FFA would show a main effect of faces and could, indeed, show a face by familiarity interaction that is mediated by backward connections from the FRA. The proper conclusion here is that the FFA is functionally selective for faces and face recognition. However, the inference that the FFA is specialized for facial recognition would be wrong because of the anatomical bias imposed by the fROI. This face-recognition study is not a thought experiment. It was reported in Gorno-Tempini et al. (1998):

The areas specialised for the perceptual analysis of faces (irrespective of whether they are famous or non-famous) are the right lingual and bilateral fusiform gyri, while the areas specialised for famous stimuli (irrespective of whether they are faces or names) spread from the left anterior temporal to the left temporoparietal regions. One specific area, the more lateral portion of the left anterior middle temporal gyrus, showed increased activation for famous faces relative to famous proper names.

Note that Gorno-Tempini et al. are entitled to talk about specialization because they used an SPM analysis to characterize functional selectivity throughout the ventral stream.

The preceding example highlights the difficulties fROI-based characterizations contend with, when a cognitive process relies on several areas. This is particularly relevant to visual processing hierarchies in which the FFA and VWFA reside. The responses of these areas are subject to both bottom-up and top-down effects (Friston 2003) and call for an analysis of selective responses that is not constrained to a single region. It had already been shown that face-selective responses were subject to top-down influences from as far away as the parietal cortex before the FFA was described (Dolan et al. 1997).

In short, to reduce functional anatomy to fROIs and their functional selectivity assumes we know a priori the parcellation and segregation of function within the cortex. Furthermore, it assumes that the voxels comprising the fROI do not change with neuronal context (McIntosh 2000) or the level of task analysis. Some might argue it is premature to invoke fROI to characterize functional anatomy. The equivalent agenda for *Areae anatomicae* (Brodmann 1909/1994), using anatomic criteria, is still incomplete after more than a century's work (Kötter and Wanke 2005).

Background to ROI   The imaging community has already entertained the debate about ROI in the early days of brain mapping with positron emission tomography (PET). Initially, in the late 1980s, people reported their results using ROIs defined by structural anatomy, perfusion, or receptor binding. Note that these ROIs were based on defining characteristics of the underlying tissue and did not reflect any functional role of that region (i.e., were not fROIs). These ROIs were assumed to be a useful summary of the distributed patterns of activity evoked. However, the problem was that ROIs preempted the questions they were supposed to answer, namely, where are region-specific responses expressed? Put simply, an ROI was the result, not the hypothesis.

One example of the pitfalls of ROI is the study of ventricular enlargement in schizophrenia. Because the ventricular ROI is easy to measure, it was the focus of imaging research in schizophrenia for almost a decade. The ventricles have no role in the pathophysiology of schizophrenia and, not surprisingly, this research went nowhere. The ad hoc and unprincipled basis for the parcellation of functional anatomy into ROI prompted the development of voxel-based approaches, namely, statistical parametric mapping. The reprise of ROI in the form of fROI, many years later, raises the same issues in a somewhat more subtle way. Now, the ad hoc nature of fROI lies in the choice of the localizer that defines the region. For example, is the only appropriate definition of the FFA the contrast of faces versus houses? If this is so by convention, what if the convention is wrong?

On a more positive note, fROI have utility in well-established research programs focusing on a specific part of the brain. Operational constructs such as FFA or VWFA play an important role in focusing experiments and enabling scientific exchange at a colloquial level. For example, the adoption of a "standard" definition of the FFA (as the set of voxels more active for faces than, say, houses) allows researchers to compare directly the effects of different manipulations. This can proceed without relying on anatomical criteria and ameliorating the effects of differences in the spatial properties of their functional images. Another virtue to arise from the fROI tradition is the emphasis on replication (focus on activations that are evident in multiple separate experiments) and refinement (the use of increasingly subtle comparisons to establish selectivity).

In summary, a fixed operational definition of fROI provides a strict and rigorous way of accumulating evidence across studies. However, it must be remembered that such operational definitions make assumptions about context invariance and functional ontology that may not turn out to be true.

fROI Averaging   One reason for averaging within an fROI is the assumption that it increases the signal-to-noise ratio. Unfortunately, this assumption is not necessarily true. The most efficient averaging depends on how the signal and noise are deployed within the fROI. Generally, the best (minimum variance) unbiased estimate of the fROI response would involve spatially whitening the data, accounting for spatial correlations and inhomogeneity in both signal and noise. Simple averaging assumes the noise is uncorrelated and uniform. Furthermore, it assumes the signal is expressed identically at every voxel. This is a strong assumption. It is possible that functionally heterogeneous responses within the fROI cause half the fROI to activate and the other half to deactivate (this is not an uncommon architectural principle in the brain. Common examples here are surround inhibition in receptive fields and lateral interactions that mediate winner-take-all mechanisms in the brain. An average, in this case, will suppress signal-to-noise. We generally deal with this by taking the first eigen variate of an fROI, which uses the temporal covariance of voxels in the fROI, to find coherent spatial modes of activity (see spm_regions at http://www.fil.ion.ucl.ac.uk/spm). The principal eigen variate is, like the average, simply a summary of the responses within an fROI. Unlike the average, it does not assume homogeneous responses within the fROI. It should be noted that if one gets a significant result using the average, then it is valid. The point made here is that the average is not the most principled measure of a regional response.

Smoothing and the matched filter theorem address the equivalent issue in conventional voxel-based analysis. Under the assumption that the spatial dependencies of signal and noise are stationary, the most effective filter weights match the spatial scale of the signal. On the basis of optical imaging experiments, we know that hemodynamic response has a spatial scale around 4 mm. Usually, single-subject data are smoothed between 4 and 6 mm. This smoothing effectively transforms the data into an ensemble of fROI averages at every point in the brain. The implicit fROI corresponds to the smoothing kernel centered at each voxel. In this sense, a standard SPM analysis can be regarded as an analysis of all possible fROIs, whose spatial scale is physiologically informed and determined by smoothing. In the context of this discussion, the signal-to-noise of a single voxel (e.g., maximum of a localizing contrast) can be made the same as the fROI average, provided the smoothing kernel and spatial scale of the fROI are comparable.

We have not distinguished between analyzing the average response of an fROI and averaging the estimated responses (i.e., contrast of parameter estimates, regression coefficients, etc.) it encompasses. This is because the two procedures give the same result. Averaging and response estimation with the general linear model are both linear operations and are commutative.[1] This means that the order of averaging and estimation is irrelevant. Furthermore, the same results will be obtained irrespective of whether or not the images are spatially normalized. This is because the fROI is subject to the same transformation as the underlying data. We mention this because one argument made in favor of fROI is that they can accommodate between-subject variations in functional anatomy, if the fROI response of each subject is taken to a second (between-subject) level for inference.

Intersubject Averaging   In multisubject studies, one has to account for between-subject variations in functional anatomy. The precise anatomical location of the FFA, for example, may vary over individuals. Conventionally, with voxel-based analyses, one assumes that most of this variability can be removed by spatial normalization (Ashburner and Friston 1999). Residual variability in functional anatomy that persists after anatomical normalization is usually accommodated by further smoothing the data according to the matched filter theorem. This matches the spatial dispersion induced by this residual variability (see above). In other words, smoothing is used to increase the probability that responses from different subjects overlap.

Clearly, this approach reduces spatial resolution. Furthermore, the degree of spatial dispersion of responses over subjects is unknown and is an active area of research. This means the choice of smoothing is motivated rather anecdotally. An alternative to smoothing, in a standard anatomical space, is to pool data from different subjects using functional criteria. Specifically, the average responses of an fROI, defined for each subject, enter an analysis of variance (ANOVA), thereby discounting between-subject variations in anatomy and eschewing any need for spatial normalization. This may be another reason why localizers have become so popular in the literature. However, even though this seems to be an important motivation for fROI, this motivation does not require fROIs to be defined from a localizer session. The same approach can be taken within a voxel-based analysis of single-subject data (with or without spatial normalization). In other words, it is very simple to perform an ANOVA on contrasts selected from the maxima of an orthogonal localizing contrast in a subject-specific fashion.

The advantage of this procedure over fROI averages is that the subject-specific maxima can be reported, providing a quantitative and useful characterization of intersubject variability in functional anatomy. Furthermore, this avoids defining fROI using ad hoc threshold criteria and the assumption of functional homogeneity with the fROI. Having said this, one could argue that any attempt to define an irregular cluster of activated voxels with a few measures (e.g., size, Talairach coordinates of maximum response) is not fully adequate for informed meta-analyses.

Summary   The advantages of fROI responses include the following:

• They provide a simple way of summarizing functional anatomy with a small number of well-defined areas that enables colloquial exchange and clarity, when addressing response properties.
• They enable a careful and comprehensive assessment of functional selectivity (of the fROI).
• They enforce reproducibility and provide a rigorous way of accumulating evidence across studies.

The disadvantages are as follows:

• They preclude inferences about function specialization because of their inherent anatomical bias (i.e., failure to characterize anatomically distributed responses and, implicitly, their anatomical specificity).
• They may provide unnatural constraints on functional anatomy because they may have no structurally invariant properties (i.e., the voxels constituting the FFA under passive viewing may change under a familiarity judgment task).
• Their definition is sometimes ad hoc, in terms of both the paradigm used in their definition and the statistical criteria determining their extent. One practical caveat is the subjective component involved in specifying an fROI. Specifically, when considering the variability in anatomical location, the definition of an fROI and its borders might be observer-dependent.
• fROI averages are a poor surrogate for mass-univariate (e.g., voxel-based) or full multivariate characterizations (e.g., eigen- or canonical-variate analyses) of responses within the fROI. Eigen variates are an important alternative to averaging and are used extensively in studies of effective connectivity because they allow for functionally heterogeneous but statistically dependent responses over the fROI.
• Their anatomy is difficult to report simply and quantitatively (i.e., for meta-analysis). This is because a meaningful meta-analysis would require a list of all the voxels comprising the fROI.
• There are no principled anatomical constraints on their intersubject variability.

In summary, there are good reasons to use fROI or maxima to constrain statistical searches for the effects of other factors. However, the analysis of fROI responses per se has many disadvantages and is probably best motivated when other summaries of regional responses, such as eigen variates, are inappropriate. Although fROI are sufficient to study functional selectivity, they cannot be used to comment on functional specialization and therefore have a limited role in characterizing functional anatomy. We now turn to the second question posed earlier and ask whether it is necessary to perform the functional localizer separately from the main experiment.

Why Use Separate Functional Localizers?

As noted previously, any orthogonal contrast can be used as a functional localizer that is embedded in the main experiment. So why acquire data for a localizing contrast outside the main experiment? We start by considering the advantages of factorial designs over localizer designs:

- First, localizers introduce inevitable confounds of both time and order. If the contrast of interest shows an effect of time (e.g., reduced activation in some areas and increased activation in others, due to perceptual learning), the localizer will be inappropriate because the activation pattern will have changed. This is particularly important in studies of visual categorization, where perceptual learning may suppress activation in lower regions and increase them at higher levels (e.g., Dolan et al. 1997). More generally, one cannot look for interactions between the localizer factor and other factors because the localizer and order factors are confounded. For example, differences in response between the localizer and main experiment can be confounded by subject movement between sessions, differences in the cognitive or physiological status of the subject, difference in acquisition parameters such as temperature, and so on.
- If the main experiment comprises n factors, the use of a localizer that preserves balance requires the localizer to be n-factorial. If it is not, the design is unbalanced, precluding a full analysis of the interactions (see lower panel of figure 1.1). In this example, a balanced $(2 \times 2 \times 2)$ design has been replaced with a (2) localizer and a (2×2) main experiment. The ensuing loss of balance precludes the analysis of three-way interactions because a factor is missing from the localizer. The inability to test for interactions is important because it prevents inferences about functional specialization or category specificity. For example, one can never say that a face-selective region does not respond to houses because this would be accepting the null hypothesis. However, within a balanced (2×2) design, one could use the "face versus nonface × house versus nonhouse" interaction to say that some object-responsive regions respond significantly more to faces than to houses. This would not be an option with a single face versus house localizer because of the implicit loss of balance.
- The localizer and main experiments are often different in many aspects: scanning parameters (e.g., number of scans), design (e.g., blocked versus event-related), task (e.g., passive viewing versus one back,) or stimuli used (e.g., expanding circles versus

moving dots). This means that the precision with which localizing and experimental effects are estimated can differ profoundly. This can have a number of detrimental consequences. For example, a quick functional localizer may fail to disclose significant responses because of low sensitivity. The effects of the experimental factors in these missed areas may have been extremely significant. However, they are precluded from analysis by the localizer, leading to biased reporting of the results.

• Factorial designs are more efficient because several orthogonal effects can be estimated using the greatest degrees of freedom. Put simply, factorial designs allow one to use the same degrees of freedom to make several inferences with no loss of statistical efficiency. Splitting the design into two sessions reduces the degrees of freedom for variance component estimation and reduces sensitivity to the effects in each session. For studies in which the localizing contrast is replicated in the main experiment, it is more powerful to combine the two sessions into one long session and use a contrast testing for activation in the first half of trials as a localizer for responses in the other half. This is because the statistical model can assume that the error variances are the same for both halves and can estimate them more precisely than for the replication or split model.

• Finally, if the experiment conforms to a multifactorial design, a separate localizer is unnecessary and represents a waste of resources and unnecessary subject or patient discomfort.

So what are the potential advantages of using a localizer? We can think of the following:

• It avoids confounds that arise from interspersing the localizer contrast within the main experiment. In experiments that are perceptually or cognitively demanding, it is often important to keep the design simple to optimize performance. Embedding a localizer in the main experiment may change cognitive set, induce task-switching costs, or lead to priming of certain stimuli. There are several psychological constraints on experimental design that may be better accommodated by separate localizers. A simple example would be the use of a high-contrast stimulus to localize the processing of low-contrast stimuli. If the high-contrast stimuli are presented sporadically, theymay change the context in which the low-contrast stimuli are perceived (e.g., one implicitly creates an oddball paradigm where low-contrast stimuli become standards). Separate localizers may be essential in paradigms that involve a training phase, followed by a test or probe phase. These phases cannot be intermixed because they entail an inherent order. In short, a localizer may be mandatory if presenting localizing and main factors at the same time changes the nature of the processing under investigation.

• There may be designs that cannot be balanced. For example, imagine that the question is whether face-selective regions are also sensitive to emotional expression. The experimenter might define an "expression" factor with two levels: happy and sad. To ensure that subjects attend to the facial expression, the experimenter asks them to make an explicit expression judgment. To define "face-responsive," the experimenter has another two-level factor of faces versus houses. Since houses do not have platonic expressions, a balanced (2 × 2) factorial design cannot be formed. However, even if the experimenter sticks with only three conditions (happy faces, sad faces, and houses), the houses cannot be presented with the faces because subjects cannot perform an expression judgment on houses. Therefore, the experimenter might consider testing faces versus houses in a separate localizer, using a different task (e.g., a one-back task). Another example is attentional modulation of sensory evoked responses, where a cell with attention to no stimulus is difficult to imagine.

These examples reflect experimental design issues and the problem of balance. One can imagine potential solutions, such as blocking faces and houses in the preceding example, and changing the task between blocks. If such solutions are inadequate (e.g., owing to task-switching or attentional confounds), and a separate localizer is performed, our arguments suggest that the experimenter needs to beware of some issues. First, they are assuming there are no significant time or order confounds. Second, they are using their stimuli inefficiently. In the face example, faces are presented twice, once in the localizer and once in the main experiment. However, only half the face-selective responses are used to make an inference about emotional selectivity. Had all the stimuli been presented in a conventional manner, the same face trials could have been used to test for emotional effects (happy versus sad) and to provide the localizing contrast (faces versus nonfaces). Third, the experimenter is making the important assumption that the different tasks in the localizer and main experiment do not interact with face effects. This may not seem a big assumption to some researchers, who tend to view visual–object processing as "bottom-up" or "modular" (i.e., impenetrable by cognition). Such studies are concerned mainly with the stimulus properties (e.g., in defining fROIs like the Lateral Occipital Complex and its role in object processing; Malach et al. 1995). However, as we have discussed, there is evidence that task factors can have important effects on responses in occipitotemporal cortex (Friston et al. 1996; Henson et al. 2002). This is particularly relevant to hemodynamic measures, which integrate over several seconds of synaptic activity and are likely to aggregate exogenous and endogenous processes (e.g., both "early," predominantly stimulus-driven and "late," predominantly task-related components). The balance of advantages and disadvantages would seem to suggest that functional localizers should be avoided if the question can be addressed using a factorial design.

Summary   Before turning to the case studies, it is worth noting a few positive developments that are associated with the use of functional localizers. These developments can be viewed as going beyond simple structure–function relationships. We have already discussed the notion of pooling over subjects using functional as opposed to anatomical criteria. Although this does not necessarily require separate localizers or fROIs, it is an important development and a challenge to the focus on anatomy as the exclusive reference for function. For example, studies of ocular dominance columns in V1 would not get very far using conventional intersubject averaging procedures. However, these studies would be feasible if the voxels showing monocular bias were selected on a subject-by-subject basis. There have been parallel developments in analyses of functional integration (with dynamic causal modeling and structural equation modeling) where interacting regions are defined, not by their anatomical position, but in terms of regions expressing the greatest functional response. This trend speaks to interesting notions such as spatially normalizing with respect to a canonical localizing contrast image, as opposed to a canonical anatomical template.

Another compelling trend attending the use of localizers is a progression of questions about where a response is expressed to how functionally defined systems respond. Rather than asking where in the brain an effect is expressed, many visual scientists would ask whether (or how) an effect is expressed in a certain visual cortical region. For example, if one were interested in the role of early visual areas in perceptual awareness in a masking paradigm, it might be perfectly tenable to constrain the analysis to V1–V3 or even to the voxels within these areas that represent the stimulus retinotopically. An important advantage of these approaches is that one can increase spatial resolution and/or signal-to-noise by focusing on a specific brain region during data acquisition (e.g., using a surface coil). Again, note that these arguments do not rest on fROI, or indeed on functional localizers; however, they are easily articulated in this context.

To conclude this section, we have seen that functional localizers are used to generate constraints on searches for the effects of the main factors. These constraints range from restrictions on voxel-based searches through averaging the response of an fROI. In many cases, however, a study can be designed to comprise orthogonal contrasts that can be used as mutual constraints in searching for regional effects. This means that balanced factorial designs circumvent the disadvantages of functional localizers, rendering them unnecessary. In light of this, it seems inappropriate to regard functional localizers as standard practice.

In the next section, we take two recent studies and illustrate the preceding points in a practical setting. We want to stress that these two case studies are used as a vehicle to make our points and do not detract from the original results reported by the authors or their significance. Furthermore, we appreciate that the original authors had specific and interesting questions in mind that our didactic deconstructions do not address. Our aim is to demonstrate how adjustments to the experimental designs enable additional questions that are precluded by functional localizers.

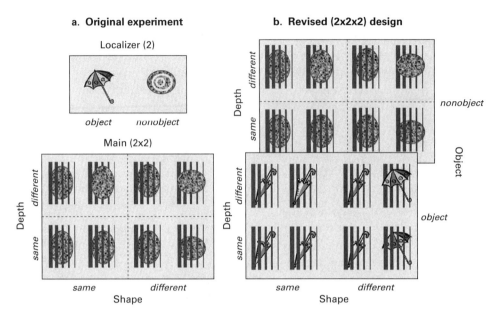

Figure 1.2
A schematic illustration of the relationship between the original (a) and revised (b) designs described in the main test for the study by Kourtzi and Kanwisher (2001). The graphics are based loosely on the original paper but are used iconically in this paper. We have simplified the presentation of the design to make our points more clearly.

Case Studies

Functional Regions of Interest in Object-Selective Regions

The first example comes from Kourtzi and Kanwisher (2001). In this study, subjects were shown objects (line drawings) and scrambled objects (arranged in circles) to define an fROI, called here the lateral occipital complex (LOC). The authors report the results of their main experiment purely in terms of the average response over all voxels within the LOC. The main experiment was an elegant two-by-two multifactorial design using the "adaptation" paradigm (in fact, there were two experiments but we will consider only one here). The two main factors were shape with two levels (same versus different) and depth (same versus different); the depth manipulation entailed a change in local contours, which were different depending on whether the object appeared in front of or behind a grid (i.e., the depth manipulation was mediated by occlusion; figure 1.2a).

Although the authors interpreted their results in terms of adaptation, for simplicity, we will regard hemodynamic responses as simple activations to a change in an attribute. Their key observation was that the LOC showed a main effect of shape change but did not show a main effect of depth change (i.e., contour change). This was an interesting and well-received observation.

So what have we learned? This study demonstrates that the average response of object-selective voxels is sensitive to changes in shape but not in depth (i.e., occlusion or local contours).[2] What we do not know are

- Where the main effects of shape changes are expressed within the LOC
- Whether a main effect of depth occurred within (subpartitions of) the LOC
- Whether there was an interaction between shape and object (i.e., Do shape-related responses depend on the stimulus being a recognizable object versus nonobject?)
- Whether there was an interaction between depth and object (i.e., Do depth-related responses depend on the stimulus being a recognizable object versus nonobject?)
- Whether there was an interaction between depth and shape (this omission is not a reflection of original experimental design, the authors simply did not report it.)
- Whether effects of depth (occlusion) or shape changes occurred outside the LOC

The first two limitations reflect the fact that an fROI average was analyzed. The remaining questions are precluded by the localizer design. We will deal with these issues using a revised analysis and experimental design, respectively. The reason that localizing information about the main effects is not available is that the effects of the main experiment were evaluated only for the averaged response of LOC. There is nothing wrong with this. However, we have learned nothing about the functional specialization of shape or contour processing per se and how it may be segregated and integrated within the ventral-processing stream. It would have been possible to address this using the following analysis.

A Revised Analysis   The effect of visually evoked responses in the main experiment could have been used to identify maxima for further analysis. This approach invokes a localizing contrast, testing for the differences between visual stimulation and inter-trial periods of no stimulation, to identify visually responsive areas. Note that this definition does not identify voxels that show larger responses to object compared to nonobjects—hence, it does not identify the LOC, but it reduces the search volume. This localizer contrast is orthogonal to the main effects of shape and depth change and their interaction. Therefore, the two main effects and interaction can be tested in a constrained and sensitive fashion at the peaks of visual responses. One would then have presumably seen that early extrastriate cortices were more sensitive to contours (i.e., depth) and that higher visual areas preferred shapes (e.g., Murray et al. 2002). It would have also been interesting to see where changes in shape interacted with changes in contour, particularly at the maxima of the main effects of shape and contour (i.e., depth) change, respectively. These interactions can usually be interpreted in terms of an integration of neuronal computations (i.e., regions responsible for integrating contour information into the representations of shape). This sort of analysis presents a very different perspective on the data from that afforded by the fROI-based analysis. Note that, in the revised analysis, the separate functional localizer is completely redundant. Inferences about the functional anatomy of shape and contour processing pertain to the systems engaged by shape and contour processing, not to the processing of the unrelated objects used in the localizer.

One potential problem with this revised analysis is that the contrast of visually evoked responses versus baseline does not isolate object-responsive areas (such as the LOC, which is traditionally defined by comparing objects versus textures, Malach et al. 1995).

Regions activated by objects relative to interstimulus baseline are likely to include early visual regions that are sensitive to any transient change in luminance and not specifically the properties of objects. A better approach would involve a revised design.

A Revised Design Let us assume that the authors wanted to understand object-selective processing in terms of its dependence on dynamic form (i.e., changes in shape and contour). One approach to this would be to integrate the localizing and main experiments to create a conventional design with three factors: stimulus category (objects versus nonobjects), shape change (same versus different), and depth change (same versus different; see figure 1.2b. The localizer contrast, in this instance, would be the main effect of object and could be used to constrain the analysis of the shape- and contour-change effects.[3] Here, the localizing contrast averages over all other factors and simply compares compound responses to paired stimuli (object versus nonobjects), irrespective of whether or not their shape or depth changed. Although addressing similar questions as the original design, this balanced factorial design properly controls the context in which objects are presented. In other words, object-selective regions are defined, operationally, in the context of changes in their shape and contours. The full design, in which the localizer factor is absorbed into the main experiment, has a number of advantages. For example, one can look at two- and three-way interactions that were precluded with the localizer design. The key interactions, from the point of view of the authors, are the two-way interactions involving stimulus category. For example, a significant object–shape change interaction suggests that object-selective responses are sensitive to changes in object shape. This inference has a much greater focus than the original design affords, where the effect of shape and contour change could not be tested in relation to the stimulus category that was changing (object versus nonobject).

Summary In summary, if the objective was to characterize shape and contour processing in the ventral stream, then the functional localizer was unnecessary. Indeed, using the localizer enforces a biased account of the underlying functional anatomy. Conversely, if the aim was to characterize the relative importance of shape and contour information in explaining object-selective responses, the original two-factor design could have been crossed with the localizer (object versus nonobject) factor to create a fully balanced three-factor design. By failing to integrate the localizer factor into the main experiment, certain cells are omitted and key interactions defining the context-sensitivity of object-selective responses are precluded. Figure 1.2 provides a schematic illustration of the relationship between the original and revised designs. We now consider another functional localizer experiment, in this case concerning visual attention.

Functional Localizers and Visual Attention Shifts

Slotnick et al. (2003) report a clever experiment showing that spatial attention can facilitate or inhibit visually evoked responses in a retinotopically specific fashion (figure 1.3a). They presented compound stimuli with sparse flickering checkerboards at the center, middle, and periphery of the visual field. In the main experiment, these stimuli were presented continuously while subjects were cued to maintain attention or shift it to specific (middle) targets on opposite sides of the visual field. Two functional localizers were used, one for labeling early retinotopic areas and the other to identify regions responding specifically to the inner (i.e., center), middle, and outer (i.e., peripheral) stimuli by presenting them separately in blocks. The results of the second localizer fROI (stimulus versus no stimuli) were used to constrain the analysis of responses evoked by shifts of spatial attention. Specifically, shifts to the contralateral field were compared with shifts to the ipsilateral field and vice versa.

The investigators showed that, within the fROIs, there was a significant difference between shifting to the contralateral field and to the ipsilateral field. These differences varied in polarity and distribution over the fROI, from area to area, confirming the author's predictions. As expected, ipsilateral to contralateral shifts of attention increased activity, and contralateral to ipsilateral shifts of attention decreased activity, in extrastriate representations of the upper–middle probe. Attentional facilitation extended to other stimulus probe representations in ventral cortex.

Inhibitory effects were also evident. Consistent with previous findings, an inhibitory pattern was seen in the outer probe representation in ventral visual area V1v. In addition, attentional inhibition dominated many of the lower visual field probe representations in dorsal visual areas, as indicated by the activity profiles in V1d, V2d, and V3.

What have we learned here? It has been shown that regions that respond to stimuli, when presented alone, show a main effect of attentional shift (contralateral versus ipsilateral). What we do not know is where the main effect of attention was expressed (because the analysis was constrained by the a priori fROI). Furthermore, because the design was not balanced, we do not know whether the effects of attention depended on the nonattended stimuli or would have been expressed in their absence (note

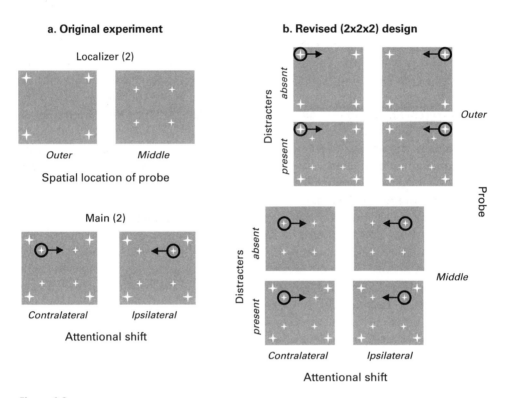

Figure 1.3
A schematic illustration of the relationship between the original (a) and revised (b) designs described in the main test for the study by Slotnick et al. (2003). The graphics are based loosely on the original paper but are used iconically in this paper. We have simplified the presentation of the design to make our points more clearly.

that the original design did not need to be balanced, because this was not the authors' question).

A Revised Design   These issues can be addressed in a revised design that brings the localizer and main experiment into the same balanced design. For simplicity, we will pretend the original experiment considered just two probes, i.e., outer (periphery) and middle (figure 1.3a).

The revised design here augments the main experiment with two additional factors (figure 1.3b): one is distracter (present versus absent) and the second is attended probe (middle versus outer). In this design, the main experiment comprises alternating blocks of continuous stimuli during which ipsilateral and contralateral attention shifts occur.

This balanced design has all the information within it to localize retinotopically specific responses to the probes and to examine the main effects of attentional shift and how these effects depend on location (middle versus outer) and the presence of distracters. For example, the simple main effect of probe, in the absence of distracters, acts as a functional localizer of the middle and outer probe locations (using a suitable contrast and the reverse contrast, respectively). Note that this localization, like the original experiment, uses attended visual stimuli. However, unlike the original experiment, the baseline for the localizer is an attended stimulus elsewhere. This ensures that nonspatial attentional effects do not confound the localizing contrast. The maxima of these contrasts can now be used to constrain tests for the simple main effects of attentional shift while attending to the middle or outer probes, respectively. Moreover, in the revised design, it is possible now to look not only for a main effect of attention, as in the original report, but also for the interaction between attention and the presence of distracters. This would enable one to partition attention-related responses into components that depended on other stimuli in the visual field and those that did not. In summary, as in the previous example, a functional localizer is both unnecessary and precludes tests of interactions among various factors that establish the context sensitivity of the inferred effects.

Conclusion

In conclusion, the apparent advantages of the fROI approach with localizer designs apply as well as or better to localizers embedded in factorial designs. The latter have many advantages, principally the ability to look at both main effects and interactions with increased statistical efficiency. If the localizer factor is an integral part of the hypothesis, then when possible, it should enter the main experiment in a balanced way. The increase in sensitivity afforded by constrained searches for region-specific effects is an important consideration, but in many instances does not call for separate functional localizers. These constraints are often implicit in multifactorial designs by virtue of the orthogonality of contrasts. The most common localizing contrast is simply a difference between activation conditions and a suitable baseline (or null event). We appreciate that in some cases there are good reasons to use separate functional localizers outside the main experiment but would like to emphasize that one should be aware of potential dangers involved in using them.

We have also addressed the use of fROIs. Although useful as constraints on statistical search spaces, their role in summarizing regional responses is less compelling. A problem with the fROI idea is that it may be self-perpetuating, in that fROI studies address only the behavior of the fROI and can never ask whether the fROI is, in itself, valid. We hope this critique will help in assessing the need for functional localizers in both experimental design and peer review.

Appendix 1.A

Two verbatim examples of anonymous reviewers' comments that refer explicitly to the lack of functional localizers in submitted scientific reports.

It will be helpful if the authors could demonstrate the relationship between their activation maps and the FFA by comparing them to more conventional localizers—e.g., faces versus buildings.

I am left wondering about the anatomical relationship between the fusiform region reported here, and the well-known fusiform face area (FFA). Why didn't the authors use an independent functional localizer for the FFA? An independent localizer would also have allowed the authors to conduct a robust and independent interaction test.

Acknowledgments

The Wellcome Trust supported this work. We thank very much Marcia Bennett for preparing the manuscript. We would like to thank Cathy Price, John Haynes, and Jon Driver for invaluable contributions. We would also like to thank Zoe Kourtzi and Scott Slotnick, for ensuring that their original findings were properly represented in this discussion.

Notes

1. This point disregards any estimation of nonsphericity, which involves second-order or nonlinear operations.

2. Clearly one cannot infer that the LOC does not show depth or contour selectivity (i.e., accept the null). One can only say there was a failure to elicit it. But this is another issue.

3. Note that the nonobjects (scrambled blobs) in our revised design are not exactly the same as those used in the localizer of the original design (scrambled objects arranged in concentric blobs). However, our purpose is not to replicate Kourtzi and Kanwisher's comparisons precisely, but rather to illustrate the form that a more general, factorial design would take.

2   Divide and Conquer: A Defense of Functional Localizers

Rebecca Saxe, Matthew Brett, and Nancy Kanwisher

Near Cape Hatteras, North Carolina, millions of cubic meters of warm salt water leave the continental shelf each second, and head northeast across the Atlantic toward Europe. This is the Gulf Stream, the most intensively studied ocean current in the world. One challenge for Gulf Stream oceanography, though, is that neither the position nor the volume of the stream remains constant from month to month, or from year to year. The location where the current leaves the coastline can vary by as much as a hundred kilometers, north or south (Mariano et al. 2003), and the stream is particularly hard to study as it approaches Europe and splits into the smaller and more variable branches. As a result of this variability, scientists wishing to take a measurement of Gulf Stream water, or mariners looking for an eastward bump, cannot simply calculate by longitude and latitude. Instead, they must first determine the path of the Gulf Stream at that moment, by measuring the water temperature or looking at satellite photographs, and then navigate accordingly.

   Much as the precise path of the Gulf Stream (measured in longitude and latitude) varies across seasons and years, the precise positions of functionally distinct regions of the brain, such as primary visual cortex (measured in Talairach or MNI coordinates), vary across individuals. So, just as oceanographers must first identify the actual path of the Gulf Stream before using water measurements to make inferences about circulation in the north Atlantic, cognitive neuroscientists often use "localizer" contrasts to functionally identify regions in the brain of a given individual (called *function regions of interest*, or fROIs) before using measurements of the activity in those regions to test hypotheses about the distribution of cognitive functions across the cortex. Here, we first sketch the advantages to using functionally defined regions of interest, and then we consider the specific concerns about this practice raised by Friston et al. (chapter 1 in this volume).

Why Use fROIs?

The goal of science is not simply to collect a list of independent facts about the world, but to organize those facts into general patterns, to test hypotheses about those patterns, and to explain them in terms of broader theories. The importance of fROIs concerns all three stages. We consider each in turn.

Knowing Where We Are

Brain imaging relates function to locations in the brain. Because cognitive neuroscience is not about specific individuals but about people in general, we need some way to specify brain locations that will generalize across individuals. The problem is that the shape of each person's brain is unique, just like the shape of her face. So cognitive neuroscientists face a serious challenge: What counts as the same place in two different brains?

One answer is to consider purely anatomical markers to align similar structures of each subject's brain. For brain regions that can be identified anatomically in vivo, such as the basal ganglia, amygdala or hippocampus, we have an excellent way to register these regions across individuals: locate them on anatomical scans within each subject individually, and collect that subject's functional data from the corresponding location. Ongoing efforts to identify cytoarchitectonic markers in individual brains may eventually enable us to extend these methods to the cortex (Amunts et al. 2004; Eickhoff et al. 2005; Schuchard et al. 2003). Promising results have also been obtained in studies using connectivity patterns to define functional areas (Johansen-Berg et al. 2004). However, for most cortical regions, we currently lack clear anatomical or connectivity markers to define specific cortical areas.

As a result, the most prevalent method of anatomical matching, since the early days of brain imaging, has been to use a standard Cartesian coordinate system such as the Talairach and Tournoux stereotaxic system (Talairach and Tournoux 1988). In this system, each individual's data are aligned to a "standard" brain, usually using an automated algorithm to match the subject's anatomical scan to an anatomical template. Increasingly, the coordinates reported in the results of individual studies are also used as input to meta-analyses (Duncan and Owen 2000; Paus 1996).

Nonetheless, the practice of normalizing individual brains to a "standard" brain space has important shortcomings. Well-known brain areas (defined functionally, or cytoarchitectonically) do not land consistently in the same place in any set of standard anatomical coordinates across individuals. One illustration of this problem is seen in the case of primary visual cortex (area V1), which lies consistently along the calcarine sulcus in all subjects, but does not land in the same location across all subjects in stereotaxic coordinates (see figure 2.1, plate 1).

Another illustration of the problem is seen in figure 2.2d, where the selectivity of the FFA is stronger when it is functionally defined individually within each subject than when it is defined from a standard group analysis, because the necessarily imperfect registration across individuals entailed in the group analysis precludes selection of all and only the FFA in each individual, thus blurring the distinctive functional profile of each region with that of its neighbors (see also Ozcan et al. 2005).

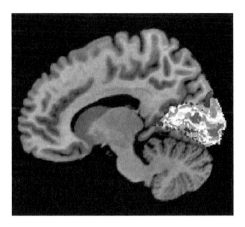

Figure 2.1 (plate 1)
Aligning V1. A sagittal slice of the MNI template brain (x = +12) overlaid with the probability map for the location of V1, determined posthumously from the cytoarchitecture of ten individuals. Color scale shows number of brains in which V1 occupies each position, from blue − 1 subject to red − 10 subjects. From Wohlschlager et al. (2005).

More sophisticated strategies for registering individual brains together use reconstructed cortical surfaces that respect sulcal locations. These systems provide better alignment across subjects for retinotopic visual areas (Fischl et al. 1999), but they do not do much better than Talairach coordinates for category-selective regions in the temporal lobe (Spiridon et al. 2005). Moreover, postmortem histology shows that sulcal borders do not reliably coincide with other, well-established anatomical divisions based on cytoarchitecture (Amunts et al. 1999; Amunts and Zilles 2001).

Thus, neither standard stereotaxic registration methods nor more sophisticated coordinate systems that respect sulcal landmarks are likely to bring distinct functional regions perfectly into register across subjects. As a result, nearby brain regions with different functional profiles will be averaged together across individuals, reducing both the resolution and sensitivity of subsequent functional analyses (Swallow et al. 2003; see also figure 2.2).

The alternative solution is for cognitive neuroscientists to use consistent patterns of functional response profiles to constrain the identification of the "same" brain region across individuals—that is, to use functional landmarks. The functional landmark approach requires using the combination of sulcal/gyral divisions (e.g., the fusiform gyrus) and robust functional profiles (e.g., strong preference for faces versus objects) in individual subjects to identify the landmark region, which can then be used to orient research in the whole patch of neighboring cortex. This practice is already nearly universal among cognitive scientists studying, for example, early visual cortex,

a)

Faces >fix

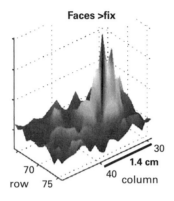

30
1.4 cm
40 column
70
row 75

c)

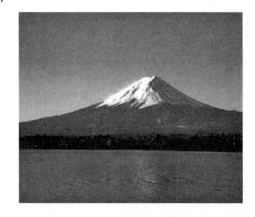

b)

Objects >fix

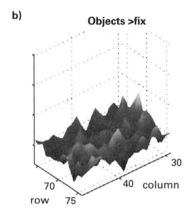

30
70   40 column
row 75

d)

Right FFA (N=14)

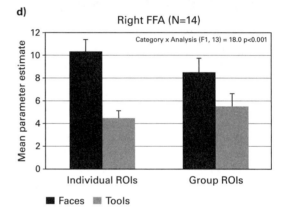

Mean parameter estimate

Category x Analysis (F1, 13) = 18.0 p<0.001

12
10
8
6
4
2
0

Individual ROIs   Group ROIs

■ Faces ■ Tools

Figure 2.2

fROI case study: the right FFA. A small section of one functional slice in one subject showing on the vertical axis the spatial profile of percent signal increase (compared to a fixation baseline) for faces in (a) and for objects in (b). Note that these displays avoid the problem of arbitrary thresholds by showing the mean response at each point in the slice; for comparable data presented on the cortical surface see figure 7 in Spiridon et al. (2005). Several of the issues concerning fROIs discussed in the text are illustrated here: (1) Why name fROIs? Despite the absence of sharp boundaries and the difficulty of defining its precise border, few would quarrel with the use of the name "Mt. Fuji" to refer to the prominent bump in (c). For similar reasons we find it useful to refer to the prominent bump in the response profile to faces shown in *a* as the "fusiform face area" or FFA. (2) Why use fROIs tailored individually to each subject rather than to the group average? Because the FFA varies in anatomical position across individuals in stereotaxic space, an FFA defined on the basis of group-aligned data will necessarily include regions outside the FFA in some or all subjects, blurring the distinctive functional profile of the FFA and weakening its stimulus selectivity ("Group ROIs" at right in d), compared to the case in which the FFA is defined for each subject individually based on that subject's own data ("Individual ROIs" at left). In both cases, data were unsmoothed, and the data used to define the ROI were separate from those used to estimate the beta weights of the response of each condition in that ROI. The analysis X category interaction is highly significant, due to a weaker response to faces in the group analysis relative to the individual analysis, and the reverse trend for all of the nonface categories. We thank Paul Downing and Annie Chan for this analysis.

where the borders of each subject's retinotopic visual areas are first identified with functional scanning before the main experimental data are collected.

Note that the use of functional landmarks, as described in this section, need not hinge on the reification of fROIs—either as the units of hypotheses about regional functions, or as fundamental theoretical entities in cognitive neuroscience. Functional profiles may be used simply as reliable guides to the "same" location from one brain to another, whether the researcher is interested in the landmark region itself or rather in a region reliably located with respect to the landmark. Once we can identify the "same place" in different brains, we are in a position to combine data across subjects, studies, and labs. Often, though, researchers use fROIs in a theoretically deeper way, to gain a richer understanding of the response profile of each region, in order to test hypotheses about the neural basis of cognitive functions.

Testing Hypotheses

For the most part, cognitive neuroscientists seek to test hypotheses about the cognitive functions of particular regions of the brain (for an exception, see Haxby et al. 2001). As we argue in this section, this work can proceed most effectively (and most easily avoid a number of common pitfalls) when researchers specify their hypotheses in advance, including both the profile of functional response that would support the hypothesis and the specific brain location(s) in which the functional profile should be tested. Although using functionally defined ROIs is just one of many ways to specify a brain location, they often serve as the regions about which specific functional hypotheses can most sensibly be framed.

First, specifying in advance the region(s) in which a hypothesis will be tested increases statistical power by reducing the search space from tens of thousands of voxels to just a handful of ROIs. Greater power allows researchers to investigate with confidence the relatively subtle aspects of a region's response profile, such as those revealed in functional magnetic resonance imaging (fMRI) adaptation studies (Grill-Spector and Malach 2001; Henson et al. 2000; see also figure 2.3). By contrast, traditional whole-brain analyses produce an explosion of multiple comparisons, requiring powerful corrections to control false positives (Nichols and Hayasaka 2003). Many researchers appear to find the necessary corrections too draconian, and it is still common for neuroimaging papers to report uncorrected statistics, which do not provide valid control of false positives. For example, in the last five years, the Brede database of published neuroimaging papers (Nielsen 2003) records that half (49%) of the 1,705 articles that report any brain location P value, report only uncorrected P values.

Blunted by the loss of statistical power entailed in multiple comparisons, whole-brain analyses are particularly poor tools for establishing the absence of an effect of interest in a given region, a real problem because the lack of difference between two tasks may be critical for testing a cognitive theory (e.g., Jiang et al. 2004). Predefined

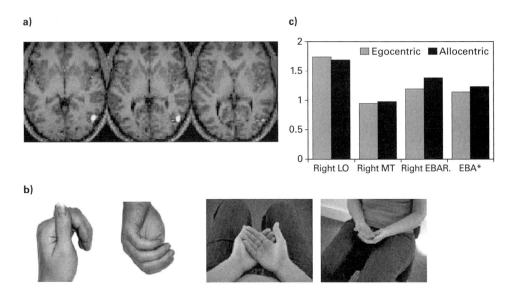

Figure 2.3

fROI case study: the right EBA. Lateral extrastriate cortex can be divided into distinct but neighboring fROIs, including the extrastriate body area (bodies > objects), MT (moving > stationary), and the lateral occipital complex (objects > textures). All three regions show a robust response to stationary photographs of human bodies, but only the right EBA shows a significant enhancement when the body parts displayed are viewed from an allocentric, rather than an egocentric, perspective. These results illustrate the strengths of fROI analyses that we have described. (1) Small effects: the small but significant preference for allocentric body parts in the rEBA fROI cannot be detected in a whole brain analysis of twelve subjects. (2) Anatomical specificity: combining multiple fROI analyses allowed the authors to show that the enhanced response to allocentric images was specific to the rEBA. Interaction tests showed that the profile in the rEBA was significantly different from that in right LO and MT. (3) Cross-lab comparisons: Chan et al. (2004) in Wales and Saxe et al. (in press) in the United States, using different stimuli and different scanners, both found evidence for the same enhancement for allocentric images in the functionally defined rEBA. The result was replicated even though Saxe, Jamal, and Powell reported the average response for all voxels in the fROI, while Chan, Peelen, and Downing reported the average response in a small cube around the peak. (a) Three slices in a single subject, showing the right EBA (red), LO (blue), and MT (green). (b) Stimuli from Saxe et al. (in press) and Chan et al. (2004). (c) Percent signal change to egocentric and allocentric images of body parts in three neighboring fROIs: right LO, MT, and EBA (Saxe et al. in press). The fourth column shows the replication of the same result from Chan et al. (2004). (For interpretation of the references to color in this figure legend, the reader is referred to the Web version of this article.)

regions of interest provide a practical, sensitive, and statistically rigorous solution to this challenge.

Second, using a predefined region of interest allows the researcher to test her hypothesis in a statistically unbiased data set. A common alternative practice that we call "voxel-sniffing" proceeds as follows: (1) hypothesize that region X will be recruited differentially for task A versus task B, (2) search for the peak voxel in the neighborhood of X that shows the predicted differential recruitment, and then (3) display the response of this voxel showing differential recruitment for task A versus task B. Since the very same aspect of the data is used to both find the region in which the hypothesis is tested and show the effect, the resulting data display is biased toward a false positive. Noise or measurement error that contributed to the measured response of the region infects both steps: finding the region and measuring its response. By contrast, when the precise voxels that will make up the ROI are determined in advance, any spurious feature of the data in the localizing step of the analysis cannot contribute to a positive result in the independent data used to test hypotheses about that region (see also Liou et al. 2006).

Finally, using a preestablished functional definition of the region at stake in a hypothesis helps researchers avoid spurious claims of contradictions or convergences across subjects and across experiments. The interpretation of one set of neuroimaging data is almost always informed by (and responsive to) a wide previous literature; the challenge is to determine whether the current result reflects recruitment of the very same brain region as in previous reports, or of a nearby region blurred together by averaging.

All of these benefits of predefined regions of interest can be garnered using anatomical markers, stereotaxic coordinates, or functionally defined ROIs. Which of these to choose is an empirical/pragmatic question: Which kind of ROI is best suited to the experimental design and the hypothesis being tested? Anatomical ROIs, defined by either stereotaxic coordinates or sulcal and gyral landmarks, may be the only means of defining ROIs in advance for comparisons between healthy subjects and patient populations, to guide hypotheses about brain damage based on functional imaging results in healthy subjects, or to make predictions about healthy brains based on analyses of selective deficits following lesions (Heberlein and Saxe 2005; James et al. 2003). Stereotaxic coordinates from prior studies may also be used to define ROIs when researchers need to be especially cautious to avoid a false negative (Jiang et al. 2004; Shuman and Kanwisher 2004).

In many cases, though, a broad consensus now exists in the literature about the locations and properties of particular regions implicated in a contrast of interest, so a pragmatic and efficient way to relate results across studies and formulate and test hypotheses about the role of brain regions identified in previous studies is to use fROIs.

Note that the use of fROIs to prespecify the region in which a hypothesis will be tested does not require a commitment to the ontological status of that region as a fundamental or homogeneous unit. Instead of assuming such a commitment, fROIs can be used to empirically test the question of whether or not a region's response profile reflects a coherent, theoretically interesting functional unit. Some robust and reliable fROIs that can be used as functional landmarks and that constrain statistical analyses turn out to have complex and disjunctive, or overly general, response profiles; for example, because the lateral frontal and superior parietal regions studied intensively with fROIs by Jiang and collaborators are implicated across a wide range of task contexts (Jiang and Kanwisher 2003), the authors explicitly argued against interpreting these fROIS as theoretical units (Duncan and Owen 2000; another example may the lateral occipital complex, Kanwisher et al. 1997a,b; Malach et al. 1995). In other cases, though, fROI analyses do reveal stable, coherent, and theoretically interesting regional response profiles that may help constrain cognitive and computational theories of the mind. It is to these cases, and these kinds of arguments, that we now turn.

Discovering Fundamental Natural Phenomena
The third and most theoretically committed reason to use fROI analyses depends on the researcher's philosophy of cognitive neuroscience—that is, on a notion of what kind of hypotheses or theories cognitive neuroscientists should be building and testing with neuroimaging data. We believe that the functional characterization of specific brain regions is a critical part of this enterprise.

The central tenet of modern cognitive neuroscience is that "different brain areas perform different information processing operations (often referred to as computations) and that an explanation of a cognitive performance involves both decomposing an overall task into component information processing activities and determining what brain area performs each" component (Bechtel 2002b). At its best, cognitive neuroscience can provide neural evidence to distinguish between functional psychological decompositions (or task analyses) of higher cognitive functions. That is, the observed division of labor across brain regions can help decide among alternative psychological theories of a cognitive capacity if the psychological components of the task are reflected in distinct and reliably localized neural components—that is, patches of cortex. In some cases, fROIs seem to pick out cortical patches of just this kind (Xu 2005; Yovel and Kanwisher 2004).

Note that such an anatomical constraint need not apply to all information processing operations the brain carriea out. First, the question of whether the cortex actually contains any functionally distinct components has been hotly debated for much of the history of neuroscience. The influential early pioneer of lesion studies, Pierre Flourens, denied the existence of any localization of function, claiming instead that all areas of the cortex served all the same functions, so that any part of the cortex could accommodate for the loss of any other region. This debate continues, in changing form (Haxby et al. 2001; Spiridon and Kanwisher 2002; assumptions of homogeneity here describes a modern version of this controversy). Second, if some functions are localized in the brain, similar computations could in principle be realized differently in each individual brain (called *multiple reliability* in philosophy). Third, in cases when functional properties do align with some anatomical properties consistently across subjects, it is still an empirical question which anatomical marker(s) will constitute the most reliable guide to function: sulcal and gyral landmarks, cytoarchitectonic divisions, or patterns of functional connectivity. Finally, even if psychological and neural components of a cognitive capacity are localized and aligned in some regions, the question of how many such neural components/entities there are in the brain (and in the mind) remains open.

For all of these reasons, the status of any given functionally defined ROI is not something to be assumed from the outset, but is rather contingent on empirical outcomes. Even the observation of robust and distinctive regularities in the response profile of a patch of cortex across individuals may not reflect a neural entity in this theoretical sense, if those regularities do not reflect any single or stable elementary computation. For each ROI, researchers must therefore assess whether the functional properties of the region are not only stable, but also theoretically coherent and meaningful. Although we make no guesses about how often theoretically important functions localized to patches of cortex will occur in nature, we believe this standard has been upheld by at least a few widely used, functionally defined ROIs including MT/V5 (Tootell et al. 1995; the FFA Kanwisher et al. 1997a,b; see figure 2.2); the region of the TPJ implicated in understanding another person's beliefs (Saxe and Powell in press); and the AIP, which is implicated in grasping (Culham et al. 2003).

In sum, fROIs are useful for specifying brain locations across subjects, for testing hypotheses concerning the function of specific brain regions, and occasionally for investigating candidate separable components of the mind. The use of fROIs is uncontroversial and indeed virtually required in any study of visual cortex involving retinotopic visual areas or MT. We see no reason why the widely accepted benefits of fROIs in research on these regions would not apply equally to other cortical regions. Nonetheless, Friston and colleagues (chapter 1) label the practice a "missed opportunity," as well as a "potentially restrictive" and even "retrograde" development in experimental design. Next, we consider and rebut their main critiques of the fROI method.

Common and Uncommon Misconceptions About fROI: Response to Friston et al.

Telescopic Vision

The most common concern about the use of fROI analyses is that they will obscure the researchers' view of the bigger picture. A small but significant effect observed in the average response of an ROI might reflect the specific engagement of the region of interest, but it could equally reflect (1) a small but consistent effect that is actually occurring across many regions of the brain, (2) the fringe or tail of a much bigger activation in the same contrast in a neighboring region, or (3) a different region, sending feedback connections to the region of interest. Friston and collegues (chapter 1) express this common concern by arguing that "anatomical specificity cannot be addressed by a single fROI." That is, an fROI-constrained analysis could lead the scientist to miss the forest for a tree.

The solution, of course, is to combine fROI analyses with each other, and/or with voxel-based whole-brain analyses. None of the advantages of independent, preconstrained functional ROIs precludes comparing multiple ROIs in the same session, or comparing the results of fROI analyses with whole-brain analyses to look for robust activity outside of the ROI. Many researchers use multiple fROIs in combination for just this reason (see figure 2.3). So the worry that the advantages of fROI analyses will lead researchers to focus exclusively on a single ROI seems unsubstantiated by the actual practice in the field. By adding fROIs to our repertoire, cognitive neuroscientists can rigorously study both the forest and the tree.

Assumptions of Homogeneity

The second basic concern about fROI analyses is that a focus on the response of a predefined region will lead researchers into the dangerous, or "untenable" (chapter 1), assumption that the neurons that compose the fROI are all homogeneous and equally well described by the average. If fROIs did lead researchers to claim the absolute homogeneity of the neurons under investigation, this would obviously be unfortunate, not to say silly. Once again, though, the solution for fROI analyses is simple: Recognize the likelihood of finer-grained structure, and treat the question of homogeneity as an empirical one. Also note that this advice applies equally to cognitive neuroscientists who do not use fROIs, but rely on the response of single voxels, each of which reflects the average activity of hundreds of thousands of individual neurons.

Inhomogeneities, or finer-grained structure, within the response of a region or a voxel may arise from any of at least three kinds of sources: (1) subgroups of neurons doing similar computations over different regions of stimulus space, as seen for example in V1 (retinotopy) and S1 (somatotopy); (2) interleaved or tightly packed groups of neurons performing distinct, even unrelated, functions; or (3) subgroups of neurons performing hierarchically arranged parts of a single computation, which are too close together to resolve with current technology, especially based on blood flow.

Researchers using fROIs have been at the forefront of empirical investigations of each of these possibilities for the organization of responses within regions. For example, several recent studies have used fROIs to explicitly test the information that is contained in the profile of response across the voxels within that fROI. Researchers using classification methods (Haxby et al. 2001; Spiridon and Kanwisher 2002) found that, although the pattern of response across the voxels within the FFA enabled discrimination of faces from nonfaces, it did not allow discrimination of one nonface category (e.g., bottles) from another nonface category (e.g., shoes), a result that reinforces the selectivity of this region for face processing. Far from assuming homogeneity, this method exploits and directly investigates fine-grained differences in the response profile of different voxels within an fROI (see also Kamitani and Tong 2005). Note further that the identification of fROIs for early visual areas using retinotopy depends precisely on the heterogeneous response profiles of different voxels within an area to stimuli presented to different retinal locations.

In all, practice in the field does not support the concern that using fROIs will lead researchers to assume, rather than to test, the finer-grain structure of neurons encompassed by a single ROI. But finally, we must concede that all fMRI investigations sacrifice some degree of fine-grained precision in favor of a broader summary view of neural responses, whether by averaging across a group of voxels or across even just the thousands of neurons that drive a single voxel. Once cognitive neuroscientists acknowledge this tradeoff, we can continue to investigate aspects of cognitive function that are shared across, and selectively recruit, whole groups of neurons.

Factorial Designs Versus Independent Localizers

Friston et al. (chapter 1) repeatedly claim that "people who like localizers should like factorial designs even more." Well, we are people who like localizers, and we are ambivalent about factorial designs. Factorial designs have important advantages, but when used to replace (rather than to complement) independent localizer contrasts, they have significant disadvantages as well.

In a full factorial design, researchers compare the effects of two or more stimulus/task manipulations on the resulting neural response of a region or group of voxels, by presenting the subject with all possible combinations of those stimuli and/or tasks. In the example discussed, Friston and colleagues (chapter 1; Kourtzi and Kanwisher 2001) compared the effects of stimulus shape (same versus different) and depth (same versus different) on the response of the LOC fROI. Since the authors presented subjects with all four possible combinations of shapes and depths, the experiment used a "full factorial" design. Full factorial designs allow the researcher to simultaneously and rigorously measure both main effects of the factors of interest, and any interactions between these factors. Undeniably, such an experimental design is the best way to test hypotheses about the relative effects of multiple factors on a regional response, especially when the factors are separable, and possible interactions between the factors are of theoretical interest.

Unfortunately, the argument of Friston et al. (chapter 1) for replacing localizer contrasts with full factorial design confuses three independent issues: (1) the relatively trivial question of whether the localizer contrasts occur within the same runs, or in separate but interleaved runs within the same scanning session; (2) whether full factorial designs are always the best experimental design for testing hypotheses in cognitive neuroscience; and (3) whether the main effects within a full factorial design should be used in place of independent localizer contrasts to identify regions of interest. We consider these three issues in turn.

First, Friston et al. (chapter 1) have emphasized the fact that fROI experiments often place the localizer experiment in a separate set of runs from the main conditions of interest. Of course, this practice is irrelevant for the logic of fROIs, as Friston et al. point out in their chapter. Whether to put the localizer contrast in the very same runs as the main experiment, or in separate runs, interleaved or counterbalanced with the main experiment (Liou et al. 2006) is just a case-specific question of experimental design. Empirical evidence suggests that the position and selectivity of fROIs is strikingly consistent both within and between scan sessions (Peelen and Downing 2005).

The second point is that full factorial designs are not the only elegant and rigorous experimental designs available to cognitive neuroscientists, and are not perfectly suited to testing all kinds of hypotheses. Other sophisticated experimental designs use parametric gradations of a single factor, or sort events by behavioral response on a trial-by-trail basis, or use classification methods to investigate the information that is represented in a given area (Cox and Savoy 2003; Haxby et al. 2001; Kamitani and Tong 2005). This is only to say that the logic of fROIs is compatible with any well-balanced experimental design in the main experiment; there is no special relationship between full factorial designs and fROIs, unless the factorial design is being used to replace fROIs as a way to constrain analyses to regions of interest.

The disadvantages of full factorial designs arise only in this final case, when a factorial design is proposed to replace fROIs. Within a full factorial design, orthogonal main effects and interactions are independent of the main effect used to define the regions of interest, and so conform to the logic of fROI analyses. In this sense, a factorial design could be used as simply one way of doing fROI analyses. The question then becomes, are factorial designs the best way?

We think not. In a factorial design, though the test of an interaction will be independent from the ROI definition, the test of the main effect will be biased, since the very same data used to find the region of interest is then used to estimate the magnitude of the main effect. Researchers using fROI analyses therefore use an independent data set—collected during a separate set of conditions—to define the region of interest, and constrain the hypothesis space, from the data that will be used to estimate the magnitude of main effects and interactions in the main experiment.

To illustrate by example, Epstein and Kanwisher (1998) used a whole-brain analysis to show that a specific area of parahippocampal cortex—the parahippocampal place area (PPA)—responded much more strongly when subjects viewed scenes (including furnished rooms) than when they viewed faces or single objects. They then used thresholded data from this experiment to define the voxels in the PPA, and performed a second experiment to investigate whether average PPA activation was better explained by the multiple objects in the furnished rooms, or by the spatial layout of the rooms. They therefore included the following conditions: furnished rooms; rooms with all objects removed, preserving only the spatial layout; and displays of the objects from the furnished rooms rearranged randomly. The inclusion of a replication of the main effect in the second experiment enabled them to show not only that spatial layout alone (i.e., empty rooms) produced a very strong response in the PPA, but further that spatial layout appeared to be alone sufficient to explain the large response to the furnished rooms, because the response to furnished and empty rooms did not differ.

Finally, Friston et al. (chapter 1) imply that there is no cost to using a full-factorial design and then testing the higher-level interactions, relative to a separate localizer (or "no loss of statistical efficiency"). On the contrary, simply multiplying the number of conditions in the experiment may produce many conditions that are of no interest to the experimenter, and simultaneously decrease the number of observations that can be conducted for the critical conditions. The result is a loss of power where it counts, and therefore reduced statistical efficiency. The basic message of this section is: People who like factorial designs should like the combination of factorial designs with an independent localizer contrast even better.

Averaging Signal in the fROI and Other Summary Measures

The fROI approach involves first identifying a candidate functional region, and then calculating some overall summary measure of response in that region. This summary measure is used for two reasons. The first is to decrease the influence of noise that varies between voxels. Of course, this is also one of the main motivations for smoothing in traditional whole-brain analyses. The second use of summary measures is to make inferences about the response of the region as a whole, rather than particular voxels within the region. Importantly, the choice of summary measure is intrinsic to the logic of fROI analyses. The same logical, statistical, and theoretical advantages of fROI analyses apply to all these summary measures.

In general, if we know the size and shape of a particular functional area, then the best (most efficient) representation of the signal from this area will be the mean from the voxels within the area.[11] There are three summary measures in frequent use, which we will call threshold-average, peak-smoothed, and first eigenvariate. All three take a weighted mean across voxels within a brain area, but differ in their method for using the localizing contrast to estimate how much each voxel contributes to the functional area.

The threshold-average method is the most common approach to region definition for fROI analyses: define the region as the set of all contiguous voxels passing a predetermined threshold, and then average the response across all voxels in the region. The threshold should be high enough to avoid noise while still detecting signal. The advantage of this approach is that it can adapt flexibly to detect regions with almost any size or shape. Friston et al. (chapter 1) appear to take particular issue with this practice, and strongly prefer the two common alternative methods—the peak-smoothed and first eigenvariate measures.

Peak-smoothed averaging uses smoothed data, and takes the time course of the voxel showing maximum activity in the localizer. In this case, the underlying region response is assumed to be a Gaussian shape with the same size as the smoothing kernel. The choice between the threshold-average and peak-smoothed methods will depend on your model of the underlying regional response. Clearly, if the region of interest is in fact a Gaussian shape of the same size as the smoothing kernel, there will be very little difference between the methods. Indeed, the results of average thresholded and peak smoothed analyses are often highly convergent (figure 2.3; Arthurs and Boniface 2003). If the region response does not fit this size and shape, though, the peak-smoothed model will be a less efficient model of the region's overall response; for example, the PPA is elongated (Epstein and Kanwisher 1998), and will therefore not be well matched by a simple Gaussian. Also, because smoothing is usually in three dimensions, rather than on the cortical surface, using smoothing for regions with complex cortical folding may lead to averaging with nearby sulcal banks, gray matter, and cerebrospinal fluid (CSF).

There is a greater theoretical difference between average thresholded and the first eigenvariate measure, which is the second approach suggested by Friston and colleagues (chapter 1). The first eigenvariate results from performing a principal components analysis (PCA) on the region data, where the time points are the observations and the voxels are the variables. The PCA returns a series of components ordered by the proportion of variance each component explains; each component is associated with a vector of weights (one value per voxel) reflecting the contribution of each voxel to that component. We can reconstruct signal proportional to the first eigenvariate by multiplying the (time by voxel) region data by the voxel weights for the first component. In this case, the model of the region shape and size is given by the voxel weights, and the time course is therefore a weighted average. The first eigenvariate reflects the time course of the main component that contributes to a region's response.

In essence, the voxel weights from the PCA can be thought of as an attempt to extract the shape and size of the underlying response from within the region activated by the localizer contrast. If the regional response is homogeneous, the average-thresholded and first eigenvariate measures will produce very similar results. If the area is not homogeneous, we need to treat the first eigenvariate measure with care; the researcher must analyze the spatial weights of the component in order to interpret the results. Because of the spatial weighting, the eigenvariate may refer to only a small portion of the localized region, rather than represent the region's overall response. There is also no guarantee that the eigenvariate will pick out the same part of the localized region for different subjects.

In sum, little practical difference is expected between the results of the different methods of summarizing the response within an fROI. Where differences arise, the standard approach of averaging across voxels above threshold has the advantages of being easy to interpret and appropriate for regions of different shapes and sizes.

Why Name fROIs?

Even granting the logical and methodological advantages of fROI analyses, some researchers continue to resist the practice of giving those fROIs names. Some worry that reifying discrete regions distorts the actual continuity of the measured blood oxygen level–dependent (BOLD) response; for others, names should be eschewed altogether because of the danger of misnaming regions before their functions are completely understood. There is merit to each of these concerns, but we believe that the pragmatic advantages of naming fROIs, when such names are treated with care and flexibility, outweigh the disadvantages.

The "activation map" images that commonly accompany brain imaging papers can be misleading to inexperienced readers, by seeming to suggest that the boundaries between "activated" and "unactivated" patches of cortex are unambiguous and sharp. Instead, as most researchers are aware, the apparent sharp boundaries are subject to the choice of threshold applied to the statistical tests that generate the image. What, then, justifies dividing the cortex into regions with boundaries based on this fuzzy, mutable measure of functional profile?

It is an empirical question whether the slopes of a given candidate fROI are shallow or sharp. For some regions, such as the FFA, these boundaries in the measured response are impressively sharp (Spiridon et al. 2005). In other cases it may still be reasonable to assume that the "real" boundaries in the underlying tissue are sharper than the edges in the measured signal, which are distorted and flattened by blood diffusion, partial-voluming, and/or smoothing during the statistical analyses. These regions will have to await technological advances to establish the true grade of their sides.

The broader point, though, is that cognitive neuroscientists need not be shy about reifying fROIs merely because the precise boundary of the region may be hard to determine. Imprecise boundaries are a feature of many scientifically respectable objects, including ocean currents like the Gulf Stream, geographical features like Mt. Fuji (see figure 2.2), and human body parts like knees and elbows. Instead, both empirical investigation and emerging conventions and consensus are needed to establish the reference of fROI names: to the region surrounding the peak, and/or to the whole area above a predetermined altitude. The second concern is that, in the absence of full knowledge, functional names may be misassigned, leading to long-term confusion.

Cautionary tales of just such confusion come from the anatomical and functional names assigned to regions of the avian brain, a confusion that generated many papers, much frustration, and eventually whole conferences dedicated to nomenclature (http://avianbrain.org/nomen).

So it is important that researchers recognize that a name is a tool, not a conclusion. Naming a region should stimulate empirical research about that region's function, and not inhibit such research. Nevertheless, the advantages of being able to talk about the results of fROI analyses outweigh the danger. A name allows researchers to precisely state both the hypotheses and the results of fROI analyses, without constant use of long ellipses (e.g., "the region of the fusiform gyrus recruited significantly more during . . ."). Also, note that the most common alternative to fROI names—the use of simple sulcal–gyral landmarks (e.g., the fusiform gyrus the temporoparietal junction)— is both imprecise and actively misleading, since the authors' claims do not apply to the whole anatomical region in question, but only to the subset of that region selected by the fROI.

Of course, fROI names should be used with precision and care. But even if, in some cases, the conventional fROI names do not capture the full truth about the function of the patch of cortex that the fROI reflects, we propose that the most powerful way for one scientist to describe this result to another is a sentence that begins with the fROI's name.

Conclusion

In sum, much is to be gained and little to be lost from the use of fROI analyses, in conjunction with other analysis methods, in many imaging studies. FROI analyses are particularly useful for studies investigating phenomena for which distinctive, well described, and anatomically restricted functional regions have been described that can be easily and straightforwardly identified in each subject in a few minutes of functional scanning, and where a broad consensus exists in the literature on how these regions are to be functionally localized.

Friston et al. (chapter 1) note that "the purpose of [their] commentary is to provide a reference for people who do not want to use functional localizers and have to defend themselves against the contrary attitudes of reviewers," and they cite in their appendix specific reviewer comments such as this one: "I am left wondering about the anatomical relationship between the fusiform region reported here, and the well-known fusiform face area (FFA). Why did the authors not use an independent functional localizer for the FFA?" We do not see an answer to this question in the commentary by Friston et al. (this volume) and we still think that many studies would benefit from the use of an fROI.

Acknowledgments

We thank Chris Baker, Giulio Boccaletti, Jim DiCarlo, Paul Downing, Jon Driver, Evelina Fedorenko, Peter Godfrey-Smith, Tania Lombrozo, Mona Spiridon, and Galit Yovel for comments and suggestions.

Note

1. Here we do not consider the effect of spatial autocorrelation, as this is rarely addressed in standard analyses, and applies to all three summary measures.

3   Commentary on Divide and Conquer: A Defense of Functional Localizers

Karl J. Friston and Rik N. Henson

We hope this exchange will clarify the different perspectives adopted by people who do and do not use functional regions of interest (fROIs). However, this debate will not be resolved here; it will be resolved only by looking at the practice of imaging neuroscientists in the years to come. We suspect that fROIs will have disappeared by then, because the questions they address are fundamentally limited. fROIs are already being subverted by the growing interest in high-resolution functional imaging and multivariate characterizations of fine-scale distributed responses. The current issue is more pragmatic: it is becoming more difficult for cognitive neuroscientists to publish imaging papers that involve extrastriate or inferotemporal areas without conforming to fROI dogma (see appendix 3.A). Our hope is to reverse this trend.

Contentious issues sometimes arise from a misconception of the other's position. It was useful to have the response of Saxe and colleagues because we realize now how proponents of fROI may miss the point of our critique. Our point was that, if one wishes to identify brain regions using functional criteria (i.e., a "localizer" contrast), then it is best to (1) embed the localizer within an explicit factorial design, in the same experimental session; and (2) use the contrast to constrain the search for brain regions showing the effects of interest (i.e., orthogonal main effects or interactions), rather than to average data over all voxels identified by the localizing contrast.

Thus, while we can imagine readers nodding thoughtfully during the first part of the Saxe et al. study (part 1A)—in which the authors describe a well-known issue in cognitive neuroscience that structure–function mappings may differ across individuals—this is not the point of contention. This intersubject variability raises questions about the validity of matching brains purely on the basis of structure (e.g., by "normalizing" to a template) in group analyses. This is independent of our critique of fROI. As we noted in our section on intersubject averaging (see chapter 1, this volume):

However, even though this seems to be an important motivation for fROI, this motivation does not require fROIs to be defined from a localizer session. The same approach can be taken within a voxel-based analysis of single-subject data (with or without spatial normalization).... The advantage of this procedure over fROI averages is that the subject-specific maxima can be reported, providing a quantitative and useful characterization of intersubject variability in functional anatomy.

In short, there is nothing to prevent one performing analyses in each subject's native space (i.e., without normalizing). Our point was simply that such analyses should not be based on averages within fROIs or need a separate localizer session.

Having clarified the focus of the debate, we will deconstruct the key advantages of fROI as detailed by Saxe et al. (chapter 2, this volume) We then address an important misconception about factorial designs. The original comments of Saxe et al. (2006) are in quotation marks. Appendix 3.B details short responses to some specific points.

The Key Advantages

"The fROI method, which resembles long established practice in visual neurophysiology, has methodological statistical and theoretical advantages."

This methodology was developed under the constraints of single-unit electrode recording. These constraints do not apply to imaging neuroscience. This is because we can measure evoked responses everywhere in the brain and do not have to specify where these measurements are taken from.

"Because functional properties are more consistently and robustly associated with fROIs than with locations in stereotactic space, functional hypotheses concerning fROIs are often the most straightforward to frame."

While it is true that fROI provide a straightforward solution, they address only a straightforward problem: the functional selectivity of functionally selective voxels. The inherent tautology precludes any questions about structure–function relationships. The most important example is specificity: It is impossible to address functional segregation (i.e., the anatomical specificity of functionally selective responses), because the functionally selective responses found in a single fROI may be expressed in many other parts of the brain that were not examined. Saxe et al. note that a solution to the problem of fROI is to "combine fROI analyses with each other or with voxel-based whole-brain analysis." However, arguing for the complementary use of statistical parametric mapping (SPM) and fROI is specious. This is because SPM (and related whole-brain analyses) is equivalent to performing all possible fROI analyses.

As noted earlier, structure–function relationships become an essential issue for fROI at the level of intersubject variability; pooling functionally defined selectivity profiles over subjects is one way to discount uninteresting subject differences in structure–function mapping. Even in this context, however, dispensing with anatomy is not always appropriate. The anatomical deployment of functionally selective responses can provide important constraints on intersubject variability (e.g., degenerate or many-to-one structure–function mappings; Henson 2005; Price and Friston 2002). For example, some subjects may activate one region, whereas other subjects activate an anatomically distinct region. This degeneracy would be revealed in conventional voxel-based analyses at the single-subject level but would be missed completely using fROI that, operationally, treat the two regions as the same. In short, fROI analyses are straightforward because they eschew deeper questions about structure–function relationships in the brain.

"Because hypotheses are tested in only a handful of fROIs, advanced specification of fROIs provides a massive increase in statistical power over whole-brain analyses".

This is nonsense. Statistical power is determined by the search volume. The power of a whole-brain analysis can be rendered identical to fROI analyses; if the search volume is suitably constrained (e.g., using the fROI). Saxe et al. are confusing the use of fROIs with the well-established relationship between sensitivity and search volume. They note later, "By contrast traditional whole-brain analyses produce an explosion of multiple comparisons requiring powerful corrections to control false-positives." This correction depends only on the volume of brain examined. It is perfectly valid to perform a search constrained to a small volume of interest, which would entail less severe corrections to P values. One can also search the whole of the remaining brain using more severe (i.e., appropriate) corrections. Whole-brain analyses enable both these extremes and intermediate searches; fROI do not. In short, one can enjoy all the advantages of a constrained search, afforded by fROI, in the context of a conventional whole-brain analysis.

"Some fROIs may serve as candidate distinct components of the mind/brain worth investigation as such."

We are not really sure what this means. Perhaps they meant that if a particular fROI is reified sufficiently, it becomes an interesting object of study. Although Saxe et al. observe that fROIs do not need to be reified, this has occurred (see appendix 3.B). And even if reification is appropriate, it should not preclude studying the rest of the brain. In their final lines, Saxe et al. focus on a question a reviewer posed to us, "Why didn't the authors use an independent functional localizer for the FFA?" Saxe et al. state "we don't see an answer to this question in the commentary by Friston et al. and we still think that many studies will benefit from the use of a fROI." The answer was that the authors of the original paper were not interested in the FFA. Differences in the way we think about functional anatomy become practically important when reviewers start prescribing the research question, focus, or analysis for their colleagues (see appendix 3.A). As peer reviewers, should we be this prescriptive? Or should we be more sensitive to the dangers of fundamentalism, be it fROI or SPM?

Factorial Designs

Saxe et al. state that "We are ambivalent about factorial designs." This is significant because localizers rest on an implicit factorial design (the demonstration of the main effect of one factor in voxels that express a significant effect of another). We wonder whether the ambivalence of Saxe et al. stems from a failure to fully understand the nature of treatment effects in factorial designs: Saxe et al. state that, "in a factorial design, though the test of an interaction will be independent from the ROI-definition, the test of the main effect will be biased, since the very same data used to find the region of interest is then used to estimate the magnitude of the main effect." This is a remarkable statement. First, only one of the main effects is the localizing effect, and clearly one would not use this effect to constrain its own search! The effects of interest comprise the other main effects and interactions. Our proposal, which is standard practice in many labs, is to test for orthogonal effects (i.e., the interesting manipulations that are combined factorially with the localizing factor), at voxels that exhibit a localizing response. Orthogonal effects are independent, up to second-order statistics. This means the test for one main effect cannot bias the test for other main effects or interactions. This can be seen simply by noting that the sum of two independent numbers is independent of their difference, despite the fact that they are mixtures of the same data. Second, it may be that Saxe et al. think there is some advantage to replicating the localizing effect with a separate localizer. There is not. Formally, localizer sessions correspond to a split-half procedure (e.g., split t test). It is well known (by the Neyman–Pearson lemma) that split-half procedures are less efficient than a single likelihood-ratio test (i.e., combining the localizer and main experimental in the same model).

Conclusion

Finally, we want to reiterate the fundamental importance of factorial designs. The use of separate localizer sessions embodies an implicit assumption that the functional selectivity of the fROI is context independent. In many situations, however, selective responses are modulated by context (e.g., McIntosh 2000; Mechelli et al. 2003). For example, a "standard" FFA-localizer that compares faces and objects in an N-back task may engage different functions and brain regions from those engaged by the task examined in the main experiment. Being unable to test for an interaction between stimulus and task factors means the main effect and interaction are confounded (i.e., one cannot partition the response into a face-selective component and its task-specific modulation). This issue becomes especially problematic when reviewers insist that authors add "standard" localizers that enforce an unbalanced design and this inherent confound.

There are clearly many issues to be resolved in the mapping of structure and function in the human brain and how this mapping varies from subject to subject. Saxe et al. provide a very nice treatment of this. However, the solution fROI offers is superficial, in the sense that it ignores structure–function relationships by focusing exclusively on function. Note that this is in contradistinction to retinotopic mapping that depends on the anatomical topography of functionally selective responses (see appendix 3.B). Although fROIs may remain the preferred practice for some investigators, they are not necessarily the most principled approach to functional anatomy.

Appendix 3.A

Since writing the target article, one of us (KJF) had a paper rejected from PLoS-B. Following is the verbatim comments of [just] one reviewer (our italics):

Analysis: ROIs. These data deserve to be analyzed using the ROI approach that is now standard in the field. Retinotopically defined early visual areas should be identified and MT should be delineated in an independent scan. *Response should be averaged within active portions of each area.*

Appendix 3.B

This appendix lists some other statements by Saxe et al. and a brief comment.

"Whole brain analyses are particularly poor tools for establishing the absence of an effect."

One can never establish the absence of an effect with classical inference (i.e., accept the null hypothesis). One can only say that there was a failure to reject the null hypothesis (i.e., one was unable to find an effect). This applies to both fROI and whole-brain analyses.

"The use of fROIs is uncontroversial and indeed virtually required in any study of visual cortex involving retinotopic visual areas or MT."

Retinotopic mapping should not be confused with fROI. Retinotopic mapping entails a careful voxel-based analysis of the topography of functionally selective responses. It does not use fROI in the sense we have been discussing. There is a fundamental distinction between using phase-encode mapping to assign a regional response to V2 and using the average of all V2 voxels as the response per se.

"So the worry that the advantages of fROI analyses will lead researchers to focus exclusively on a single ROI seems unsubstantiated by the actual practice in the field."

Though a matter of opinion, our perception is that an exclusive focus has occurred in the case of the fusiform face area (FFA). When performing "standard" localizer contrasts of faces versus objects, researchers find not only a region within the mid-fusiform (FFA), but also regions in occipital (Gauthier et al. 2000) and superior temporal (Haxby et al. 1999) cortex, among others (as also the case in single-cell recordings from the nonhuman primate). But ask a nonexpert in this domain, and a typical answer will be "faces are processed in a part of the brain called the FFA." The FFA is often reified in this sense, at the expense of other face-selective regions. This focus may be confounded by the historical accident that many initial studies used a surface coil over the occipital lobe, rendering them less sensitive to anterior regions.

"The second basic concern about fROI analysis is that a focus on the response of a predefined region will lead researchers into the dangerous … assumption that the neurons that comprise the fROI are homogeneous." There is no concern about assumptions. The point made in Friston et al. (chapter 1, this volume) was that the fROI averaging procedure provides an unbiased estimate of the activation if, and only if, the response is homogeneous.

"Other sophisticated designs use parametric gradations of a single factor …"

Of course, but there is no reason why such designs cannot be made factorial.

"Peak-smoothed averaging uses smooth data and takes the time course of the voxel showing maximum activity in the localizer."

Not quite. This time course is a weighted average of nearby voxels (cf., fROI average) determined by the smoothing kernel.

"If the area is not homogeneous, we need to treat the first eigenvariate measure with care."

While it is true that any summary measure needs to be treated with care, the reason to use an eigenvariate is precisely to deal with areas that are not homogeneous.

"Finally, Friston et al. (2006) imply that there is no cost to using a full-factorial design … (or 'no loss of statistical efficiency'). On the contrary, simply multiplying the number of conditions in the experiment may produce many conditions that are of no interest to the experimenter, and simultaneously decrease the number of observations that can be conducted for the critical conditions. The result is a loss of power where it counts, and therefore reduced statistical efficiency."

It could be argued that all cells of a factorial design are both interesting and necessary (see above). However, just absorbing the localizer cells into the main experiment increases the degrees of freedom and power; under a pooled variance assumption, the estimated variance (i.e., standard error) becomes more precise with more data, even if these data do not contain an effect of interest. In other words, pooling the data from a localizer and main experimental will always be more powerful than analyzing them separately.

Acknowledgement

We would like to thank Rebecca Saxe and her colleagues (chapter 2, this volume) for providing a comprehensive and engaging commentary on our target article (chapter 1, this volume).

4 An Exchange about Localism

Martin Bunzl, Stephen José Hanson, and Russell A. Poldrack

Contemporary neuroimaging is fraught with profound disagreements about method and its underlying assumptions. A primary goal of this volume has been to bring these disagreements and assumptions to the foreground for discussion. In the exchange that follows we attempt to do this in a way designed to provide those not in the field with a sense of what is at issue. Two points of terminology in what follows: Much of the discussion centers on localist versus holist strategies. For the purposes of this discussion, we treat modularity and nonmodularity as part of the same debate. How should "localism" be understood in this discussion? We treat it is a functional notion. A local function is a specific cognitive computation (i.e., a process that exists in our current ontology of cognition) that is performed within a region. That is, there is a one-to-one mapping between a brain region and a box in one of our box-and-arrow models of cognition.

MB: If we begin with Luria's work, there seems to be something undeniably useful in what we learn from structural damage and loss of function. Admittedly, you have to be careful. But at least this seems plausible: If injury to area A takes place and function F1 is disrupted but F2 is not, then you can conclude that A plays SOME causally relevant role in the normal functioning of F1 but perhaps none in F2. ("Perhaps" because there may be alternative causal paths for F2.) The same is true when you cut pathways in animals and look for disruption of observed behavior. The fact that not every function is disrupted by damage to any area is enough to establish that holism can't be right for the brain any more than for the rest of the body. Against that background, what is wrong with trying to associate areas and functions by imaging?

SH: Well first, in any distributed system, such as the brain, the danger of localization is that there is nothing really to localize. Even the back half of the brain, which is rife with sensory pathways that often appear localized, is involved in many different interactions with prefrontal cortex, which often appears to be opportunistic with regard to brain function. Luria and others were thinking of a kind of "lesion and factor" metaphor, which assumes the system under study to be modular and locally (maybe linearly) identifiable. Even simple distributed systems that are weakly interactive will confound the lesion strategy. Consider a classic story from computational neuroscientists from the early 1960s, also dealing with the neuroscientist's "lesion logic," the broken radio metaphor. When the radio repairman removed a tube from the radio in order to see if he could diagnose the problem in the radio, immediately on its removal, the radio began to whistle loudly. In parallel, based on what the neuroscientists are claiming, clearly the repairman had accidently found the "antiwhistling tube"!

RP: I think that Martin is correct that lesion evidence undercuts the strong holist claims, but there will always be those who come along and purport to show how one can get what appear to be dissociations out of a single unified system. Good examples of this can be found in the literatures on implicit versus explicit memory or semantic memory. The strategy of functional decomposition and localization is just that—a strategy. If the brain turns out to be a completely holistic complex dynamic system, then this strategy will fail, but as Bechtel and Richardson lay out in their book *Discovering Complexity*, this strategy has been fairly successful in the history of biology and I would argue that it has also been relatively successful in neuroscience as well. For evidence of this, look at neurosurgery. There is a reason that neurosurgeons are now using fMRI to help plan surgical resections, and it's not because they like the pretty pictures. It's because it helps them do a better job of avoiding damage to important areas of cortex. We can argue all we want about the nature of brain organization, but the success of fMRI for surgical planning suggests to me that the strategy of decomposition and localization has worked, at least to a rough approximation. I think the proper counter to the Weiner example is that, while it might properly describe the reasoning of a radio repairman (though I doubt that), it is most certainly a caricature of scientific reasoning. For example, people with Parkinson's disease exhibit akinesia (decreased voluntary movement), and we know that this arises from the death of dopamine neurons in the substantia nigra. However, to my knowledge no one in neuroscience has ever proposed that the role of dopamine is as an "antifreezing" agent. Rather, the discovery of dopamine's role in this disease led to the formation and testing of hypotheses about how this akinesia could arise from perturbation of the relevant networks when dopamine is taken away. Here, again, I would argue that the decomposition and localization approach has been wildly successful; there are no doubt very lively debates about the details of this disorder and no cure for it yet, but both drugs and surgeries exist that can help reduce or eliminate at least some of the symptoms of the disorder, and the development of these treatments arose directly from the localization of the disorder to specific neurochemical and neuroanatomical systems.

SH: I'm not saying the brain is holistic or equipotential in some Lashly-like sense, nonetheless, fMRI neurosurgery planning is more a testament to recovery of function and local equipotentiality than the success of factor and localize strategies. Lesions in V1 allow for "blindsight," whereas Wernike's and Broca's lesions, which seemed obviously related to syntax and semantics in the nineteenth century, are now hopelessly tangled up in a muddle of more specific yet–to-be-named cognitive functions.

RP: Decomposition/localization strategy is, in large part, the basis of modern biological science. As Bechtel and Richardson argue, and I agree, it's not clear what the alternatives are to this strategy. The obvious alternative is the dynamic systems approach, which abandons any hope of localization in favor of characterizing the dynamics of the entire system, but I know of few examples where that strategy has been successful in advancing our understanding of a system (motor control being an example of where it seems to have been at least somewhat useful). And a state-space equation describing whole-brain dynamics is not going to be very useful for the surgeon who wants to figure out where to cut in order to spare eloquent cortex. With regard to modularity, I think that the sensibility of this notion depends entirely on how one conceptualizes a "module." In the sense of isolated processing units that are informationally encapsulated (à la Fodor), the neuroscience clearly rules this out. However, I think there is good evidence for some milder form of modularity in brain function. I think that one strong piece of evidence for weak modularity comes from recent work on the "connectome," which has shown that both structural and functional networks in the brain exhibit scale-free characteristics, such that a small number of hubs exhibit long range connectivity as well as dense local connectivity (e.g., Sporns et al. 2004). These local, heavily connected neighborhoods would seem to me to be a reasonable approximation to a weak module.

SH: This discussion seems to have fallen into a classic tension of modularity and dynamics. Fodor distinguishes between two kinds of modularity: horizontal and vertical. As he explicates the distinction in *The Modularity of Mind* (1983):

[A] horizontal faculty is a functionally distinguishable cognitive system whose operations cross content domains. (p. 13)

   ... vertical faculties are domain specific, they are genetically determined, they are associated with distinct neural structures, and—to introduce a new point—they are computationally autonomous. (p. 21)

So, in effect, modularity might map conveniently and pleasantly onto familiar lexical concepts (vertical), and another type might map basic functions that are more universal (horizontal) but less familiar and more difficult to map. The first case was embraced in cognitive science and eventually cognitive neuroscience, partly driven by linguistic arguments and partly driven by parsimony. Unfortunately, in both cases, this first type of modularity has proven to simply be wrong in either linguistics or in leading to a simple explanation of cognitive processes, especially in the context of its potential computational nature. The second, I would say "forgotten," Fodor modularity seems closer to reality. Here, we might imagine simple pieces of code—"bubble sort," "get regular expression," "count and cumulate," "find differences," "minimize cost," and so on—simpler, compact, and more potentially distributed functions that are reused and can be recombined opportunistically, but also not familiar in some stimulus context (e.g., "faces").

Once one accepts the notion of horizontal modularity, it is easier to see how this might be reconciled with dynamics, since this type of modularity is less likely to have a specific brain area rather than an equivalence class of circuits that have an equipotential arising in numerous ways and flavors. It is possible to imagine a horizontal modularity as a type of weaker modularity. These are often considered to be structured dynamics, which are more opportunistic and yet predictable when they arise (even though they might not arise in the same circuits or geography). A serious experimental problem arises under this type of modularity in identifying the functions, universal or not, that arise when a cognitive or perceptual task is imposed on a subject. Unfortunately, the tasks we have in the cognitive/social neuroscience are unlikely to reveal very much about this type of modularity or the nature of the requisite functions underlying it. Worse, horizontal modularity can intersect with a vertical modularity, making it appear that stimulus properties have some unique relation to cortical function, despite the evidence we have to the contrary.

Consider a simple case: What does the STS do? It appears to be "activated" across numerous tasks, and contexts without a simple interpretation. Often cognitive neuroscientists refer to it processing "biological motion." But what's the potential contrast? What is nonbiological motion? It appears to some to be part of the "FACE processing network" (Grill-Spector et al. 2006b), and to others as part of the "social network," and to still others as "the mirror system." This multiplicity of function of the STS simply underscores the muddle and bankruptcy of modularity, which even Fodor found "unlikely to be very useful" and yet is now presently embraced by the neurosciences.

MB: Steve, bracketing the methodological difficulty of imaging a source of knowledge, are you saying there is nothing to be learned from the differentiated structure of the brain? If there is something to be learned from it, are you saying that functional analysis is of no value at all? For example, I am thinking of LeDoux's stimulation, tracing, and ablation studies on fear in rats.

SH: No, I am saying functional analysis, as used in the standard vertical modularity, is too simple and misleading, and does not rule out less familiar and potentially more powerful horizontal modularity explanations.

MB: If it is too simple and misleading, then why isn't the answer "no"?

SH: Because the functional analysis of something as complex as a brain doesn't lead to mutually exclusive or unique strategies. Picking the simplest strategy first is rational, even if wrong, and won't be abandoned until its completely exhausted and the last dogmatic experimentalist falls over on his talairach atlas.

RP: Steve raises two important issues here that I will discuss in turn: the issue of horizontal versus vertical modularity, and the more general issue of how our experimental data bear on modularity claims. On my reading of Fodor, there is no injunction that horizontal modules can't be localized, only that vertical modules must be. From this standpoint, a number of the cognitive processes that have been localized to specific regions are really horizontal rather than vertical. The best example that I can think of is the hippocampus, which is involved in declarative memory regardless of the domain. I thus disagree with Steve's claim that horizontal modules will be more difficult to map or that the concepts will be less familiar. In fact, to the contrary, Fodor (1983, p. 14) argues that horizontal faculty psychology is "the common-sense theory of the mind." I think that what Steve is suggesting, with the concept of basic operations such as bubble sorts and cost minimization as horizontal modules, is something completely different from both of these conceptions; it's not really modularity at all as far as I am concerned, unless one thinks that the alphabet of basic computational operations should be called "modules"—at which point the concept seems to become somewhat meaningless.

The more important issue here, from the standpoint of neuroimaging research, is what our studies tell us about localization, and here I think Steve is absolutely right. There is a strong and pervasive tendency in the field to interpret localized regions of statistically significant activation as reflecting functional localization and specialization for the mental process in question. These localizations are then reified through the use of "reverse inference," in which activation in a specific region is interpreted as reflecting the presence of a particular mental process. As an example, activation in the amygdala is often interpreted as reflecting fear or negative emotion, even though there are powerful demonstrations that the amygdala can be equally active for positive outcomes. Very rarely does one see studies that test alternative hypotheses for these activations, leading to a research program that one might characterize as "confirmation bias gone wild." The "mirror system" work that Steve mentions is one of the starkest examples of this; for a set of researchers in this domain, activation in a very broad set of regions is sufficient to proclaim that the mirror system is engaged, write a paper demonstrating yet another cognitive domain in which the mirror system is involved, and move onto searching for involvement of the mirror system activity in another domain.

MB: Russ, if you don't think this kind of localization work gives us an understanding of the human brain and mind, what would?

RP: One strategy that I can envision is laid out in a recent paper that Steve and I have written (Poldrack Halchenko and Hanson, 2009). What we do is take a number of imaging datasets (eight, in this case) and first code each of the tasks according to a coarse mental ontology. We then perform dimensionality reduction on the fMRI data, so that we end up with a small number of dimensions that we can analyze for each subject (six dimensions in this case). We can then project the cognitive ontology X task matrix onto the task X neural dimension matrix, to get a mapping of the cognitive ontology onto these neural dimensions. The neural mapping here is similar in spirit to much of the work that has used multivariate approaches to characterize functional and effective connectivity in neuroimaging data. The use of a task ontology, however, allows a more direct mapping of mental processes onto these patterns of activity. The next step is then to characterize these networks using computational models that explicitly incorporate the structural connectivity and functional dynamics of the system; because fMRI can provide only a very limited view of the dynamics, we will need other neuroscience techniques to fully characterize those aspects of the system.

SH: Close, but not quite. I think there is localization of function in the Fodor horizontal sense of modularity, that is, basic computational functions that we don't understand and have no good language at this point to completely describe, but are "opportunistic" and "combinatorial." So I do believe there are local functions. For example, I think the IPL does something computationally promiscuous and is part of kinds of cognitive functions. On the other hand, describing the IPL in some familiar and yet vague folk psychological terms creates a hopeless muddle of claims and agendas that get fossilized in the journals and training of graduate students.

RP: So I think we agree that the fundamental problem is our stone age psychological ontology.

5 Multivariate Pattern Analysis of fMRI Data: High-Dimensional Spaces for Neural and Cognitive Representations

James V. Haxby

Functional magnetic resonance imaging (fMRI) produces a deluge of data about neural activity in the entire brain. A typical fMRI study collects data from 20,000 to 100,000 locations every two to three seconds over periods ranging from five minutes to a full hour. The resulting data set consists of 10 million or more measures. Analyzing such a data set so that it provides a clear and easily communicated answer to a research question is a major challenge for fMRI investigators. The necessary data reduction is shaped by assumptions about the organization of the functional architecture that produces patterns of neural activity and by the goal of removing unrelated and noninformative complexity. Consequently, different methods of analysis reflect more than a mathematical preference; they reflect different assumptions about the basic structure of brain organization.

In this chapter, I discuss the difference between two approaches to fMRI data analysis. These approaches are univariate analysis based on the general linear model (GLM) (Friston et al. 1994) and multivariate pattern (MVP) analysis based on machine learning pattern classifiers (Haxby et al. 2001; Haynes and Rees 2006; Norman et al. 2006; O'Toole et al. 2007). The comparison will not focus on the differences in computational procedures but rather on the underlying assumptions about the functional architecture of the brain and the difference in kinds of scientific questions that these analytic approaches can address.

Whereas conventional univariate analysis casts local neural activity in a one-dimensional space in which activity is characterized as high or low, MVP analysis casts local activity in a high-dimensional space in which activity is characterized as a vector. Consequently, univariate analysis can only compare conditions on the single dimension of activity strength. Due in part to the limited representational space, univariate analysis usually makes the implicit assumption that stronger activity reflects more engagement in a cognitive state. By contrast, MVP analysis compares conditions in terms of the discriminability or distances among the vectors associated with each condition. Consequently, MVP analysis investigates the structure of the high-dimensional representational space that a brain region supports, whereas univariate analysis asks a much simpler question—namely, which perceptual or cognitive functions "activate" a region.

I argue that the representational framework provided by MVP analysis is more powerful in terms of both capacity—the number of different brain states that can be distinguished—and explanatory power. In particular, I argue that distances among vectors in a high-dimensional space provide a framework for investigating the similarity structure of multiple brain states. This neural similarity structure can be related to stimulus and cognitive similarity. Finally, I argue that multivariate analysis brings fMRI investigation closer to investigating the codes for how functions are represented in neural population responses, whereas univariate analysis limits fMRI mostly to function localization.

Conventional Univariate Analysis of fMRI Data

Conventional analysis of fMRI data is based on univariate analysis of the time series at each brain location. The goal of this analysis is to find brain locations that show a significantly different level of activity for different experimental conditions, for example, a greater response while viewing faces compared to viewing houses. Consequently, the representational capacity of a brain location can be characterized as "on" or "off" or somewhere in between, like a neural dimmer switch. With this analytic tool, the function of a brain location is characterized by the experimental conditions that activate it. If one condition, such as face perception, activates a brain location more than another, such as body parts perception, then one infers that the location is more involved in the perception of faces than in the perception of body parts.

The brain locations identified by univariate analysis with GLM are called brain areas, with the implicit assumption that all locations within a brain area have similar response profiles across different experimental conditions. This assumption is embodied in two common features of univariate analysis with the GLM. First, the data from neighboring voxels are smoothed, generally with a filter that has a full width at half maximum (FWHM) of 6 to 12 mm. The size of the smoothing filter reflects the assumption that the functional areas to be identified have a cortical area of approximately 1 cm^2 or greater. Second, the functional response of a location is expressed either as the response of the maximally responsive voxel, which reflects a large cortical area after smoothing, or by the average response in a region of interest (ROI) that is defined on either a functional or anatomical basis.

These choices for analytic methods direct the investigator to assumptions about the functional architecture of the brain:

1. The brain is divided into areas with cortical areas of 1 cm^2 or greater that each performs a distinct function.
2. The nature of an area's function can be determined by finding the experimental condition that evokes the maximal response in that area.

3. Weak levels of response suggest that an experimental condition was suboptimal and, therefore, less related to the function of that area.

4. Local variability of response within an area is irrelevant noise.

Multivariate Pattern Analysis

MVP analysis uses machine learning pattern classifiers to analyze patterns of activity in fMRI data. A pattern of activity is characterized as an n-dimensional vector, n referring to the number of features or voxels[1] in the pattern. The goal of MVP analysis is to detect distinct patterns that are associated with each experimental condition and characterize the relationships among those patterns. For example, MVP analysis may detect distinct patterns of activity in primary visual cortex for viewing gratings with horizontal, vertical, and 45-degree orientations and show, further, that the patterns of response for vertical and horizontal gratings are more different from each other than they are from the patterns of response to 45-degree gratings (Kamitani and Tong 2005).

The representational capacity of a brain area is analyzed in a high-dimensional space, affording the power to distinguish numerous brain states. The representational capacity for a brain area in a univariate analysis essentially collapses this high-dimensional space onto a single dimension, either by averaging the responses across voxels or by characterizing a brain area's response as the response of the maximally responsive voxel, thus discarding all other voxels. Retaining information from all voxels in the representational space for a brain area has two important consequences. First, it assumes that local variation in voxel responses can carry information about the brain state. This assumption implies that the features of functional brain organization that can be identified with fMRI have a higher spatial frequency—local bumps in the patterns of response—than that of whole brain areas. Second, it assumes that weak responses in some voxels for a given condition can carry information.

The use of multivariate pattern analysis for fMRI, therefore, directs the investigator to different assumptions about the functional architecture of the brain:

1. A brain area has the capacity to represent a variety of stimuli or cognitive states.

2. Local variation of response strength within a brain area is signal that reflects changes in the representational state.

3. Weak activity, as well as strong activity, can be important in specifying the representational state of a brain area.

Thus, MVP analysis is based on a different model of functional brain organization in which the local neural code is a distributed population response that produces different patterns of activity for different brain states and local activity therefore encodes information in a high-dimensional space with high capacity for encoding a large variety of brain states. As I make clear in a later section, these assumptions lead naturally to relating regional patterns of response in fMRI data to distributed population responses for encoding perceptual and cognitive brain states.

The remainder of this chapter focuses on multivariate pattern analysis, This review will focus on studies of visual representation. MVP analysis also has been applied successfully in studies of other cognitive domains such as audition (Raizada and Poldrack 2007), semantic representation (e.g., Mitchell et al. 2008), memory (e.g., Norman et al. 2006), and intention (e.g., Haynes et al. 2007).

What Is Multivariate Pattern Analysis?

Multivariate pattern analysis treats each observation as a high-dimensional vector. An observation in such an analysis can be a single timepoint (TR), a single event with activity measured by a small number of timepoints, or a series of events in a block-design experiment with activity averaged across the duration of the block. The vector is composed of the activity level or image intensity in each voxel and, thus, is a compact representation of a pattern of activity.

The vectors that represent observations for different conditions can be analyzed in a variety of ways that address different scientific questions. These analyses can be grouped into three categories: classification, similarity analysis, and model-based prediction. Classification demonstrates whether each condition, compared to other conditions, is associated with a distinct pattern of neural responses. Similarity analysis investigates the degree of similarity of the neural response patterns to different conditions, allowing the comparison of the neural similarity structure to other measures of the similarity of conditions, such as cognitive attributes and physical stimulus properties. Model-based prediction recasts the dimensional structure of the original feature space into the dimensional structure of a neural or cognitive model, thus allowing one to predict the response to new stimuli or conditions.

MVP analysis has proven to be far more sensitive than conventional analysis for all of the questions these three types of analysis address (Hanson et al. 2004a; Haxby et al. 2001; Haynes and Rees 2005; Haynes et al. 2008; Kamitani and Tong 2005; Kay et al. 2008; Kriegeskorte et al. 2008; Mitchell et al. 2008). Both MVP analysis and conventional analysis aggregate data across multiple voxels to increase statistical power. Conventional analysis uses spatial smoothing for data aggregation, which suppresses noise but also eliminates any signal that may reside in between-voxel response differences. MVP analysis, on the other hand, aggregates data across voxels without discarding between-voxel response differences. If between-voxel response differences carried no information, that is, if they were simply statistical noise, MVP analysis would be no more sensitive than conventional analysis.[2] The fact that MVP analysis is substantially more sensitive than conventional analysis indicates that the between-voxel differences conventional analysis discards carry substantial information. Later, I discuss the probable source of this information in between-voxel differences.

Pattern Classification

Pattern classification is applied to fMRI data to determine whether different experimental conditions are associated with distinct patterns of neural response. In other words, classification determines whether the vectors associated with responses to one condition can be distinguished reliably from vectors associated with responses to other conditions. A variety of methods exist for determining a decision rule for distinguishing the vectors for different experimental conditions.

Pattern classification is almost always done within subject (a notable exception is Poldrack et al. in press). The data are divided into training and test sets. The decision rule is derived based solely on the data in the training set. It is critical that the test data are not used in any step of this derivation to maintain the validity of generalization testing. All decision rules involve defining sectors of the high-dimensional vector space that are associated with each condition. The validity of the decision rule is tested by classifying the test data. Each observation or vector in the test data is classified as the condition associated with the sector in the high-dimensional space in which it is located. If the test data are classified into the correct categories at a rate higher than expected by chance, the decision rule is judged to be valid.

The key innovation represented by the use of pattern classification for the analysis of fMRI data lies in the capacity of a high-dimensional vector space to represent a large number of different states. Conventional univariate analysis rests on representation in a one-dimensional space. Consequently, the representational capacity in conventional analyses is severely limited and, in practice, is usually restricted to attempts to find a single condition that best characterizes the function of a region, as indicated by a maximal response to that condition compared to other conditions. By contrast, pattern classification leads the investigator to examine a number of conditions that can be represented by activity in a single region.

In our original paper (Haxby et al. 2001), we found that activity in ventral temporal (VT) cortex (or in functionally specified subregions in VT) could produce distinct patterns of response for eight categories of faces or objects. Previous work using conventional analysis methods had attempted to find regions that represented single categories (e.g., Downing et al. 2001; Epstein and Kanwisher 1998; Kanwisher, McDermott, and Chun 1997). Subsequent work using pattern classification methods has corroborated our finding that, in fact, even these putatively single-category regions actually carry discriminative information about multiple categories (Hanson et al. 2004; Reddy and Kanwisher 2007).

A second demonstration of the power of pattern classifiers came from work on the representation of the edge orientation in early visual cortex. Two research reports appeared back-to-back in *Nature Neuroscience* in 2005 (Haynes and Rees 2005; Kamitani and Tong 2005), both showing that viewed gratings with different orientations produced distinct patterns of response in early visual cortex (V1, V2, V3). This demonstration was surprising because the topography for orientation-selective columns in early visual cortex is well-understood but has a much higher spatial frequency than that of conventional fMRI voxel size. Every orientation is re-represented every millimeter in a well-organized topography. Consequently, a 3-mm voxel will contain numerous columns for all orientations. Before the reports by Kamitani and Tong (2005) and Haynes and Rees (2005), it was believed that orientation selectivity in early visual cortex could be detected only using fMRI adaptation (Tootell et al. 1995), a method that uses conventional analysis to show a response reduction for repeated compared to novel stimuli (Grill-Spector et al. 2001). Both Kamitani and Tong (2005) and Haynes and Rees (2005) concluded that the sensitivity of MVP analysis could be attributed to low spatial frequency features in the orientation-selective topography. A lumpy topography produces a subtle orientation bias in each voxel, reflecting overrepresentation for some orientations and underrepresentation for others. These subtle biases are too small to be detected by conventional univariate statistics because they vary voxel by voxel. Pattern classifiers, on the other hand, can aggregate the information in an early visual area like V1 across a large number of voxels with different orientation biases without smoothing the data.

Subtle biases in the response tuning curves of individual voxels could also underlie the sensitivity of MVP analysis to other types of visual information. In the inferior temporal (IT) cortex of monkeys, individual cells have tuning curves that reflect differential responses to complex features (Tanaka 2003) and whole objects (Kiani et al. 2007; Logothetis and Sheinberg 1996) that can produce distinct population responses for categories (Kiani et al. 2007). The topographic distribution of cells in IT cortex with different tuning functions is poorly understood, but low spatial frequencies in this topography could produce subtle biases in voxel responses. The category-selective regions FFA and PPA represent very low spatial frequency features in the functional topography of ventral temporal cortex. MVP analysis has shown, however, that information about nonpreferred categories can be detected even within these regions (Hanson et al. 2004a; Haxby et al. 2001; Reddy and Kanwisher 2007), indicating that the information that discriminates multiple categories is not attributable solely to these regions. In other words, the low spatial frequency features in the topographic organization of category-selective response tuning are not found only at the very coarse scale of these category-selective regions but also at a finer scale, even within these regions. In fact, although single-unit recording in the putative monkey homolog of the FFA shows a very high concentration of cells that respond maximally to faces, the weak responses in these cells to nonface objects carry enough information to classify the population responses at both the category and the individual stimulus levels.[3]

Similarity Structure Analysis

MVP analysis can also quantify the similarity of patterns of response, in addition to detecting whether the distinctions among patterns are simply significant. There are several ways that dissimilarity can be quantified. One is the frequency of misclassifications. This measure is valid only if obtained from generalization test data. A more direct measure can also be obtained by simply calculating the distance between the vectors for different conditions. Distance can be measured as a Euclidean distance or with correlation, which reflects the polar angle between vectors and factors out differences in overall magnitude.

Measures of similarity can be used to examine the similarity structure of neural representations, namely, the set of similarities among all pairs within a set of experimental conditions. The complete similarity structure is the full matrix of pairwise similarities. The similarity structure can be compressed, or projected into a lower dimensional subspace, to permit illustration—for example, with multidimensional scaling or a dendrogram—but these illustrations distort the original similarity structure.

The similarity structure of neural responses to different categories of objects and faces was first analyzed by Hanson et al. (2004a; figure 5.1a). In their reanalysis of the data of patterns of response in human VT from the Haxby et al. (2001) study, they performed a cluster analysis on the intermediate layer weights a neural network classifier generates. The results of this analysis were illustrated with a dendrogram. This analysis showed that the dominant distinction in this representational space was between animate and inanimate categories. Within the inanimate domain, houses were most different from the other categories, which were all small manmade objects. In a subsequent, independent analysis of the same data (O'Toole et al. 2005), in which the similarity structure was illustrated with multidimensional scaling (figure 5.1b), the similarity structure revealed the same features as those found by Hanson et al. (2004a).

Kiani et al. (2007) analyzed the similarity structure of population responses in monkey IT (inferior temporal) cortex using similar methods applied to single-unit recording data (figure 5.2, plate 2). They recorded responses from a large number of IT cells during perception of a large variety of images of faces, animals, and objects. As in the analyses of human fMRI responses, the major distinction was between animate and inanimate entities. Moreover, the similarity structure of population responses to animate entities reflected category relationships that resemble human semantic knowledge. Faces formed one major cluster, with greater similarity between human and monkey faces than with the faces of other animals. Animal bodies formed the other major cluster, with three subclusters for (1) human, four-legged mammals, and

a)   b)

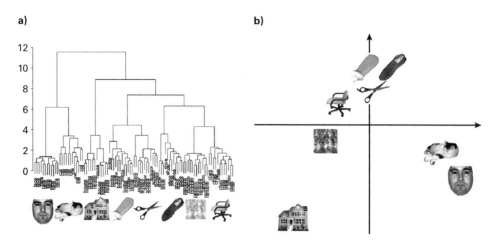

Figure 5.1
Similarity structure of neural responses in Haxby et al. (2001) in reanalyses by Hanson et al. (2004) and O'Toole et al. (2005). (a) Hanson et al. (2004a) analyzed the data with a neural network and examined the similarity structure by doing a cluster analysis on the intermediate layer weights, illustrated as a dendrogram. Note the major distinction between animate and inanimate categories and the distinction between houses and all other categories of inanimate objects. (Adapted from Hanson et al. 2004a) (b) O'Toole et al. (2005) analyzed the data with a linear discriminate analysis and displayed the similarity structure using multidimensional scaling on the distances based on classification errors. Note that the same distinctions between animate and inanimate categories and between houses and other objects are evident in this analysis. (From O'Toole et al. 2007)

birds, (2) butterflies and other insects, and (3) fish and reptiles. In an fMRI study in humans, Kriegeskorte et al. (2008) used a subset of the images from Kiani et al. (2007) and found that the similarity structure revealed in fMRI patterns in human ventral temporal cortex showed many of the same features as the similarity structure revealed in population responses consisting of single-unit recordings in monkey IT cortex. The major distinction was between animate and inanimate stimuli, with a second major division within the animate domain between faces and bodies. By comparing the similarity structures in VT and early visual cortex, Kriegeskorte et al (2008) were able to show that neural similarities based on visual features carried over from early visual cortex to VT, but greater neural dissimilarities due to category distinctions were found in VT only.

An intelligible similarity structure also is apparent in the response patterns seen in early visual cortex to a simple visual feature, edge orientation. In Kamitani and Tong (2005), classification errors for patterns of response to different grating orientations almost always falsely identified a similar orientation as that being viewed rather than

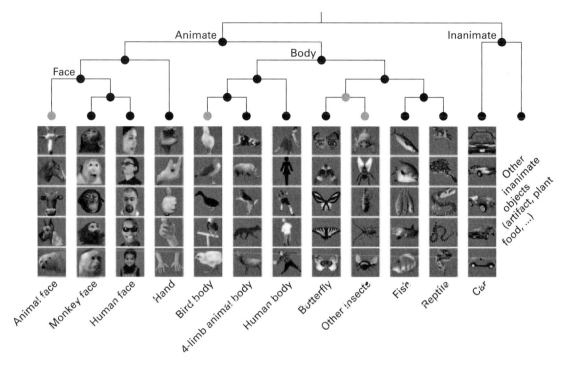

Figure 5.2 (plate 2)

Similarity structure of population responses measured in monkey IT during viewing of a wide variety of images of faces, animals, and objects (from Kiani et al. 2007). Similarity was indexed as $1 - r$, where r is the correlation between the pattern of response strengths across IT neurons. Results are displayed as a dendrogram produced with hierarchical clustering.

an orthogonal orientation (figure 5.3). In addition to knowledge of the topographic organization of orientation-selective columns (see above), the tuning function for orientation-selective cells is also known.

Orientation-selective cells respond maximally to one orientation but also respond significantly above baseline to neighboring orientations, showing a gradual decline in response strength related to dissimilarity between the viewed and preferred orientation. The predicted fMRI response patterns to orientations, based on the model of subtle bias in voxel-by-voxel orientation selectivity based on a lumpy topography, predicts the similarity structure seen in fMRI MVP classifier performance.

The single-unit recording results in Kiani et al. (2007) suggest that the similarity structure of population responses to different categories of faces and objects is also a result of coarseness in the tuning functions of individual cells to different categories. They found that the tuning functions of most cells revealed significant responses to

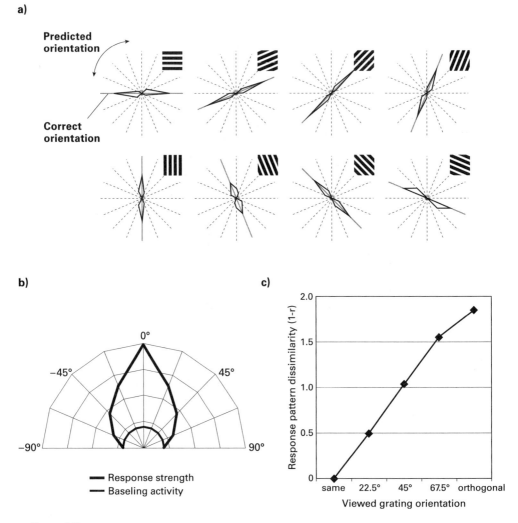

Figure 5.3
(a) Classification performance for identifying the orientation of viewed gratings based on patterns of response in V1. The correct orientation is indicated by the red line. Classification performance is indicated by the blue line in the polar plot. Note that nearly all classification errors misidentify the orientation as the one most similar to that being viewed. (From Kamitani and Tong 2005) (b) An idealized tuning function for an orientation-selective cell that responds maximally to vertical edges. (c) Similarity of simulated patterns of fMRI response to different orientation differences based on orientation tunings similar to that shown in (b). Voxel response biases were simulated by assigning variable numbers of units tuned to each of eight orientations to each simulated voxel. The responses to each orientation in all simulated voxels was calculated and similarity was indexed by the correlation between response patterns.

multiple categories and significant differences among the responses to nonpreferred categories. Such coarse tuning can produce voxel-by-voxel subtle biases to categories that, in aggregate, will produce a similarity structure showing greater similarity for categories that tend to coactivate individual cells than for categories that show less shared activation of cells.

Thus, analysis of similarity structure reveals a high-dimensional representational space that reflects the coarseness of tuning functions for neurons that participate in population codes for simple and complex stimuli. By contrast, univariate representational schemata do not accommodate or address these aspects of neural representation.

These results demonstrate the power of a high-dimensional framework for understanding neural representations. In addition to detecting distinctions among representations, which are afforded by classification, similarity structure analysis quantifies the magnitude of those distinctions. The similarity structures for representations vary for different brain regions in the visual pathway, allowing examination of how the representations change as processing progresses. In early visual cortex measures of dissimilarity reflect low-level visual features, such as edge orientation, spatial frequency, and retinotopic location. In VT cortex, measures of dissimilarity among representations of faces and objects reflect the semantic relationships among categories. Moreover, these measure of dissimilarity appear to reflect the coarseness of tuning functions for neural populations. Greater similarity between the neural representations of two visual features or two categories reflects cells that respond significantly to both. Thus, MVP analysis of neural representations appears to progress toward understanding the relationship between neural population responses, on the one hand, and perceptual and cognitive representations, on the other.

Model-Based Prediction

MVP analysis is based on building a classifier for each individual subject, and all of the studies described thus far have limited classification and similarity analysis to the stimuli that were included in the training data set. The similarity structure of neural representations was related to simple physical stimulus dimensions (orientation) (Kamitani and Tong 2005) or notions about semantic relations among categories that are not in a formal model (Hanson et al. 2004; Kiani et al. 2007; Kriegeskorte et al. 2008; O'Toole et al. 2005). Recent work, however, has cast information about stimulus conditions into more formal, computational models that allow the dimensions in these models to be recast into the dimensions in fMRI voxel space (Kay et al. 2008; Mitchell et al. 2008). Consequently, these models allow prediction of the expected pattern of response to novel stimuli, that is, stimuli that played no role in the construction of a classifier.

Kay et al. (2008) analyzed natural images—grayscale photos of natural scenes—with a model based on knowledge of the tuning properties of V1 cells. The model was based on Gabor wavelet pyramids that varied along the dimensions of orientation, spatial frequency, and location. They then built a model of response patterns, as measured with fMRI, for each subject's V1 cortex. The response of each voxel was modeled as a weighted sum of the power of the Gabor wavelet filters. The model was based on measured responses to 1,750 images. After the model was built for an individual subject, the pattern of response could be predicted for any novel image by analyzing the image with the Gabor wavelet model and calculating the predicted response for each voxel. The results show that these predictions were remarkably accurate. Responses were measured for 120 novel test images. The image being viewed was identified correctly (1 out of 120) with 92% accuracy for one subject and 72% accuracy for the other. Expanding the set of modeled images to 1,000 decreased accuracy only slightly to 82% (chance was 0.1%).

Mitchell et al. (2008) modeled the meaning of nouns using latent semantic analysis. Each noun was modeled as the rate of co-occurrence with a small set of verbs (25 verbs) in a large corpus of text. This analysis produces a semantic representational space with 25 dimensions. The response of each voxel could then be modeled as a weighted sum of the value on each of these dimensions. To test whether this model could predict the pattern of response to novel stimuli (picture-noun pairs) that were not used in the training data set, they built a new model repeatedly, based on all stimuli except two, and then test whether the model accurately discriminated the two out-of-sample stimuli. The results showed that the model accurately predicted which of two novel stimuli was shown, even when the test stimuli were from categories not represented in the training data set.

These two studies show that MVP analysis integrated with a high-dimensional model of a stimulus space is generative, insofar as the responses to novel stimuli can be predicted accurately. This prediction is accomplished by calculating correspondence rules that convert coordinates in stimulus space into coordinates in voxel space.

The success of these studies cannot lead to the conclusion that the neural representational space is using the same features that were used as dimensions in the model of stimulus space. In the case of V1, the model in Kay et al. (2008) is based explicitly on models of V1 neuron response tuning functions. Nonetheless, a more powerful demonstration would contrast the effectiveness of their V1 model to alternative models of stimulus space, for example, Fourier analysis or other types of wavelet decomposition. Similarly, the model of semantic space in Mitchell et al. (2008), which implies that the meanings of nouns are represented by coactivation of the meanings of frequently co-occurring verbs, needs to be tested against other models of semantic meaning that are computationally specified.

Conclusion

Analytic methods carry assumptions about what one expects to find. Univariate analysis and multivariate pattern analysis are based on markedly different assumptions about how neural activity encodes information. Stepping back to examine these assumptions is important for advancing our understanding of neural representation and what functional brain imaging can contribute. Univariate analysis casts representations in a one-dimensional space, limiting the number of states that can be distinguished to "on," "off," or somewhere in between. By contrast, MVP analysis casts representations in a high-dimensional space, making the number of states that can be distinguished virtually unlimited. Thus, local representation is not a matter of whether a function simply is engaged but is, instead, a matter of how neural population activity encodes information.

MVP analysis has changed the role of functional neuroimaging in the investigation of neural representation. It allows the investigation of local neural representation in a high-dimensional space. The high-dimensional patterns of response can then be related to high-dimensional representations of neural population codes, on the one hand, and to high-dimensional representations of stimuli and cognitive processes, on the other. The similarity structure of patterns of response is related to the coarseness of the tuning functions of individual cells in population codes and to stimulus and cognitive similarity. These correspondences allow a much more direct investigation of how stimulus and cognitive features are represented in neural population codes. Explicit, computational models of stimulus and cognitive spaces allow a more formal correlation of neural and psychological spaces that can be generative. In other words, these models are not limited to the stimuli and conditions that are presented in the experiment but can be extrapolated to make explicit predictions about an arbitrarily large set of new stimuli and cognitive states.

MVP analysis is not simply a new method for analyzing the same types of neuroimaging experiments that can also be analyzed with conventional univariate statistics. Rather, the experimental designs that will take greatest advantage of MVP analysis will require a large number of stimulus variations or conditions to map out the high-dimensional stimulus space. Early experiments with MVP analysis classified moderate numbers of conditions, such as eight categories of faces and objects (Haxby et al. 2001) or eight grating orientations (Kamitani and Tong 2005). More recent experiments, however, have included much larger numbers of conditions, such as 92 distinct images of faces and objects (Kriegeskorte et al. 2008), 60 noun-picture pairs (Mitchell et al. 2008), or 1,750 images of natural scenes (Kay et al. 2008). The increase in noise for the measurement of each individual condition, resulting from less signal averaging over blocks or repeated trials, is more than compensated for by the sophistication of methods for mapping out the high-dimensional representational spaces for complex objects, semantic meaning, and low-level visual features.

Notes

1. MVP analysis can be applied to whole brain data. In this chapter, however, I focus on the application of MVP analysis to studying patterns of response within brain areas. These brain areas can be as restricted as a conventional brain area, such as primary visual cortex (V1) or visual-motion-selective cortex (MT), or more broadly defined based on anatomical boundaries, such as ventral temporal cortex. Whole-brain MVP analysis can be quite powerful, but for the present discussion, it blurs the distinction between MVP analysis and conventional analysis of regional response magnitudes (cf. Pessoa).

2. Some methods of MVP analysis discard overall response magnitude differences (e.g., nearest neighbor methods that use correlation as a distance metric; Haxby et al. 2001), which is precisely the signal that conventional analysis exploits. If most of the information-bearing signal resided in these overall response magnitude differences, such MVP analyses would be less sensitive than conventional analyses, but, in fact, they appear to be more sensitive.

3. The classification accuracy for nonface objects in the study by Tsao, Freiwald, et al. (2006) can be calculated from the data presented in their figure 3. Nonface objects were classified into the correct category 111/320 times, which differs from chance (53/320) at $p < 10^{-14}$ (binomial probability), and were classified correctly at the level of individual stimulus 55/320 times, which differs from chance (4/320) at $p < 10^{-47}$.

II Inference and New Data Structures

6 Begging the Question: The Nonindependence Error in fMRI Data Analysis

Edward Vul and Nancy Kanwisher

You sit with a deck of fifty-two cards in front of you, face down.

You flip the first card: a 10 of diamonds.

What are the odds of that? One out of fifty-two.

Remarkable.

You flip the next card: a queen of hearts.

Unbelievable! The odds of this sequence were 1/52 * 1/51 (less than 1 in 2,000).

You continue flipping cards: a 4 of clubs follows, then an 8 of diamonds, then an 8 of hearts. Once you have flipped them all over you stare in disbelief; the particular sequence of cards you just observed happens one out of every $8*10^{67}$ (52 factorial) times. Every person in the world could shuffle a deck of cards and flip through it every minute of their entire lives, and even then, the odds of the world seeing your particular sequence of cards will be less than $1/10^{50}$!

Extraordinary.

Something is very wrong here. The conclusion is absurd. Yet similar logic is prevalent in both lay and scientific reasoning. Some have used variants of this argument to account for the origins of humans on earth: Proteins could be randomly shuffled for eons before humans emerged in all their glory. Since the likelihood of human existence by pure chance is so slim, surely intelligent design is the most parsimonious explanation. The card example was introduced to illustrate just how preposterous this objection to evolution is.

Unfortunately, this logical fallacy, which we will call here the "nonindependence" error, is not restricted to arguments from the scientifically unsophisticated. It is prevalent in cognitive neuroscience as well. For instance, of the eight papers in a recent special issue of *Neuroimage*, five contained variants of this error (den Ouden et al. 2005; Gillath et al. 2005; Harris et al. 2005; Mitchell et al. 2005; Sander et al. 2005). The prevalence of this error is troubling because it can produce apparently significant effects out of pure noise (figure 6.1). In this chapter, we describe the error formally, consider why it appears to be more common in fMRI than in other fields, provide examples of this

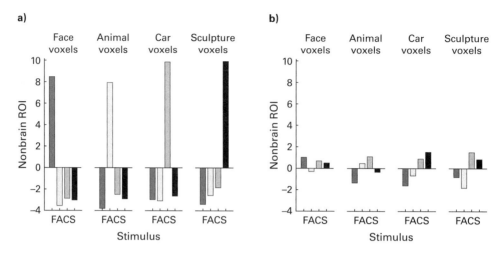

Figure 6.1

A portion of the graph from Baker et al. (2007). (d) A nonindependent analysis and (e) the suggested independent analysis were performed on nonbrain fMRI data (the nose). With a nonindependent analysis, even the nose may be shown to contain face-, animal-, car-, and sculpture-selective voxels. A sound, independent analysis does not produce such spurious results.

error in its most common guises, and propose a few heuristics that may help lay people and scientists alike avoid the error.

Formal Description of the Nonindependence Error

What exactly is the error that leads to the absurd conclusion in the card example?

We can describe it in different theoretical frameworks: statistical hypothesis testing, propositional logic, probability theory, and information theory. These frameworks are rarely discussed together, and never connected in the context of the nonindependence error. In this section we describe the error in the context of statistical hypothesis testing; in the appendix we consider it from the three other perspectives.

In statistical hypothesis testing, the most common nonindependence error is referred to as "selection bias." Essentially all statistical models used for hypothesis testing assume that the sampling (selection) process is independent of the relevant measure. Selection bias is a violation of this independence assumption.

If we assume that our deck of cards is a random sample from the population of all decks of cards, and we are evaluating the likelihood that such a deck of cards will have a particular order specified in advance, we would be surprised to find such a coincidence (indeed, $p < 10^{-67}$). However, our sampling process is very different. Our sample was not drawn from the population of all random decks; instead, it was a sample from all decks that we just observed to have the particular order in question.

Statistics textbooks often describe selection bias via simplistic examples of samples that are not representative of the population (e.g., drawing data exclusively from the NBA when assessing the height of Americans). Obviously, in such cases, the sample will be different from the population, and generalizations to the population would be unjustified because they rely on the assumption that the sampling process is independent of the measure. This classical form of selection bias effectively conveys the intuition that a sample ought to be representative of the population. However, "representative of the population" is loosely defined. If we seek to test whether a particular group (say, people who are taller than 6 ft 5 in.) somehow differs from the population (say, have higher salaries), then, if such an effect truly exists, the process of selecting our population of interest necessarily gives us a sample different from the global population, and there is nothing wrong in this case.

We can define selection bias more formally than "not representative of the population" as follows: If our selection criteria are applied to a sample from the null hypothesis distribution, the selected subset of that sample must also be a sample from the null hypothesis. For example, if we seek to evaluate whether a sociology class is more difficult than a psychology class, we might find a sample of students who have taken both, and evaluate the difference in this group's average score in the two classes. Let's imagine that the average grades for sociology and psychology are identical in this sample (thus, we have a sample from the null hypothesis distribution—there is no effect in the sample). Now imagine that, from this sample, we choose only students who had a better grade in sociology than in psychology. This newly selected subsample will have a higher average grade in sociology than in psychology. So our analysis procedure "(1) select all students with a higher grade in sociology than psychology, and (2) evaluate average scores for sociology and psychology in this sample" violates the requirement that the selection criteria not alter the null hypothesis distribution when applied to it. Thus, our selection is biased.

This definition of selection bias can be expressed in terms of independence in probability theory: if X is a random variable representing our data, and $P(X)$ reflects the probability distribution assumed by the null hypothesis, then $P(X|C)$ where C is the selection criteria, must be equal to $P(X)$, the null hypothesis distribution. Thus, selection bias is a violation of independence between selection and the subsequent statistical measure. Though this point may appear obvious or trivial, it is crucial when considering examples further removed from our intuitions about circular reasoning or population representativeness.

Examples of the Nonindependence Error in fMRI

The nonindependence error arises in fMRI when a subset of voxels is selected for a subsequent analysis, but the null hypothesis of the analysis is not independent of the selection criteria used to choose the voxels in the first place. Take the simplest practical case: If one selects only voxels in which condition A produces a greater signal change than condition B, and then evaluates whether the signal change for conditions A and B differ in those voxels using the same data, the second analysis is not independent of the selection criteria. The outcome of this nonindependent second analysis is *statistically guaranteed* and thus *uninformative*: A will be greater than B, since this conclusion is presumed by the selection criterion (Culham 2006). Furthermore, this outcome will be *biased*: given that the data will be perturbed by random noise, selecting voxels in which A > B preferentially selects voxels in which the random noise is positive for A and negative for B.

There are many ways for the combination of voxel selection and subsequent analysis to produce a nonindependence error and thus biased results. However, neither a particular selection method nor a particular analysis method is alone sufficient for a violation of independence; the violation results from the relationship between the two. We will describe a few situations in which the particular combination of selection method and subsequent analysis results in nonindependence. We start with the simplest cases, where the error will be most obvious, and go on to more elaborate cases where nonindependence is harder to spot.

fMRI analyses that contain the nonindependence error often jeopardize the conclusions of the study for two reasons. First, the nonindependent analysis will be statistically biased, rendering its conclusions limited (at best) and completely invalid (at worst). Second, because researchers often rely on the secondary analysis to support their claims, the initial analysis used to select voxels is often not statistically sound because it is not properly corrected for multiple comparisons. Insufficient correction for multiple comparisons guarantees that some number of voxels will pass the statistical threshold, and offers no guarantee that they did so because of some true underlying effect rather than fortuitous noise. In cases when both a lax multiple-comparisons correction is employed and a nonindependent secondary test is used, all of the conclusions of the experiment are questionable: The lax selection threshold may have only selected random fluctuations, and a seemingly significant result may have been produced literally out of noise (figure 6.1, reprinted from Baker et al. 2007).

Testing the Signal Change in Voxels Selected for Signal Change

The most damaging nonindependence errors arise when researchers perform statistical tests on nonindependent data. In these cases, the nonindependent tests are explicitly used in support of a conclusion, while the nonindependence renders the test biased, uninformative, and invalid.

One such example can be seen in a recent paper by Summerfield and colleagues (Summerfield et al. 2006). The authors sought to identify category-specific predictive codes. Subjects were exposed to "face set" blocks in which they had to identify faces, and "house set" blocks in which, for identical stimuli, subjects had to identify houses.

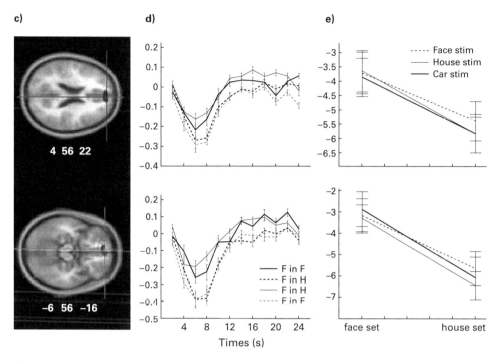

Figure 6.2
Voxels selected for having a main effect of set (at a low, uncorrected threshold) are reported as having a very significant main effect of set. Reprinted by permission from Summerfield et al. 2006.

In figure 6.2 Summerfield et al. show the voxels that are more active for face set blocks than house set blocks (selected at a low, uncorrected threshold: $p < 0.01$). The authors then take the maximally significant voxel in this contrast and run post hoc ANOVAs. The ANOVAs are defined with two factors: face set versus house set and stimulus (which *is* independent of face or house set because different stimuli types were equally distributed in the two set conditions). The result of this ANOVA is a significant main effect of face set, with remarkably high F statistics reported.

However, these ANOVAs were run only on the maximally active voxel in the face set minus house set contrast, defined by the same data. This means that the voxels are guaranteed to have a significant main effect of face set greater than house set. The statistics reported for the main effect in the ANOVA add no new information, and do not bolster the authors' claims in the slightest. The ANOVA results were presupposed by the selection criteria.

These statistics are misleading. The ANOVA results are used to bolster the whole-brain analysis that identified the regions. The whole-brain analysis itself used a particularly low threshold ($p < 0.01$, without multiple comparisons correction), and as such could not stand on its own. However, it effectively imposes a bias on the subsequent ANOVA. It is quite possible that the results displayed in figure 6.2 may be entirely spurious: the results of the whole-brain analysis may be due to chance (false positives), and the results of the ANOVA are guaranteed given the selection criteria. This is exactly the sort of analysis that has motivated us to write this chapter: The numbers reported (F values greater than 20) appear convincing, but they are meaningless.

Nonindependent statistical tests appear in numerous other high-profile articles (e.g., Cantlon et al. 2006; Grill-Spector et al. 2006b; Piazza et al. 2007; Ruff et al. 2006; Todd and Marois 2004). Although nonindependent tests are prevalent in the literature, the conclusions of an entire paper do not always depend on that biased analysis. In some cases (Summerfield et al. 2006), however, the researchers may have produced their main significant result out of nothing.

Plotting the Signal Change in Voxels Selected for Signal Change

The most common, simple, and innocuous instance of nonindependence occurs when researchers simply plot (rather than test) the signal change in a set of voxels that were selected based on that same signal change.

Selecting an Interaction   Take for instance a classic article about the effect of load on motion processing (Rees et al. 1997). In this study, the researchers sought to test Lavie's load theory of attention—that ignored stimuli will be processed to a greater degree under low-load than high-load attended tasks. Subjects performed either a difficult or an easy linguistic task at fixation (to make load high or low, respectively), while an ignored dot field either moved or did not move in the background. The authors predicted a greater difference in activation between motion and no motion conditions during low load compared to high load. Thus, Rees et al. found the peak voxel within some distance of area MT in which this interaction was greatest, and plotted the time course in that voxel. The conclusions of Rees et al. relied on the whole-brain analysis that identified the cluster of interest, not on the time course of the peak voxel; however, for our purposes, it is useful to ask what the reader might have gained from the graph of the time course (see figure 6.3).

This graph appears informative of the hypothesis under investigation, but it is not; the presence of the predicted interaction was a prerequisite for data to be included in this graph. Of all voxels that could be processing motion, only the one with the most significant interaction is displayed. So, of course an interaction will be apparent in this plot. This graph, however, may be used to evaluate other, orthogonal aspects of the data. We discuss this in the section on information gleaned from nonindependent data. For now, it is important to note that the average activity of voxels that were selected under some hypothesis is not diagnostic of the hypothesis, and should never be used as implicit evidence.

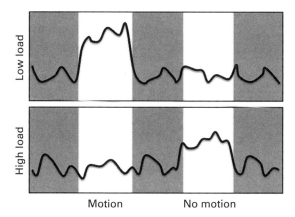

Figure 6.3
Time course from the peak voxel selected for an interaction is biased toward implausible activation patterns (no motion > motion in MT; under high load). This image is an artist's rendition of figure 1d and e from Rees et al. (1997).

This graph of signal change in the peak voxel selected for an interaction is also an excellent example of how nonindependence introduces bias. The hypothesis used for selection was that the difference (motion–no motion) will be greater under low load than high load. Imagine that the ground truth about V5 (the area being tested in this experiment) is what Lavie's theory predicts: Under low load, motion produces greater activation than no motion, but under high load, there is no difference. The measured activity in each voxel will be perturbed by noise around this ground truth. If we then select only the voxels for which low load(notion–no motion) is much greater than high load(motion–no motion), we will be preferentially selecting voxels in which the noise that corrupts ground truth causes motion–no motion to be *negative* under high load conditions (as this will maximize the interaction). This is precisely what we see in the data that were selected by this interaction test—under high load, MT, a motion-processing region, is more active under the no motion condition than under the motion condition. This otherwise unintelligible result perfectly illustrates the effects of noise selection, that is, how the selection criteria favor certain patterns of noise over others.

Barcharts of Selected Effects   Although one can plot the time course of nonindependent data, the most common variant is to plot a bar chart of the selected area. Take, for instance, a recent article by De Martino, Kumaran, Seymour, and Dolan (2006). In this study, the researchers sought to identify regions that respond to framing effects—in their experiment, regions that respond similarly to the "sure" option in the gain frame and the "gamble" option in the loss frame (while responding differently to the

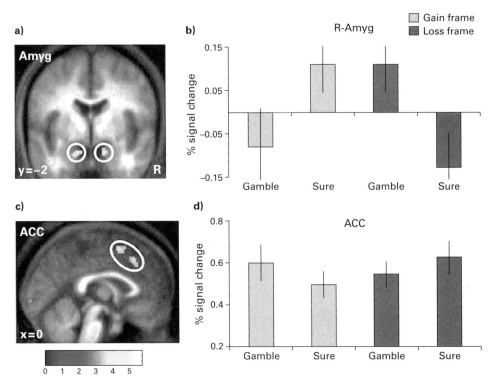

Figure 6.4
The percent signal change in areas selected for each of those percent signal change profiles. Despite the error bars, these bar graphs do not contain any information about the main claims of the paper. Reprinted with permission from De Martino et al. 2006.

opposite combinations). Regions were selected if they showed this interaction: (a) responded more to (Gain-Sure + Loss-Gamble) than (Gain-Gamble + Loss-Sure), or (b) responded more to (Gain-Gamble + Loss-Sure) than (Gain-Sure + Loss-Gamble). Figure 6.4 (p. 686) shows the regions that were selected based on either of these contrasts, and to the right of the pictures of these regions the authors plot the percent signal change within that region for each of the four conditions.

What exactly could one learn from these plots and what aspects of the plots can not be trusted? For regions that were selected for the positive interaction, we are sure to find the effect. Similarly, for regions that were selected for the negative interaction, we are guaranteed to find that as well. We are also guaranteed to find that these differences will be greater than the noise fluctuations in the data—such is the definition of statistical significance. Furthermore, the magnitude of the guaranteed effects cannot be trusted, because the selection process will select voxels with random noise favoring these effects. What we might learn from these data, however, are whether or not the percent signal changes are greater than zero; however, that is certainly not the point the reader is asked to take from these graphs.

Despite the fact that plotting nonindependent data provides little new information, this practice is very common—it is rare to find an issue of a neuroimaging journal in which none of the articles have plotted nonindependent data. Indeed, even one of the authors of this chapter has done this previously (Culham et al. 1998; Kanwisher et al. 1997b). This leaves us with several questions: What can plots of this sort contribute? Just how damaging is the practice of plotting the data that were used for selection?

What Information May One Glean from Nonindependent Data?   In general, plotting nonindependent data is misleading, because the selection criteria conflate any effects that may be present in the data with those effects that could be produced by selecting noise with particular characteristics. On the other hand, plots of nonindependent data sometimes contain useful information orthogonal to the selection criteria. When data are selected for an interaction, nonindependent plots of the data reveal which of many possible forms the interaction takes. In the case of selected main effects, readers may be able to compare the activations to baseline and assess selectivity. In either case, there may be valuable, independent, and orthogonal information that could be gleaned from the time courses. In short, information is often lurking in graphs of nonindependent data; however, it is usually *not* the information that the authors of such graphs draw readers' attention to. Thus, we are not arguing against displaying graphs that contain redundant (and perhaps biased) information, we are arguing against the implicit use of these graphs to convince readers by use of nonindependent data.

How Damaging Are Plots of Nonindependent Data?   In cases where no inferential statistics are computed on the selected data conclusions are explicitly based on the voxel selection process itself, and not the displayed ROI analyses. In such cases, plotting these graphs is a problem only because they may mislead readers. The reader is presented with graphs that appear informative (insofar as they show data exhibiting effects that the paper is describing), but the graphs are not informative of the primary claims, and are distorted by selection bias. Authors who show such graphs must usually recognize that it would be inappropriate to draw explicit conclusions from statistical tests on these data (as these tests are less common), but the graphs are presented regardless. Unfortunately, the nonindependence of these graphs is usually not explicitly noted, and often not noticed, so the reader is often not warned that the graphs should carry little inferential weight.

Just as in the case of testing for a selected effect, a particularly troublesome situation arises when voxels are selected at a low threshold—a threshold too low to effectively correct for multiple comparisons. In these cases, the displayed graphs falsely bolster the reader's confidence in the reliability of the effects, while in such cases, the reader's confidence in the result should be based only on the threshold used to initially select the voxels.

Because the most damaging consequence of plotting nonindependent data is to mislead readers, a good antidote is full disclosure. Authors should explicitly state whether the plot corresponds to the same (nonindependent) data used for the selection criteria or different, independent data. Furthermore, if nonindependent data are plotted, this should be accompanied by a description of which effects are biased and statistically expected due to the selection criteria. Ideally, any such graph would also feature an illustration of these biases (Baker et al. 2007).

Reporting Correlations in Voxels Selected for Correlations

A recent methodological trend, especially in social cognitive neuroscience, is the correlation of evoked activity with some traits of the individual. One such example is Eisenberger, Lieberman, and Williams (2003). In this study, participants played Cyberball, a video game in which subjects tossed a virtual ball with other agents in the game. Subjects were told that the agents were other human participants, while in reality they were simulated computer characters. On some runs, subjects watched the other agents play the game; in another run, subjects watched the other agents play the game while apparently intentionally excluding the subject. The researchers identified regions in the anterior cingulated cortex (ACC) that were more active during trials when subjects were excluded from the game than during trials when they were included (excluded-included contrast). Within this contrast, the researchers then found brain regions where activity was correlated with ratings of distress elicited from each subject after the experiment. The authors report two sets of coordinates in the ACC that correspond to a positive correlation between BOLD and self-reported distress. They also report impressively high correlations at each of these coordinates: $r = 0.88$ and 0.75.

What do these correlations mean? They are the correlations of voxels selected for having correlations significant at the $p < 0.005$[1] level. The significance of a correlation may be assessed by a t-test with a t-value of $r^2/(1 - r^2)/N - 2$. Given that there were 13 subjects in the experiment, we can compute the minimum correlation necessary for voxels to be selected. This minimum possible r value is 0.7,[2] so we know we will see an average r value greater than 0.7 in any voxels that were selected, even if the null hypothesis holds true for those voxels (these would be voxels selected due to noise that aligned with the selection criteria).

Surely, you might suppose, since some number of voxels were above the critical correlation values necessary to reach significance, activity in the ACC must truly be correlated with self-assessed distress. We do not aim to question this finding—if the assumptions of the minimum cluster size method for multiple-comparison correction were met in the multivoxel analysis undertaken in this paper, there may indeed be a true correlation. We object, however, to the prominent display of average correlations from voxels that were selected for having significant correlations.

Imagine that ACC activity is correlated with subjective distress. This means that all voxels in the ACC (as identified by the excluded-included contrast) have some greater than zero correlation with subjective distress. The correlations in each of these voxels will be perturbed by noise; by chance, some voxels will cease to have detectable correlations, while other voxels, by chance, will become more correlated. All of the voxels in the ACC will follow some distribution of correlation values. An independent analysis of these correlations could have averaged the correlations across all voxels in the ACC, and computed statistics on this quantity. Instead, however, the authors found regions within the ACC that were significantly correlated with subjective distress. Thus, from the distribution of all voxels and their respective correlations, the authors chose only those that had correlations greater than 0.7, then averaged them. Such a procedure is guaranteed to find an average correlation greater than 0.7, even if the true correlation between evoked ACC activity and subjective distress is substantially lower. Again, if the multiple-comparisons selection was done appropriately, it is still likely that the ACC does contain such a correlation; however, the magnitudes of the average correlations the authors report are spuriously elevated.

We have dwelt on this example because, unlike the post hoc displays of signal change described previously, biased post hoc displays of correlations seem to be substantially more convincing to audiences and readers, and appear to appeal to high-profile journals (Dapretto, et al. 2006; Kennedy et al. 2006; Mobbs et al. 2005; Yoo et al. 2007). Since biased analyses and results such as these have a greater impact on audiences, it is more important to be aware of them, and to curb their use.

Multivariate Correlations

Another newly popular class of analyses is even more conducive to hidden non-independence errors: multivariate analyses. In these analyses (e.g., Haxby et al. 2001), researchers assess the multivariate pattern of voxel activation for any given condition (this volume, chapter 5). That is, to what extent is the pattern of increased and decreased BOLD signal across voxels in a particular region (a measure independent of the mean signal in that region) diagnostic of a particular condition? In Haxby's analysis, this was measured as the correlation of voxel activations across two sets of identical conditions compared to two sets of different conditions. When correlations between identical conditions are greater than correlations between different conditions, those conditions may be distinguished by the pattern. This intuition has been extended into more elaborate machine learning methods that explicitly classify conditions based on the evoked patterns of activation.

Just as in standard analyses, researchers typically select some subset of voxels on which to perform a multivariate analysis (to characterize a particular cortical region, gain power, or remove uninformative voxels). Unfortunately, in the original Haxby paper, the method used to select voxels was not fully independent from the subsequent analysis. While this is not likely to have strongly affected the main results of that study, it is worth explaining the problem as an illustrative case.

Haxby et al. selected voxels based on significance in an omnibus ANOVA across all stimulus conditions, which was computed on all data (to be split into odd and even runs for the pattern analysis later). An omnibus ANOVA is significant insofar as one or more of the group means is different from the others. Effectively, this selection criterion biases the final correlations one might obtain: voxels will be selected if their mean activation is significantly different in one condition from another (and this would have to be reliable, across both data sets). If one condition is reliably different from others within this voxel, this means that activation across split halves will be better correlated for identical than different conditions.

Of course, the strength of this bias depends on how much the conditions differ from fixation. In the Haxby et al. paper, most of the reported effect is likely driven by true underlying effects. However, the fact that the analysis could be biased is a nontrivial problem that can produce spurious results (Simmons et al. 2006).

Summary

We have described four classes of analysis that are tainted by the nonindependence error. In some of the case studies, the error undermined the main claims of the paper, in other cases, it simply resulted in the display of redundant information. Our goal in this section was not to single out these particular papers—many other examples are available. Our goal was to illustrate the many faces of the nonindependence error in fMRI research. We hope that in describing these cases, we have provided a broad enough spectrum that readers may be able to generalize to new instances and spot these errors when planning experiments, writing papers, and reviewing for journals.

Why the Nonindependence Error Is Prevalent in fMRI

The nonindependence error we have outlined is not novel and has been committed in many other disciplines; however, it seems to be especially prevalent in fMRI. For example, five of the eight fMRI studies in a recent special issue on social cognitive neuroscience (in *Neuroimage*, 2005, 28) included nonindependent analyses (den Ouden et al. 2005; Gillath et al. 2005; Harris et al. 2005; Mitchell et al. 2005; Sander et al. 2005). There are three circumstances of neuroimaging that put the field at high risk. First, fMRI researchers work with massively multidimensional data sets, in which only a subset of dimensions contain information that may be relevant to the experiment. This situation encourages researchers to select some subset of their data for analysis, thus to use nonindependent selection criteria. Second, fMRI analyses are complicated, involving many steps and transformations before the final statistics may be computed, resulting in confusion (and thus a diminished ability to identify such errors) not only on the part of the researchers themselves, but also on the part of reviewers. Finally, fMRI research usually asks binary qualitative, not quantitative, questions—data are presented as binary values (significant or not significant), further veiling any biases that may lie behind the analysis.

fMRI Data Are Massively Multidimensional

A typical low-resolution scan on a low-field magnet will produce an imaging volume every 3 seconds. The imaging volume will contain twenty 3-mm slices, each of which is divided into a 64×64 (3 mm $\times$ 3 mm) grid, producing 81,920 measurements every 3 seconds. A high-resolution scan on state-of-the-art scanners might produce an image volume every 2 seconds, and this volume may contain thirty 1.5-mm slices, each of which is divided into a 128×128 (1 mm $\times$ 1 mm) grid, producing a staggering 491,520 measurements every 2 seconds. Thus, a single scan session could easily produce more than one billion measurements, and often multiple sessions are combined in the analysis.

Statisticians are not known to complain about an overabundance of data, and the problem here is not the raw number of measurements, but rather the fact that usually only a small proportion of the measurements are informative about the experimental question. In a fortuitous and skillfully executed experiment, one may find 5% of voxels to be of experimental interest. This poses a difficult multiple comparisons problem for whole-brain analyses. In this chapter, we have only indirectly discussed this problem, because the applications (and misapplications) of the many technical methods used to correct for multiple comparisons are a considerable topic on their own. Instead, we have discussed a consequence of this problem: selection.

When experimenters ask subtler questions than "Which area lights up under condition X?," they invariably select some subset of the enormous fMRI data set to avoid correcting for multiple comparisons and losing statistical power. Therefore, most modern fMRI analyses proceed in two stages: (1) identifying a subset of voxels that play an interesting role in the experiment (a region of interest—ROI),[3] then (2) assessing some additional measure in those voxels. Obviously, the criteria used for selection in step 1 are a condition one puts on the measure in step 2; in this chapter, we have discussed whether the conditions from step 1 satisfy the assumption of independence necessary for the statistical analyses in step 2.

The nonindependence error arises from the relationship between the ROI selection method and the statistical test. If the conditions imposed by the selection process alter the distribution assumed by the null hypothesis of the subsequent statistical test, then this secondary test is nonindependent. Naturally, this will mean that some combinations of ROI selection methods and analyses do satisfy the independence assumption (and are hence legitimate), and different combinations of the same techniques may not (and are not).

Selecting small subsets of large data sets is an integral part of most fMRI analyses to a much greater degree than in behavioral studies. Since selection (biased or not) is more common in fMRI, then, even if selection biases are inadvertently introduced equally often in analyses in other fields, we would expect to see a greater proportion of reported results tinged by selection bias in fMRI.

fMRI Analyses Are Complicated (Both to Do and to Review)

There are many steps between acquiring fMRI data and reporting results. Before the final analysis, a staggering variety of preprocessing techniques are applied to the data. The four-dimensional image (volume by time) obtained from the scanner may be motion-corrected, coregistered, transformed to match a prototypical brain, resampled, detrended, normalized, smoothed, trimmed (temporally or spatially), or any subset of these, with only a few constraints on the order in which these are done. Furthermore, each of these steps can be done in a number of ways, each with many free parameters that experimenters set, often arbitrarily. The decisions an experimenter makes about preprocessing are less likely to be crucial for the issue of nonindependence.[4] However, these steps play an important role in the final results, and must be specified when describing an experiment.

After preprocessing, the main analysis begins. In a standard analysis sequence, experimenters define temporal regressors based on one or more aspects of the experiment sequence, choose a hemodynamic response function, and compute the regression parameters that connect the BOLD signal to these regressors in each voxel. This is a whole-brain analysis (step 1 described in the previous section), and it is usually subjected to one of a number of methods to correct for multiple comparisons (false detection rates, minimum cluster size thresholds, Bonferroni, etc.). Because it is difficult to gain enough power for a fully corrected whole-brain analysis, such analyses are rarely done in isolation. Instead, in conjunction with anatomical assumptions, the whole-brain analysis is often the first step in defining a region of interest in which more fine-grained, technically sophisticated, and interesting analyses may be carried out (step 2 in the previous section).

The analyses within selected ROIs may include exploration of time courses, voxel-wise correlations, classification using support vector machines or other machine learning methods, across-subject correlations, and so on. Any one of these analyses requires making crucial decisions that determine the soundness of the conclusions. Importantly, it is the interaction between a few of these decisions that determines whether or not a statistical analysis is tarnished by nonindependent selection criteria.

The complexity of the functional magnetic resonance imaging (fMRI) analysis has two consequences, each of which can only increase the likelihood that experimenters will inadvertently use nonindependent selection criteria. First, with so many potential variables, it is difficult to keep track of possible interactions that could compromise independence. Second, and perhaps more important, to fully specify the analysis in a publication requires quite a lot of text—text that high-profile journals prefer not to use on Methods sections. So editors (and publication policies) encourage authors to exclude details of the analysis on the assumption that they may be trivial or unimportant. The result is a hamstrung review process in which reviewers are not given the full information necessary to evaluate an analysis. The complexity of fMRI analyses is not inherently bad; however, it offers opportunities for researchers to make mistakes and diminishes opportunities for reviewers to spot the errors.

fMRI Analyses Are Usually Qualitative

The qualitative nature of the questions asked and results obtained in fMRI also contributes to the prevalence of the nonindependence error. An area is said to respond differently, or not; to contain some information, or not; to predict behavior, or not. Of course, the brain states underlying the effects observed are quantitatively different, and we draw arbitrary lines to produce qualitative answers. Why does this matter?

As our examples have shown, the nonindependence error in fMRI analyses usually does not guarantee a particular result. Instead, the results are biased to favor a particular outcome. The extent to which results are biased is usually unclear. Since results are displayed as binary outcomes (significant or not), it is substantially more difficult to evaluate whether the significance of an effect is due to the bias. One might ask what proportion of an effect is suspect, but such a question arises less naturally for results with binary outcomes. By drawing hard thresholds, the practice of significance testing further muddies the results of an analysis, and complicates evaluation.

Summary

Functional MRI is not the only field to contain biased results and nonindependent selection criteria, and it is also not the only field to suffer from the conditions previously described. Gene sequencing involves massively multidimensional data. Electrophysiology experiments require complicated time-series analysis. Most behavioral experiments in psychology evaluate results via a statistical test with a binary outcome. Although these factors are shared by other fields (and result in nonindependence errors in those fields), fMRI data and analyses are subject to all of these factors, thus increasing the odds that any one analysis may be tainted.

Heuristics for Avoiding Nonindependence Errors

How might one avoid committing variants of the nonindependence error when conducting fMRI analyses? For independence of selection and analysis, we require that selection criteria, if applied to a distribution from the null hypothesis, will produce another distribution drawn from the null hypothesis. Three classes of solutions seem intuitively reasonable. The best option is to safeguard against nonindependence by using different data sets for the selection and analysis. Another possibility is to determine a priori whether the analysis and selection criteria are independent. Rather than deducing this independence analytically, a third option is to assess such independence by simulation.

Each of these strategies has advantages and disadvantages, and none can be guaranteed to be effective. Although we advocate the use of independent data, it is important to note that even then, some degree of the other two approaches may be required of the researcher.

Ensuring Independence by Separating Data Sets

Perhaps the most intuitive precaution against nonindependent selection criteria and analysis is the use of completely different data sets. Voxel selection would be based on a subset of the data (specific trials, blocks, runs, experiment halves, etc.), while the analysis would be performed on the remaining data. If the data are truly independent, selection bias cannot be introduced when selection and analyses are executed on different subsets of the data.

However, certain divisions of the data and physiological factors may render superficially independent data actually nonindependent. Imagine that we decide to separate our data into odd- and even-numbered columns of the fMRI image. We will select a subset of even-numbered columns for further analysis based on what would be otherwise a nonindependent criterion imposed on paired odd-numbered voxels. The data set used to define a region of interest and that used for the subsequent analysis are *nominally* independent. However, in this case the data are not really independent because of the spatial correlation intrinsic to fMRI (as should be expected from either explicit spatial smoothing or the correlation induced by vasculature, blood flow, and MR image construction).

One could imagine a different example, in which alternating image acquisitions (TRs) are used to select voxels, and the interceding images are used for the subsequent analysis. Explicit temporal smoothing of the data is quite rare in fMRI, so nonindependence is not likely to be introduced from preprocessing. However, again, physiology introduces bias: Because of the temporal delay and extent of the hemodynamic response function, temporally contiguous images are far from independent.[5]

These two examples demonstrate that the use of distinct data sets for selection and testing does not guarantee independence. Data may be rendered more or less independent in myriad ways, by preprocessing, nonrandom experimental sequence, and so on.

Evaluating Independence by Analytical Deduction

One might attempt to deduce, a priori, whether the conditions one imposes on the sample of voxels selected for further analysis are orthogonal to the analysis itself. Since analytical solutions to this problem are often intractable, and assumptions about the joint probability distribution of all of the data unjustified, we do not consider the possibility of attempting to derive independence through pure mathematics. That said, the only method we know for determining independence a priori is to try very hard to find reasons why the selection criteria might not meet this criterion, and fail to find any. It seems perilous to advocate such a subjective use of statistics (after all, some people may not find failures of orthogonality where others succeed). Indeed, the cases we have described, more likely than not, reflect a failure to come up with a reason why the orthogonality condition is not met.

Assessing Independence by Numerical Simulation

Rather than producing armchair arguments about the independence of selection from the subsequent analysis, one may run numerical simulations to measure mutual information between the conditions and the null hypothesis distribution (described earlier). This approach occurs in the literature most frequently as a post hoc illustration of a failure to meet the nonindependence criterion (Baker et al. 2007; Simmons et al. 2006). Such post hoc refutations of biased analyses are useful in weeding out spurious results from the literature and advancing science. However, we hope that authors will take it upon themselves to use such approaches to determine the soundness of their own analyses before they are published. Permutation tests are one particularly effective method when analyses are particularly complicated. Researchers can randomly permute the condition labels for their data and undertake the same analysis. If this is done enough times, it is possible to empirically estimate the probability of the outcome observed with the true data labels. Unlike simpler (and faster) white noise simulations, this permutation analysis includes the non-Gaussian structure of the BOLD signal noise, and is thus more accurate.

Summary

All in all, we would advocate using one data set for voxel selection and a different, independent data set for subsequent analysis to decrease the likelihood of the nonindependence error. However, because of spatiotemporal correlations in fMRI data, even in these cases, independence is not guaranteed, and researchers ought to use caution to make sure the two data sets are in fact independent.

It is worth noting that we are explicitly advocating the use of independent data, not necessarily alternative stimulus sequences for use in localizers. This advice is orthogonal to the "ROI debate" (Friston et al. 2006; Saxe et al. 2006) about the role, and meaning, of functionally defined regions. However, we do depart from Friston et al. in advising that independent data be used. Friston advocated the use of a "factorial design" such that voxel selection and a subsequent analysis are achieved with the same data set (with the condition that voxel selection and the analysis are orthogonal). In principle, if these analyses are truly orthogonal, then they are independent, and we agree. Unfortunately, orthogonality of selection methods and analyses seems to be often wrongly assumed.[6] Though it is more economical to use one data set for selection and analysis, it seems much safer to use independent data sets (indeed, if spurious results are published because of failures of orthogonality, the entire research enterprise ends up substantially more costly).

Conclusion

We have described a common error in fMRI research: the use of nonindependent selection criteria and statistical analyses. This error takes many forms, from seemingly innocuous graphs that merely illustrate the selection criteria rather than contribute additional information, to serious errors where significant results may be produced from pure noise. In its many forms, this error is undermining cognitive neuroscience. Public broadcast of tainted experiments jeopardizes the reputation of cognitive neuroscience. Acceptance of spurious results wastes researchers' time and government funds while people chase unsubstantiated claims. Publication of faulty methods spreads the error to new scientists. We hope that this chapter finds itself in the hands of the authors, reviewers, editors, and readers of cognitive neuroscience research and arms them with the formalism and intuition necessary to curtail the use of invalid, nonindependent analyses.

Appendix: Formal Description of the Nonindependence Error

What exactly is the error that leads to the absurd conclusion in the card example from the introduction? Here we describe it in three additional theoretical frameworks: propositional logic, probability theory, and information theory.

Propositional Logic

In formal logic, the nonindependence error goes under many names: *petitio principii,* "begging the question", or "circular reasoning."[7] A distilled example of begging the question will read as follows:

p implies p;
suppose p;
therefore p.

In practice, of course, the fallacy is usually cloaked by many logical steps and obfuscatory wording, such that the assumption of p is rarely obvious. In the card (or evolution) example, we start with the outcome (the particular arrangement of cards or genes: "suppose p"), and then marvel that we have found the same outcome ("therefore p"). Thus, these cases exemplify "begging the question"—a condition when the conclusion is implicitly or explicitly assumed in one of the premises.

In the opening example, and throughout the chapter, we concern ourselves with statistics and probability, so this fallacy is best fleshed out in terms of probability theory and statistics. However, the essence of the problem is still simple question begging: evaluating the truth of a statement that has been presupposed.

Probability Theory

We can also analyze begging the question in a probabilistic framework by evaluating the implicit and explicit assumptions in the deck of cards example. It is true that a fully shuffled deck of cards has one of fifty-two factorial possible arrangements. It is also true that a deck of cards randomly sampled from a distribution over all possible shufflings will be unlikely to have any one particular arrangement (a probability of 1/52 factorial). So if we were to choose a random arrangement and then shuffle a deck of cards until we found that arrangement, we would probably find ourselves busy for a long time.

However, we are not evaluating the prior probability of a random deck of cards having a random arrangement. Instead, we are evaluating the probability that a deck of cards will have a specific order—the order we just observed the deck of cards to have. Thus, the probability distribution we should be evaluating is not the prior probability $P(X = x)$, but the conditional probability $P(X = x \mid X = x)$. Of course, this probability is 1.

One of an enormous number of outcomes was possible, but if we condition on the observed outcome, that particular outcome is guaranteed. In the formalism of probability this difference between prior and conditional probabilities may be described as a violated assumption of independence: $P(X)$ is not equal to $P(X \mid C)$, where C is our condition.

The deck of cards case is an extreme example where the disparity between the assumed prior probability and the relevant conditional probability is particularly large—the prior probability is impossibly low and conditional probability is 1. These probabilities make the scenario easy to describe in terms of predicate logic, but the same violation of independence arises if the probabilities are not 1 and (near) 0.

Information Theory

Finally, we can formalize the nonindependence error in the framework of information theory to appeal to another intuition about a desirable quality of statistical analyses: how much information they assume of, or add to, the data. If we specify the null hypothesis of our statistical test as $P(X)$ and the selection criteria as imposing a condition on the data, producing $P(X \mid C)$, then we can derive how much information the selection criteria (condition C) give us about X.

The Shannon entropy of a random variable reflects the uncertainty present in the probability distribution of that random variable.

$$H(X) = -\sum P(X) \log_2 P(X)$$

Intuitively, this number expresses how many bits would be necessary to encode a sample from that distribution, thus expressing uncertainty in terms of information.

With this measure, we can describe how much information (H) a selection condition gives us about a random variable by evaluating how much less uncertainty there is in the conditional distribution compared to the prior distribution. This is expressed as mutual information: $I(X; C) = H(X) - H(X \mid C)$.

To return to our example of a deck of cards, we can assess how many bits of information it takes to encode the order of a random deck of cards:

$$H(X) = -\sum_{i=1}^{52!} \frac{1}{52!} \log_2 \frac{1}{52!} = -\log_2 \frac{1}{52!} = 226$$

And we can calculate the amount of information necessary to encode a deck of cards sampled from the distribution of all decks of cards that we have observed to have a particular order (index 1):

$$H(X \mid C) = -1 \log_2 1 - \sum_{i=2}^{52!} 0 \log_2 0 = 0$$

This means that, given the selection criterion, we get no additional information.

The mutual information is thus 226 bits ($226 - 0$). This is an enormous number, reflecting the huge disparity between $P(X)$ and $P(X \mid C)$. It is also useful to express the information gained from our selection criteria as a proportion of all the information one could have gained:

$I(X; C)/H(X) = 226/226 = 1.$

In this extreme example, our selection criteria have given us all the information available about a sample from the prior distribution. Our sampling process has thus fully constrained our data by giving us full information about it. Obtaining full information about the outcome from the starting conditions is identical to begging the question in propositional logic: starting with full information about the outcome means that the outcome was presupposed.

Summary
We formalized the nonindependence error from the opening example in terms of propositional logic, probability theory, statistics (in the first section of the chapter), and information theory. This allowed us to describe violations of assumed independence in probability theory as a generalized case of "begging the question" in propositional logic. Similarly, the error of selection bias in classical statistics is formally equivalent to a violation of independence in probability theory. We then used

information theory to quantify violations of independence as the mutual information between the measurement and the selection criterion. Finally, by taking the limiting case wherein the mutual information between the measure and the selection criterion is 100% of the total information available in the measure, we again produce the case of explicitly begging the question in propositional logic. By describing this error in different frameworks, we hope that readers can apply their intuitions from any of these domains to actual fMRI examples.

We use the term *nonindependence error* throughout this chapter in favor of "begging the question" to convey the idea that the selection criteria need not be so restrictive as to guarantee the outcome (as is the case in propositional logic). Instead, if the selection criteria applied to a null hypothesis distribution alter the distribution in any way, they are introducing some degree of sampling bias, providing some amount of information about the outcome, and thus will produce biased results because of the violation of independence.

Notes

1. This was the threshold used in conjunction with a minimum cluster size constraint. The assumptions and validity of this particular correction for multiple comparisons may be disputed, but here we are concerned with how the selection criteria this method imposes on the data affect the subsequent analyses.

2. If one computes the inverse of the Fisher Z-transform method for ascertaining significance of a correlation, the numbers work out even less favorably.

3. Note that defining a region of interest need not be done with a priori functional localizers (for a discussion of this controversy, see Friston et al. 2006; Saxe et al. 2006); this may be done with orthogonal contrasts from the present experimental manipulation, or even anatomy.

4. However, an often ignored fact is the key role played by voxel size and smoothing parameters in the assumptions behind minimum cluster size methods for multiple-comparisons correction; thus, smoothing, at least, alters the conditions imposed by the ROI selection analysis.

5. See Carlson, Schrater, and He (2003) for an example of such an analysis, as well as some discussion about the magnitude of the presumed bias.

6. Consider the case of selecting voxels based on two main effects and testing for the interaction. Although the two main effects and the interaction appear orthogonal, they are not. If we select random noise in which two main effects are significant ($[A1 + A2] > [B1 + B2]$, and $[A1 + B1] > [A2 + B2]$), the mutual constraint of both main effects will preferentially select positive noise in the $A1$ cell and negative noise in the $B2$ cell, thus biasing results toward an interaction.

7. In our discussion, we consider these three interchangeable, but some differentiate "begging the question" as an error that occurs within one argument, whereas "circular reasoning" involves two mutually dependent arguments.

7 On the Proper Role of Nonindependent ROI Analysis: A Commentary on Vul and Kanwisher

Russell A. Poldrack and Jeanette A. Mumford

The chapter by Vul and Kanwisher is centered on a statistical point that is incontrovertible: Region of interest (ROI) analysis using nonindependent ROIs can lead to inflation of type I error rates when those analyses are used for inference, and inflation of effect sizes in the resulting plots. Reminding the field of this point is a beneficial service. However, we believe that there is still an important place for nonindependent analyses in neuroimaging research.

Why Are Nonindependent Analyses So Prevalent?

The Vul and Kanwisher chapter points out just how widespread the use of nonindependent analysis is in the field of neuroimaging. The first question to ask is why. One cynical answer might be that it is used exactly because it provides inflated and thus more impressive effects. However, in our experience, this is not the reason for most nonindependent analyses. Instead, they are usually presented in order to assure the reader that an effect in a whole-brain analysis is "real," that is, not driven by some odd pattern or outlier. In many cases this assurance is illusory. For example, reviewers will often ask to see plots of hemodynamic responses in a region of interest that was obtained using a whole-brain analysis. However, if this analysis was performed using hemodynamic basis functions (as is very often the case in fMRI analysis), then it is guaranteed that the active regions will have signals that conform more or less to the shape of those basis functions.

In some cases, however, there are very good reasons to want to see the raw data, particularly when correlations are involved. We have on a number of occasions been presented with what looked like astoundingly strong results from whole-brain correlation analyses (of the form that Vul and Kanwisher discuss in the context of social neuroscience). On several of these occasions, a nonindependent ROI analysis showed that the effect was driven by a single outlier. This problem is so prevalent that we now try to use robust analyses whenever possible (e.g., Wager et al. 2005; Woolrich 2008), though there are some cases where robust analyses may not be feasible. Thus, we believe that whereas nonindependent ROI analysis should play no role in inference, it can play a critical role in quality control.

Another example where plotting the data can be useful is in the context of interaction effects. Since one can focus on only a single parameter at a time in the mass univariate setting, and the sign of the interaction term itself does not supply enough information to describe the pattern of effects, understanding interactions requires further visualization, and plotting signal within nonindependent ROIs can provide important insights into the nature of interactions. For example, in Poldrack et al. (2005) we examined motor sequence learning using a three-way (pre/post × single/dual task × sequence/random trials) design. The only way to understand the complex pattern of activity reflected by a significant interaction in such a design is to plot activation in regions of interest. In this case, the goal is not inference, but instead exploring the data that underlie a significant effect. The interpretation of an interaction becomes even more difficult in the case where one or more of the regressors involved in the interaction are continuous and a careful plot should be provided to help interpret the interaction. Of course, as Vul and Kanwisher's examples illustrate, plotting the trends of the single-peak voxel of an ROI will only exacerbate any biases that descriptive plots may illustrate, so one should at least use ROI averages and clearly direct the reader away from any misinterpretations the plots may imply.

Throwing Out the Data with the Bath Water?

As discussed by Vul and Kanwisher, one approach to solving the problem of nonindependence is to use ROIs that are defined either anatomically or using a completely independent localizer scan. Anatomical ROIs can certainly be useful, but they do pose some problems for analysis of functional MRI data (cf. Poldrack 2007). First, anatomical ROIs are often large, such that the truly active voxels will make up a relatively small proportion of any anatomical region. This means that purely anatomical ROIs will almost always be biased toward the null hypothesis. Second, if one does not have a preexisting anatomical hypothesis, then it is necessary to correct for a relatively large number of tests (e.g., 110 regions in the *Harvard-Oxford Probabilistic Atlas* that accompanies FSL), which will also reduce sensitivity. Thus, anatomical ROIs don't seem to be a suitable general solution to the problem of regional interrogation.

The functional localizer approach has been used to very good effect in visual neuroscience, and when available can be very useful. However, the use of functional localizers presupposes localization of function that is often not present, for example, for regions such as prefrontal cortex. Thus, though very useful in some domains it does not seem to offer a general solution.

One other potential solution is the use of split-half or cross-validation strategies, wherein an ROI is created with one portion of the data from each subject that is then used to interrogate the other portion of the data. Because the noise is stochastically independent across runs (even though the same subjects are involved), this leads to independent data sets such that the estimates on the test data set are unbiased. In principle, this approach is appealing. However, there are several problems. First, in many cases there are learning or habituation effects across runs, such that one would not expect the runs to have exactly the same functional architecture. Second, and more important, this approach sacrifices statistical power in order to achieve an unbiased ROI analysis. For example, we previously carried out a power analysis using the methods of Mumford and Nichols (2008) to find the appropriate number of runs for an event-related paradigm and found that reducing a study from two runs to one greatly reduces power. A sample size of 14 subjects yielded 80% power to find a particular effect with two runs per subject, but with only a single run the power to find the same effect was reduced to 57%. In order to split the two runs across subjects, a total of 20 subjects will be necessary to achieve 80% power in the analysis of each split. Thus, whatever inferential or descriptive benefit is provided by an independent analysis comes at the cost of a substantial increase in sample size. This is a decision that each investigator will have to make, but we remain unconvinced that the benefits of independent ROI analysis over whole-brain corrected analysis plus nonindependent ROI analysis will be worth the cost for most studies.

Challenges for the Field

The Vul and Kanwisher chapter raises two important challenges for the field. First, the impact of nonindependent analysis is heavily mitigated by the use of strict correction for multiple tests at the whole-brain level. Any statistic that passes this criterion is guaranteed to be significantly different from the null value with a specific error rate; in the case where the measures from the whole-brain and ROI analyses are the same, the worst that can come of nonindependent analysis is that it can inflate the observed effect size, making the effect appear larger than it actually is.[1] It is difficult to know how large this bias is and whether it can be strong enough to inflate an effect from a level that is not biologically important to one that is. A reanalysis of data from one of our papers that used nonindependent ROI analysis following whole-brain analysis corrected for multiple comparisons (Tom et al. 2007) suggests that the bias due to nonindependent analysis is moderate, on the order of 0.3 inflation of correlation coefficients (Poldrack and Mumford 2009). It is unfortunate that too many journals still allow publication of papers that do not employ strict correction for multiple tests. Many papers are published using small-volume corrections, in which multiple comparisons are corrected within a smaller region; this is appropriate when the region was chosen in a completely unbiased way, but there is some concern that the regions for correction may sometimes be chosen after seeing the initial data, which introduces a bias and may inflate type I errors.

Second, the concerns outlined in this chapter make clear just how important it is to present the details of statistical analyses clearly in neuroimaging papers. We (Poldrack et al. 2008) have recently published a set of guidelines for describing methods in fMRI publications, which includes details about how ROIs were defined. We hope that concerns about the nature of ROI analyses will drive researchers toward greater transparency in describing their methods.

Finally, we note that the issues discussed in this chapter would be much less worrisome if data from all fMRI studies were available for sharing and reanalysis by the community. We hope that such debates will lead to increased interest in and support for the development of new data sharing mechanisms that can potentially overcome some of the social and technical problems that have doomed previous data sharing efforts (cf. Toga 2002).

Note

1. When the measures are different, if they are independent, there is an unlikely chance of bias, and if they are not independent, strong biases are likely.

8 On the Advantages of Not Having to Rely on Multiple Comparison Corrections

Edward Vul and Nancy Kanwisher

'We agree with Poldrack and Mumford's commentary about potential valid uses for nonindependent displays of data: Although those data should not (and cannot) be used to make inferences, they may be used as quality control on the effects of interest (e.g., by checking for outliers in correlations and what may be driving interactions). We also agree that collecting additional independent data is not necessary if one does not care to measure effect sizes and the original whole-brain analysis has adequately established the significance of the effect, including solving the crucial problem of correcting for multiple comparisons. However, we think that correcting for multiple comparisons is less straightforward than often acknowledged, that misunderstandings of correction methods are widespread in the field, and that many papers do not provide sufficient information to determine whether the correction was done adequately. Given this situation, we think the simpler and more transparent method of replicating one's results with independent data may be worth the cost of collecting additional data.

A wide array of methods exist for correcting for multiple comparisons in fMRI data analysis. Classical stringent corrections like Bonferoni have given way to modern methods designed to increase power. Small-volume corrections are designed for finding effects within independently defined subsets of the fMRI data. False discovery rate corrections consider the distribution of p-values across the volume to control the proportion of detected signals that should be attributed to chance. Cluster-size correction methods use an estimate of the spatial correlation in the data to define a null hypothesis distribution over the probability of detecting a number of spatially contiguous voxels, each of which exceeds a particular per-voxel p-value.

These methods are effective at increasing statistical power; however, they come with a cost of complexity, and they make additional assumptions that may not be satisfied. Often, readers are not given sufficient information to evaluate the appropriateness of particular correction parameters: How was the small volume selected? What was the spatial correlation of the data? What was the brainwise distribution of p-values? It might not be a problem that readers and reviewers are not given sufficient information to evaluate the soundness of multiple-comparisons correction procedures if they were never misapplied. However, this is not the case. Vul et al. (2009) pointed out one common error: choosing clusters that exceed a height threshold of $p < 0.005$ and an extent threshold of 10 voxels. These numbers were taken from Forman et al. (1995), who derived them from simulations in two-dimensional slices, not three-dimensional volumes, where they are now applied. Thus, these numbers result in false alarm rates that are orders of magnitude higher than researchers assume.

We think that these misapplications of multiple-comparison corrections have sneaked through the review process because of their complexity and because reviewers and readers do not know any better or simply assumed they were right. This seems a poor state of affairs.

Using independently selected ROI approaches (like split-half analyses) removes the additional complexity of multiple-comparison corrections and produces a transparent false alarm rate. Replicating your own results is, after all, the most straightforward way to strengthen your findings, and we think that, given the complexity of the multiple-comparisons problem in fMRI, a replication with a transparent false alarm rate is often worth the cost of extra data collection. Moreover, if you are going to replicate your results anyway, doing so with independent ROIs confers the added benefit of unbiased measures of the effects in those ROIs.

9 Confirmation, Refutation, and the Evidence of fMRI

Christopher Mole and Colin Klein

For some researchers, expanding the range of topics that neuroimaging techniques are used to address is a more or less explicit goal. Ellis, for example, claims that "Delusions (or at least some forms of them) are eminent candidates for imaging analysis" (Ellis 2006, 146); Bartels and Zeki use fMRI to study romantic and maternal love (Bartels and Zeki 2000, 2004); Holstege et al. (2003) use neuroimaging techniques to study the orgasms of male undergraduates.

Neuroimaging research is now expected to help us in answering once-intractable questions, some of them with long philosophical pedigrees. Houdé and Tzourio-Mazoyer (2003), for example, claim that "Brain imaging techniques have made it possible to explore the neural foundations of logical and mathematical cognition" and they trace this topic back to Aristotle (p. 507). Berns et al. (2005) "bring functional magnetic resonance imaging (fMRI) to bear on the problem of social conformity," and note that this topic "has been debated contentiously" since Jean Jacques Rousseau's *The Social Contract* (1762). If there are any remaining fields of psychology to which imaging techniques have not yet been applied, we may be sure that there are psychologists working in those fields who are looking for ways to apply them.

The question we wish to address here is the question of how far this boundary pushing can go. Where are the bounds to the sorts of questions neuroimaging techniques can be used to answer? We approach this question as a special case of a general question about what sort of theory can be confirmed by data from a given source. We begin by formulating some general principles about what is required for data from neuroimaging (or from any other source) to provide informative evidence regarding hypotheses in cognitive science. We then identify some examples of neuroimaging research that, in various ways, fails to respect those principles. We conclude by outlining a positive but modest account of the role neuroimaging data can play in the cognitive sciences.

Refutation and Confirmation

Our question—What can neuroimaging tell us?—may be reconstrued more approachably as "Which hypotheses can neuroimaging data provide us with a reason to believe?" When asked in that form it is clear that our question about neuroimaging data is a special case of a more general and more philosophical question, one that is usually discussed under the rubric of "confirmation theory."

Suppose we have a body of data, *d,* and are interested in the truth or falsity of a hypothesis, *H.* Confirmation theory is an attempt to answer the question, "What conditions have to be met in order for the data to provide a reason to believe the hypothesis?" One tempting but mistaken answer to this question would be that *d* provides a reason to believe *H* if and only if *d* is just what one would expect to find if *H* were true. It's easy to see why this is tempting, but also easy to see that it is mistaken.

The mistake is clearest in the case where *d* is a body of irrelevant data. Suppose (following Hempel 1945) that the hypothesis we are interested in is the hypothesis that all ravens are black, and suppose the data come from observations of objects that are neither black nor ravens. Those data might be just what one would expect to find *whether or not* all ravens are black. In that case, they are, a fortiori, just what one would expect to find if all ravens are black. But observations of nonblack nonravens might be observations of almost anything. Data *consistent with* the hypothesis that all ravens are black might come exclusively from observations of red herrings. In that case, they provide no reason at all for thinking that the hypothesis is true. The fact that a body of data is *consistent with* a hypothesis is not enough to show that the data provide a reason to believe the hypothesis is true. As Karl Popper realized (Popper 1959), something more is required.

We can begin to see what more is required by reflecting on the fact, important in the thinking of Fred Dretske and others (see Dretske 1981), that an informative body of data is a body of data that enables us to rule out certain possibilities. The problem with observations of nonblack nonravens is that they don't rule out any of the possibilities that we are interested in. They are compatible with the hypothesis that all ravens are black and also compatible with the contradictory of that hypothesis. That is why they are uninformative. To provide evidence for a hypothesis, the data must not only be consistent with the hypothesis, they must also count against the contradictory of the hypothesis. They must, as we say, refute the null hypothesis.

When properly understood, this point is relatively uncontroversial. It is something that we all sign up to when we use the familiar statistical tests for ascertaining when our data are significant. Indeed, "incompatible with the null hypothesis" is more or less what "significant" means in the context of significance testing.

Although we usually speak of data "refuting" null hypotheses, this way of talking may be misleading if it suggests that the relationship between data and null hypothesis must be one of absolute incompatibility. In a science such as psychology, the data (and the subject matter) are typically noisy. It is a consequence of this that data rarely refute a null hypothesis absolutely or unconditionally. They merely weigh against it. For some purposes, it is useful to represent the weighing of data against a null hypothesis as a conditional probability. Using that notation, we can state the principle linking evidence and refutation in the following form, familiar in so-called Baysian epistemology: The data, d, provide a reason to believe the hypothesis H only if $P(H \mid d) < P(\sim H \mid d)$.

Such formal apparatus is often useful, and it will be used from time to time in what follows; but the points to emphasize here can be made without it, and without incurring commitments to any of the contentious claims that go under the name of Baysianism. We have seen, as a fully general point about confirmation, that data provide us with a reason to believe a hypothesis only if they weigh against the contradictory of that hypothesis (that is, if they refute the corresponding null hypothesis). Applying this general principle to the case of neuroimaging research gives us the result that neuroimaging research can tell us about hypotheses only when the data from that research weigh against the corresponding null hypotheses.

There are two lessons to be learned from this. The first, which is an immediate consequence of the result just stated, is that to have found neuroimaging data that are consistent with a hypothesis is not yet to have found any reason for believing the hypothesis to be true (or even probable). The second slightly more precise result is that the easier it is for a null hypothesis to accommodate a body of data (the higher the value of $P[d \mid \sim H]$), the less support the data provide for the hypothesis.

When the first of these lessons is ignored, neuroimaging data that are merely consistent with a hypothesis will mistakenly be thought to provide evidence for it. This, as we shall see in the following section, is a mistake that is often made, sometimes overtly, sometimes in more concealed form. When the second lesson from confirmation theory goes unheeded, neuroimaging data will be taken to provide evidence for hypotheses even though there are relatively straightforward ways in which those data can be accommodated by the corresponding null hypotheses. In the section on accommodating null hypotheses, we will see some examples of research that falls into this trap, and we will see some of the reasons why it is a difficult trap to avoid.

Mere Consistency

Because data that are merely consistent with an hypothesis may fail to provide evidence for that hypothesis, a fallacy is committed whenever a researcher moves from claiming that his or her neuroimaging data are consistent with a hypothesis to claiming that those data show the hypothesis to be true (or even probable). Evidence for a hypothesis comes only from data that weigh against the null hypothesis. Data that are merely consistent with the hypothesis are no sort of evidence for it.

An unusually clear example of the fallacy that results from treating compatibility of data with a hypothesis as evidence for that hypothesis is found in the recent work of Joel Winston and his collaborators (Winston et al. 2007). The authors of this work claim, quite correctly, that the data from their scans of amygdala responses to attractive and unattractive faces are *"in keeping with the idea that the amygdala is tuned to the detection of events of emotional value, irrespective of valence, in the sensory environment"* (p. 203, emphasis added). They go on to conclude, on that basis alone, that "the response profile of the amygdala *demonstrates* a role for this region in encoding value (a non-linear function of valence) from stimuli in the environment" (p. 206, emphasis added, parentheses in original).

We have seen that this is a fallacy. As is clear when thinking about the logic of significance tests, there is a gap between having found some data that are *in keeping with* an idea and having *demonstrated* that the idea is correct. You can't demonstrate that an idea is correct by finding data that are merely in keeping with it. Because Winston et al. have not shown that their data weigh against the null hypothesis, they have not provided a reason for thinking their hypothesis is true. It is quite possible, given all that Winston et al. have said, that their neuroimaging data are accurate, but that their hypothesis about amygdala function is false.

Winston et al.'s work is a particularly clear example of what we might call *the consistency fallacy*. Further cases of the same mistake are easy to find. Look, for example, at Thein Thang Dang-Vu et al.'s (2005) interpretation of their neuroimaging data from subjects in dream sleep:

[The neuroimaging results] may also explain several hallmarks of dreaming experience that are found in dream reports after awakening from REM sleep. For instance, amygdala activation is consistent with the predominance of threat-related emotions. Temporo-occipital activation is in keeping with visual dream imagery. Prefrontal deactivation is suggestive of the lack of orientational stability, the alteration in time perception, the delusional belief of being awake, the decrease in volitional control and the fragmented episodic memory recall. Inferior parietal deactivation may contribute to the lack of distinction between first- and third-person perspectives. (p. 418)

Dang-Vu et al. may be right to say that their neuroimaging data are "consistent with," and "in keeping with," and "suggestive of" these features of dreaming. What our lessons from basic confirmation theory show us is that they are mistaken in thinking that being consistent with those phenomena makes their data explanatory of them.

Not all examples of the consistency fallacy are so easy to spot. A less manifest instance of the fallacy is found in the work of Luiz Pessoa et al. (2002). Pessoa et al. use neuroimaging data to argue against the view that the emotional expressions of faces can be detected when we are not paying attention to them. They claim that "neural processing of emotional faces requires attention" (p. 11458). They make that claim on the basis of imaging neural responses in the following situation. Subjects were either given the task of recognizing the gender of a face, or of recognizing whether two concurrently presented bars were of the same orientation. The faces, together with the bars, were presented for 200 ms. In this situation, the neuroimaging data show that "all brain regions responding differentially to emotional faces, including the amygdala, did so only when sufficient attentional resources were available to process the faces." That finding is, to be sure, *consistent with* the hypothesis that neural processing of emotional faces requires attention. But it is also consistent with a plausible version of the null hypothesis, which says that emotional faces *can* be processed without attention, but that, *when the faces are presented for only 200 ms*, their processing makes no discernible difference to levels of neural activation unless attention is being paid. Pessoa's data are consistent with their hypothesis and with this version of the null hypothesis. Since the data do not require that a low probability be assigned to the null hypothesis, they provide little reason for thinking the hypothesis is true.

Accommodating Null Hypotheses

We established, in the first section, that the easier it is for a null hypothesis to accommodate a body of data, the less support the data provide for the hypothesis. When the null hypothesis can accommodate the data (that is, when $P(d|{\sim}H)$ is high), those data provide only weak support for the hypothesis.

There are various ways in which cognitive null hypotheses can find room in which to accommodate the data that neuroimaging experiments provide, and which therefore keep $P({\sim}H|d)$ high. These are partly owing to the tactics that must be adopted to deal with the noisy BOLD signal, and partly owing to the difficulties of moving between the different levels of description involved in accounts of neural activity and claims about cognitive phenomena. We explain each of these difficulties with reference to some notable examples.

Dramatic Stimulus Differences Suffice to Explain Differences in Data

Neuroimaging is a noisy business, and the brain is a noisy place. To prevent all of this noise from creating problems, neuroimaging experiments typically compare the neural activity elicited by task conditions that differ from one another in substantial ways. Clear contrasts between task conditions are needed if there are to be significant differences in the BOLD signal. Using task conditions that are clearly different, however, means that one should *expect* differences in the resulting neural activation. The likelihood of the null hypothesis conditional upon such data might therefore differ little from the likelihood of the hypotheses. The resulting image, while cleaner, will end up being less informative.

The well-known work of Joshua Greene and his collaborators examining the engagement of emotions in moral judgment (Greene et al. 2001) illustrates this point. Greene et al. required their subjects to make judgments about dilemmas of three sorts. One set of dilemmas involved nonmoral decisions about matters such as whether a journey is best made by train or bus. The second set contained moral dilemmas with an "up-close and personal" aspect, and involved asking such things as whether, in suitably dire circumstances, it would be acceptable to throw people off a sinking lifeboat. The third set of dilemmas were again moral, but had no "up-close and personal" aspect. These involved decisions such as whether one should vote for a policy with life and death consequences.

What Greene et al. found was that subjects showed patterns of neural activation when considering up-close and personal moral dilemmas that were quite different from the patterns shown in the other conditions. In particular, the up-close and personal moral dilemmas elicited activation in medial frontal gyrus, posterior cingulate gyrus, and angular gyrus, all of which areas tend to be activated in emotional situations. Greene et al. take these results to support the hypothesis that the emotionally engaging nature of up-close and personal moral situations affects our judgments in a way that accounts for our tendency to judge certain acts as not permissible in those situations, even though we judge acts with similar consequences to be permissible in other situations.

The patterns of activation observed by Greene et al. are certainly just what one would expect to find if their hypothesis were true. As the preceding discussion of confirmation theory reminded us, however, that isn't to the point. If we want to know whether the findings provide good evidence for the hypothesis we need to know the value of $P(d\mid{\sim}H)$—that is, we need to know whether one should expect those findings if the hypothesis were *false*. The null hypothesis here is the claim that it is *not* the subject's emotional response to up-close and personal dilemmas that accounts for his judgment about what is permissible. In order to estimate the extent to which Greene et al.'s findings support their hypothesis, we must make an assessment of the probability of those findings conditional on the null hypothesis.

This conditional probability might, on the face of it, be rather high. If so then the data do not provide much support for the hypothesis. Some dilemmas are certainly more emotional in their contemplation than others. That is not at issue. Nor is it at issue whether there are some brain areas that are more active in emotional contemplation than in nonemotional contemplation. Both of those claims are parts of the background that Greene et al. assume in the design of their experiment, and are not a part of what that experiment is intended to establish. But the clear contrast between the emotional engagingness of their different task conditions means that Greene et al.'s null hypothesis can accommodate their neuroimaging data. Given that the up-close and personal dilemmas are more emotionally engaging, and given that emotional engagement, per se, will be reflected in neural activation, it would seem quite likely that the contemplation of up-close and personal moral dilemmas will activate those parts of the brain that are typically active in emotional situations, *whether or not* that activity constitutes an emotional influence that accounts for our ethical judgments. It therefore seems that Greene et al.'s findings are quite likely given their hypothesis, *and that they are quite likely given the null hypothesis.* If that is right, then, with our lessons from confirmation theory in mind, we can see that the neuroimaging results provide little evidence for the hypothesis. (Of course, Greene et al. can bring in nonimaging considerations at this point, and they would be quite right to do so: Our concern here is not to assess the truth of Greene's claims, but to assess the usefulness of neuroimaging data for establishing them.)

The problem with taking Greene et al.'s data as evidence for their hypothesis is one that applies with some generality. Their hypothesis concerns the factors that contribute to moral judgments. Their experiment involves task conditions that differ in ways that are apt to make clear differences to the sorts of judgments people make. The differences need to be big ones, since only this will ensure that comparisons of noisy BOLD signals reveal recognizably significant patterns. But one big psychological difference between task conditions brings other differences with it: The differences between the task conditions may make for a difference in the subjects' approach to making moral judgments, but they also make for differences in the extent to which the subjects are emotionally engaged. That difference, together with its diverse psychological ramifications, may be sufficient to explain the observed difference in neural activation. This is true even if, as the null hypothesis would have it, we credit none of the difference in neural activation to differences in ways of making judgments about the dilemmas presented.

In general, the clear differences between task conditions that neuroimaging requires may make for differences in the subjects' attention, readiness, interest, degree of expertise, beliefs, surprise, enjoyment, perception, verbal and nonverbal thinking, desires, inclinations, mood, confidence, and so on and on. All of the psychological differences that different task conditions beget must be reflected somehow (perhaps each in its quite different way) in the patterns of neuronal activation recorded in the neuroimaging data. Each of these differences therefore provides a potential uncontrolled variable, and so a potential way in which the defender of the null hypothesis can explain away the differences between the neural activation patterns that different task conditions elicit. The clear differences in the task conditions that neuroimaging experiments employ thereby make room in which the null hypotheses can accommodate neuroimaging data, and so they make it difficult for neuroimaging data to support cognitive hypotheses.

High-Level Null Hypotheses are Noncommittal About Low-Level Data

Striking contrasts between task conditions are not the only sources of space in which null hypotheses can accommodate neuroimaging data. Another way for null hypotheses to accommodate such data is by exploiting the difference between the level of description at which cognitive hypotheses are stated and the level of description at which imaging data are described.

Hypotheses in cognitive psychology typically make claims about the functional architecture underpinning a particular mental phenomenon. Such hypotheses place constraints on what the underlying anatomical architecture must be like. But those constraints are neither especially specific nor especially precise. Several different anatomical arrangements might implement any given functional architecture. Even when hypotheses in cognitive science require particular anatomical arrangements for their implementation, they do not imply clear commitments about the patterns of neural activation those arrangements must display. This means that the null versions of cognitive hypotheses are compatible with a considerable range of data about patterns of activation. Data about patterns of activation are correspondingly ill suited to refuting those null hypotheses. From the basic confirmation theory previously outlined, it follows that those data are ill-suited to confirming cognitive hypotheses.

Since the problem here arises from a mismatch between the relatively high-level vocabulary of cognitive hypotheses and the relatively low-level descriptions that neuroimaging data provide, the clearest examples arise in cases where the neuroimaging techniques being employed give particularly fine-grained information. The use of neuroimaging techniques to study face perception is exemplary in this regard, being a field in which very sophisticated imaging techniques have been employed and in which the hypotheses at issue pertain to high-level claims about the basic structure of the cognitive architecture. In a recent survey of the face processing literature Nancy Kanwisher and Galit Yovel (Kanwisher and Yovel 2006) make clear the way in which their claims about the mechanisms of face perception are related to higher-level hypotheses about the modularity and localizability of cognitive functions:

One of the longest running debates in the history of neuroscience concerns the degree to which specific high-level cognitive functions are implemented in discrete regions of the brain specialized for just that function.... Despite [the] currently popular view that complex cognitive functions are conducted in distributed and overlapping neural networks, substantial evidence supports the hypothesis that at least one complex cognitive function—face perception—is implemented in its own specialized cortical network that is not shared with many if any other cognitive functions. (p. 2109)

The evidence that Kanwisher and Yovel adduce in support of this claim is drawn from a number of sources, but their discussion focuses "particularly on functional magnetic resonance imaging (fMRI) investigations" (p. 2110). A great deal of neuroimaging research, employing a great many techniques of data analysis, has been devoted to the hypothesis that face perception is, as Kanwisher and Yovel say, "implemented in its own specialized cortical network" (p. 2109). (There has also been a great deal of research using other methods—that work is not the focus of Kanwisher's discussion and is not our present concern.)

A considerable portion of the neuroimaging research devoted to the hypothesis that there is a face-specific cortical mechanism is an attempt to gather a body of data showing that no stimuli other than faces elicit a consistently strong response from the so-called fusiform face area (FFA) (see Grill-Spector et al. 2004; Kanwisher et al. 1997b). The claim that the FFA is the site of a module responsible for the perception of faces is taken as showing that at least one cognitive function is implemented by a localized module, and so, as the preceding quotation from Kanwisher and Yovel makes clear, as counting against a thoroughly nonmodularized view of cognition. The thoroughly nonmodular view, according to which the mechanisms responsible for face perception aren't specialized and aren't localized, is the null hypothesis that needs to be ruled out.

Data showing that faces alone elicit strong responses from the FFA are just what one would expect to find if the modularity hypothesis were true; as before, that fact alone does not entail that such data provide evidence for that hypothesis. To assess the extent to which the modularity hypothesis is supported by data showing that no stimuli other than faces elicit a consistently strong response from the FFA, we must assess the probability of those data, conditional on the null hypothesis. It is, however, very far from obvious what that conditional probability is. The null hypothesis says that the same distributed system is responsible for the processing of faces and of other stimulus types, but this does not imply that the different stimulus types must elicit the same patterns of activation from that distributed system. Different tasks can load an unmodularized system in different ways, leading to different patterns of activation in that system. It is therefore consistent with the nonmodularized hypothesis that some areas of cortex are more strongly activated in response to some stimulus types than to others. The localized patterns of activation need not indicate the sites of distinct processing modules, they may indicate which parts of a general unmodularized system are working the hardest.

Since the null hypothesis is compatible with the claim that a region of cortex is activated more strongly by faces than by other stimuli, and is therefore compatible with the finding that the FFA is activated more strongly by faces than by other stimuli, it is not at all clear that $P(d \mid \sim H)$ is low. It is far from clear, therefore, that neuroimaging data of the sort that Kanwisher and Yovel cite can provide evidence supporting the modularity hypothesis. (A more detailed discussion of this point is given in Mole et al 2007.)

The work of James Haxby and his collaborators makes vivid the difficulties that are faced here. Haxby has made important contributions to the development of increasingly sophisticated techniques for extracting information from the BOLD signal that fMRI procedures measure. Such techniques give us an increasingly accurate picture of where information-carrying neural activity is taking place. But even with that accurate picture before us, the question about the cognitive architecture responsible for face perception remains open.

O'Toole et al. (2005) took the raw data from Haxby et al.'s (2001) scans of subjects viewing several objects from eight various categories (faces, shoes, chairs, houses, bottles, etc.). They determined which voxels in the scan contained data that, when added to the analysis, increased the accuracy of pattern-based classification algorithms, and they thereby gauged the extent to which different neural regions encode information about the object viewed. What they found was that accuracy was highest when *all* available voxels contributed to the classification. This shows that information about the category of the objects viewed is carried by patterns of activation distributed throughout the ventral temporal cortex. O'Toole et al. also found that, when considered by themselves, the patterns of activation in the regions responding most strongly to faces carried rather little information about the other categories of objects (and, *mutatis mutandis*, for the regions responding most strongly to the other categories). The first of these results is consistent with, and suggestive of, a nonmodular architecture. The second result is consistent with, and suggestive of, a modular one. But, as we have been emphasizing, data that are consistent with a hypothesis—even *suggestive* data consistent with a hypothesis—may not provide any reason for believing the hypothesis to be true. O'Toole's work makes vivid the fact that one set of data can be consistent with two radically opposed hypotheses. It cannot, of course, provide evidence for both.

The problem is *not* that fMRI data fail to show there are "partially distributed representations of faces and objects." O'Toole et al. are quite right to claim they have shown that, *if*, by "representations of faces and objects," they mean "states carrying information about faces and objects." But not every state that *carries information about* faces (or objects) need play any role in underpinning our ability to perceive faces (or objects). This is made clear in recent work by Haynes and Rees (2005), which shows that in some situations the patterns of activation in visual cortex *carry information about* the features of visual stimuli, even when the subject whose cortical activity carries this information fails to have any experience of the features in question. (In Haynes and Rees's experiments the information "represented" concerns the orientations of masked gratings). The claims about representations that O'Toole et al. have established, like Kanwisher's claims about patterns of activation, do not immediately entail anything about the subject's psychology. They are no more than suggestively consistent with any claims about the distributed nature of the mechanisms responsible for our ability to perceive faces.

The general problem here is analogous to one that Tim Shallice has emphasized in the case of making inferences from data concerning deficits: Careful analysis is always required to move between functional and anatomical hypotheses (see, e.g., Shallice 1998, especially chapter 11). Although it is true that differences between cognitive mechanisms will tend to be manifested in different patterns of activation (or different patterns of deficits), there is plenty of variation in the activation patterns that any given arrangement of mechanisms might display. There is also plenty of variation among the mechanisms that might account for any given activation pattern. Any inference from claims about patterns of activation to claims about cognitive architectures requires knowledge of the probability of the observed patterns of activation, given a particular cognitive architecture, and that sort of knowledge is difficult to come by.

The use of neuroimaging data to support cognitive hypotheses depends on an assessment of the probability of claims at the cognitive level conditional on data at the level of neuronal activation. Judgments about such probabilities depend on a background theory of how these different levels of description are related. According to one such background theory, there is a mapping from distinct regions of elevated neural activity to distinct cognitive modules. If we adopt that theory as a working hypothesis, then some of the required conditional probabilities linking imaging data and cognitive hypotheses can be assigned. We could *presuppose* that the cognitive architecture is modular, and, having taken this as an assumption, the way would then be clear for using Kanwisher's imaging results as evidence for the hypothesis that the FFA is the site of a module specialized for face perception. But that is not the direction in which Kanwisher's argument is intended to go. The question of the modularity of the cognitive architecture is the large-scale question that Kanwisher's neuroimaging research is intended to help us *answer*. But the modularity hypothesis is the sort of claim that needs already to be in place before one can make the assignments of conditional probability needed to interpret neuroimaging data as evidence for cognitive hypotheses.

Conclusion: Imaging as Normal Science

Neuroimaging data are often presented as if they gave us a way of looking directly at the working brain. Claims of "mind-reading" are common in the popular press (see Adler and Carmichael 2004), and even sneak into the work of careful researchers (Leopold and Wilke 2005; Norman et al. 2006). This creates the impression that those neural events which could previously be known only through tortuous inferences can now be observed directly. This, we have seen, is a mistake.

The epistemology of neuroimaging is not the straightforward epistemology of direct looking. Interpreting imaging data requires complex inference even in simple cases. We have shown in this chapter some common obstacles to this interpretive process. These obstacles do not make it impossible for carefully designed neuroimaging experiments (or, more likely, sets of those experiments) to confirm interesting hypotheses

about either functional or anatomical architecture; the pitfalls can be avoided if sufficient care is taken. But the disanalogy between imaging and looking reveals a more
fundamental limitation on the sorts of things that neuroimaging will tell us. We conclude by saying a bit more about this.

What is not possible, even when great care is taken, is for imaging to have a revolutionary effect on cognitive psychology. Neuroimaging has become popular because it
provides "faster, safer, or more cost effective information than was previously available" (Owen et al. 2006b). The information so provided, however, has no higher evidential standing than data provided by slower, riskier, more expensive techniques.
Imaging does not give us a qualitatively different kind of evidence for believing large-
scale hypotheses about the explanation of cognitive phenomena.

Neuroimaging is, in fact, in worse shape than many other techniques in an important respect: Its correct application nearly always relies on facts drawn from the very
theories that it is called upon to adjudicate. In this regard, imaging is quite unlike,
say, Galileo's telescope. Telescopic observation could be revolutionary precisely because its epistemic credentials were underwritten by a science (i.e., optics) independent
from the astronomical claims in question. Not so for imaging.

For imaging data to serve as evidence for cognitive hypotheses, we must assume a
good deal of intimately related hypotheses about cognitive function. Again, this is necessary in order to correctly assign probabilities to the cognitive hypotheses conditional
on the neuroimaging data. We saw, in the case of Kanwisher's research, that the bits of
theory we need to use to get to these conditional probabilities are bits of theory that
come from domains close to, or overlapping, the domains we are trying to investigate.
They are substantive cognitive hypotheses. Neuroimaging data provide evidence about
cognitive topics only when we already have substantiated theories about those very
topics. It is for this reason it cannot be revolutionary.

This is not a reason for thoroughgoing pessimism, of course. There are many exemplary cases in which neuroimaging research is applied to cognitive hypotheses. One
telling case is the use of fMRI to map patterns of functional retinotopy in V1 (Tootell
et al. 1998; Warnking et al. 2002). This work is illustrative for several reasons. There is a
large body of well-confirmed data about the cytological and functional anatomy of V1
that supports the background theory, on the basis of which conditional probabilities
linking neural activation patterns and cognitive claims can be assigned. Tootell et al.
point out that their study "benefited greatly from the wealth of previous data in area
V1 of humans and other mammalian species" (p. 815). They also emphasize that
many of their assumptions—about the location, retinotopic precision, monocular
dominance, and polar organization of retinotopic maps in V1—derive from other,
nonimaging studies (p. 816). These assumptions are so embedded in the experimental
design, and so crucial to the confirmation process, that the conclusions of these experiments would be greatly weakened without them.

Tootell et al.'s study is in part a confirmation of previous results, in part an extension to new hypotheses about function. It is fantastically useful and important, but it does not constitute a radical break with results obtained with nonimaging techniques. We suggest that the best—indeed, probably the *only*—use of imaging is as a tool in this process of slow accumulation of results, a slow accumulation that Thomas Kuhn characterized as ''normal science'' and famously contrasted with the dramatic paradigm shifts that take place during scientific revolutions (Kuhn 1962).

The problematic uses of fMRI are the ones that try to decide between dramatic, large-scale hypotheses. Dramatic hypotheses include most of the really interesting problems in psychology, of course, but they are also precisely where there is too little knowledge to expect imaging to confirm anything much at all. Imaging is a valuable tool for doing normal science, and a poor tool for doing revolutionary science. The logic of confirmation demands that it be so.

10 Words and Pictures in Reports of fMRI Research

Gilbert Harman

I want to briefly note three worries by philosophers about how functional magnetic resonance imaging (fMRI) research results have sometimes been presented.

First, Mole and Klein (this volume) argue that some of these reports commit serious fallacies, for example, confusing (a) the data's being *consistent* with a hypothesis with (b) the data's *confirming* the hypothesis.

This is indeed a fallacy, if the relevant sort of consistency is *logical* consistency. However, the expression "is consistent with" is often used by scientists to mean something much stronger, something like *confirms* or even *strongly confirms*. Compare Mole and Klein's worry with the following passage from Johnson-Laird (2001):

[I]ntelligent individuals make mistakes in reasoning in everyday life. A lawyer in a civil action, for example, got an opposing expert witness to admit the following two facts concerning a toxic substance, tricholoroethylene (TCE):

If TCE came down the river (from other factories), then TCE would be in the river bed.
TCE was not in the river bed.

At this point, the lawyer asked the witness:
The pattern is consistent with the fact that no TCE came from the river, isn't it?

What he should have pointed out is that this conclusion follows necessarily from the premises. Neither the lawyer nor the author of the book from which this report comes appears to have noticed the mistake (see Harr 1995, 361–362). (p. 85)

Johnson-Laird, like Mole and Klein, apparently supposes that "consistent" in this sort of context must mean "logically consistent." One might instead conclude from the transcript that "consistent" in such a context means something much stronger. Indeed, a Web search for documents containing the phrase "is consistent with" appears to show that a stronger meaning is often intended in scientific contexts, something like "implies or confirms," as in Fisher et al.'s (2006) "Evidence from Amazonian Forests Is Consistent with Isohydric Control of Leaf Water Potential," to take a random example.

It is true that this use of "consistent" may confuse logicians, philosophers, and psychologists, perhaps even judges and members of juries. That may be something to worry about.

Second, Mole et al. (2007), relying on Haxby et al. (2001) and Hanson, Matsuka, and Haxby (2004), argue that Kanwisher (e.g., Kanwisher and Yovel 2006) overstates the implications of fMRI research for whether "the fusiform face area ... is the site of cognitive resources that are specialized for and dedicated to the processing of faces" (p. 199). One problem is that activity elsewhere in the brain can *carry information about* perceived faces and activity in the "fusiform face area" can *carry information about* other things perceived. Furthermore, "the locus of maximum activation need not be the place where the processing is done. It might simply be an indication of the place at which the load is greatest.... The fact that some manual tasks, such as hammering, lead to blisters on the palm of the hand does not show that it is the palm that performs the task of hammering" (p. 203).

On the other hand, Mole et al. reject Haxby's conclusion that faces must receive some sort of "distributed representation" in a relevant sense. They argue it has not been shown that the relevant activity represents anything except in the sense of "carrying information" in a statistical sense. This does not imply that the relevant activity *determines the content* of associated mental states.

Third, I noted previously that a scientific use of the term "consistent" might confuse certain readers for whom that use is relatively unfamiliar. Roskies (this volume) argues that presenting the results of fMRI research in the form of what look like photographs can be very misleading in a somewhat different way, because of great differences in the ways in which photographs represent what they are photographs of and in which fMRI pictures represent what they represent. To the reader, it may appear that one can see the result of the fMRI experiments just by looking at the picture, much as one can see what the camera was pointed at by looking at a photograph. This is a complete illusion, because of the large amount of more or less controversial interpretation used to come up with the fMRI picture. As Roskies puts it, the "inferential distance" between a photo and what it depicts is normally quite small compared with the inferential distance between an fMRI picture and what it depicts.

In summary, readers of research reports may be subject to various *cognitive illusions* that go beyond those discussed by psychologists like Kahneman and Tversky. Readers may misunderstand the ways certain words are being used—words like "consistent" for example—a misunderstanding that may negatively affect their appreciation of the research reported. They may fail to distinguish different ways in which activity might or might not represent something. And they may fail to appreciate the "inferential distance" between a picture and what it depicts, a misunderstanding that may lead them to read more into the results than they should.

11 Discovering How Brains Do Things

Stephen José Hanson and Clark Glymour

The aim of psychology is to learn to how the brain produces thought, feeling and action. Those are fundamentally *causal* questions about the brain and its parts. Traditional cognitive neuropsychology relied on brain damage and autopsies to obtain limited (but once upon a time, revolutionary) information about such mechanisms and parts. Cognitive psychology has used an ever-growing collection of behavioral semi-regularities to support various theories about the "computational architecture" of the brain. Computational models are indirectly specified causal hypotheses, which the behavioral data of conventional cognitive psychology radically under-determines. The only way to understand how a black box works is to peer inside the box. Functional magnetic resonance provides our best currently available method of peering inside the human brain while its owner is doing simple tasks. The fundamental methodological problem is to discover how to extract the most correct causal information from such observations.

We met some years ago at a McDonnell Foundation workshop in Dallas, that, as usual, had brought a diverse and interesting set of players together to ask how Bayesian graph theory might inform cognitive neuroscience. We both agreed at that point there was probably no simple application of graph theory to neuroimaging because of many obvious and less obvious problems. Years later, we (Martin Bunzl and I) had invited Glymour to the Rutgers' meeting that resulted in this volume. Following that meeting, Glymour and Hanson, after some debate, decided to join forces to investigate graphical modeling and neuroimaging with other researchers (James Haxby from Dartmouth and Russell Poldrack from UCLA), thanks again to the McDonnell Foundation. This chapter is about that collaboration at the time of writing (about a year before publication), and perhaps the less obvious problems we both expected to encounter—and some we did not.

Over the last decade, brain imaging has focused on matching specific functions to local brain structure and neural activity. Despite the apparent success of this program in identifying brain areas associated with memory, attention, executive control, action-perception, language, and the like, it is typical for many other areas to be engaged during basic cognitive/perceptual tasks that are often considered "background," "secondary," or just irrelevant and consequently ignored. As the neuroimaging field matures, interest in understanding how one brain area may influence another—that is, the "effective connectivity" (Friston et al. 1994) of brain areas during performance of a given task—is increasing. Whether we consider language processing, working memory, or simple detection tasks, cognitive and perceptual processes are likely to include networks of regions that operate interactively to uniquely define a kind of local computation. The localized regions of brain activity *do* something, and part of what they do is to influence one another. This kind of local computation might have at least two properties: (1) A sequence of brain regions are activated jointly in a particular dynamic—and causal—sequence; and (2) allowing in the small what everyone allows for the brain as a whole, a network, depending on its state and transmission sequence, may serve multiple functions, and overlapping (or even identical) brain regions may be components of multiple networks serving several distinct cognitive functions. These ideas are in no way original with us. McIntosh (1999; 2000) in particular has been notably committed to network analysis of brain imaging data, and groups from around the world have begun publishing proposed methods for turning imaging data into causal models using a variety of statistical/machine learning methods. This shift from merely identifying punctuate regions of interest (ROIs) to inferring causal relations among them pushes the edge of current measurement technology and statistical methodology, and uncovers issues that we think are frequently buried under an avalanche of technical papers.

Here we consider the following questions: (1) What are variables and how are they to be formed? (2) What might it mean, quantitatively and qualitatively, to claim that one region of activity influences another? (3) What do experimental or other interventions do, quantitatively and qualitatively, to change a system of brain region interactions? (4) In view of several difficulties (about which more below), what methods will find what information about a system of interactions among brain regions in a cognitive task? (5) How are methods that aim to identify novel relationships to be tested and evaluated?

What Are the Variables?

In physics and chemistry and biology, nature is sorted into stable kinds of things and stable kinds of relationships that behave according to stable regularities—even if only statistical regularities. The natural kinds of science are generally not the kinds that seem natural to us without science. They had to be discovered, and in many cases discovery amounted to creation. No one ever saw a force. That reflection should make it less shocking that in causal analyses of fMRI signals, the variables are constructed, almost on the fly, from the data.

The construction of variables from fMRI signals has a lot of steps, some of which are essentially hidden nowadays. The raw signals have to be given a spatial interpretation, and mapped to a surrogate brain, and the individual recordings by voxels have to be statistically cleansed of variation caused by head movements and other factors. Sets of voxels, often called ROIs, are either identified by statistical thresholding after general linear model (GLM) fits (say, selecting peaks) or constructed (often based on a centroid or whatever voxel or sets of voxels the user choses) in a brain map with software (e.g., SPM5-DCM). This determination could be based on prior anatomical or functional information as to which areas of the brain are most probably related to the task. This has many risks, but the largest involves the specific assumptions the algorithm implemented makes about the selected voxels representing the ROI. There is no a priori reason, for example, that local brain tissues acting coherently in a task would form a convex space, and forcing any such shape (a ball, for example) could reduce coherence of activity over time. A key challenge, therefore, is to define an ROI that has both meaningful spatial density and functional coherence.

One approach to the ROI problem is statistical clustering methods. Statistical clustering, or "parcellation," generally involves three choices: a distance metric, defining distance between voxels and clusters of voxels; a group membership rule, which defines the rule for combining voxels with clusters; or clusters with clusters. The methods often fall into one of three categories: single linkage (distance to the nearest neighbor), complete linkage (distance to the farthest neighbor), and centroid (distance to the centroid of the cluster based on chosen distance metric.) Finally at issue is whether the search is divisive (starting with all voxels in the same bag), or agglomerative (starting with each voxel in its own bag). All clustering methods fall into some combination of these choices. Common methods include k-means analysis (a divisive method using centroid membership), ward's method (an agglomerative method using variance as a distance measure) and single-linkage (an agglomerative method using nearest neighbor rule), which tends to "chain" voxels, creating large spindly and sparse clusters often shown in brain maps as spanning the whole brain. Another challenge in graphical analysis is to define a clustering method that can be combined with prior anatomical or functional assumptions and maximizes both cluster density and temporal coherence of cluster voxels. Recent work in our (Hanson et al. 2007a) laboratory provides a new method called *dense mode clustering* (DMC), which is discussed later.

A ROI is not a variable; it is a collection of voxels, each with an estimated signal at various times. Time-dependent variables can be formed from a ROI in any number of ways, and which way is chosen can make a good deal of difference downstream in understanding what is going on in the brain. For example, the voxel recordings with a ROI are often "spatially smoothed"—individual signal values are replaced by an average or weighted average of the values of their spatial neighbor signals. The extreme form of spatial smoothing determines a variable that is the average over all voxels in a

ROI of the fMRI signal. This procedure disables some potentially useful data analysis procedures, about which more later. One could, instead, take the maximum voxel value in a ROI at a time; in our experience this choice does not lead to a stable causal model, but sometimes it might. One could treat the voxel signals in a ROI at different times as separate sample cases and estimate a "naive Bayes model"—in other terms, a one-factor latent variable model in which the several voxel records in a ROI are functions of a fictitious latent variable. The ROI variable value is then the estimated value of the latent common factor in the naïve Bayes model. (Naïve Bayes models are not intended to be realistic models of causal relationships, but they turn out to be excellent classifiers in many applications.) A related strategy, sometimes called *eigenvalue analysis*, is to treat the time records of the voxels in a ROI again as cases in a sample and take some principal component of the variation. First principal components are commonly used in other applications, such as climate dynamics, but arguments have been made for using higher-order principle components in fMRI analysis on the grounds that first components are confounded with heart rate and other physiological variables. Such effects should create harmonics that can be removed prior to causal analysis, and may even be removed to some extent by thresholding. There seem to be no good a priori arguments for defining variables from ROIs in one of these ways (or possibly still others). We can only recommend trying alternative variable definitions and seeing which lead to hypotheses that are conformable to prior knowledge, show some stability over time and subjects, and, one would hope eventually, are independently confirmed.

What Is Causal Influence between Brain Regions?

Here is an interesting social fact: many universities around the world have departments of statistics, but to our knowledge no university has a department of causality. The reasons are historical. The notion of cause was at the center of the ideas in play in the seventeenth century, when science as we know it emerged in Europe. Aristotelian notions of cause, and Aristotelian terminology, were replaced by notions of constitution—as in the constitution of visible bodies and their properties—by invisible corpuscles and their properties, and by the notion of a cause as a change in some local condition that brings about changes in other local conditions. Newton assimilated the notion of cause into the notion of force, which, like "cause," was a kind of placeholder for many specific kinds of lawful relationships. So, by the beginning of the eighteenth century, one might have expected a mathematical theory of causality to develop, but it did not. The mathematics told against it. Mathematicians were focused on the calculus, including its application to probability theory, and algebra as well combinatorics. Graph theory played a minor role, and then only for undirected graphs. Causal relations between events are two-place, asymmetrical relations. A mathematical theory of

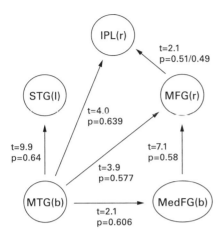

Figure 11.1
Graphical model of event perception task. See Hanson et al. (2007) for more detail.

causality required a joint understanding of directed graphs and probability, and that understanding did not emerge until nearly the end of the twentieth century, even while particular probabilistic causal theories, *implicitly* combining directed graphs and probability, were propounded in almost every subject from physics to psychology. The delay in the development of a mathematical theory of causality is explained in part by the evil influence of philosophy on statistics, but we will defer that discussion to another time. Let's now focus on the problem of causility in neuroimaging data.

In recent years, and in the fMRI literature in particular, causal hypotheses have routinely been represented by directed graphs. Figure 11.1 provides an example of a particular linear graphical causal model expressing a hypothesis about influences of activities in specific regions on one another in the course of a cognitive task activity (Hanson et al, 2007b). Abstractly, a directed graph G is a pair, $\langle \mathbf{V}, \mathbf{E} \rangle$, consisting of a set of objects $\mathbf{V}$ called vertices or nodes, and a set $\mathbf{E}$ of ordered pairs of members of $\mathbf{V}$, called directed edges and denoted, for example, by $v_1 \rightarrow v_2$. In our discussion, $\mathbf{V}$ will always be a set of brain regions, and a directed edge $v_1 \rightarrow v_2$ will signify the hypothesis that it is possible for activity in v_1 to cause activity in v_2 even if all other members of $\mathbf{V}$ were forced to be constant.

What can "cause" mean here? We follow a lesion model, where to say that a piece of brain tissue, X, causes a behavior phenomenon, or influences other brain tissues, implies that an ideal intervention that altered or removed X would alter the behavior or the other brain tissues, *if* that intervention were to influence behavior and other tissues only indirectly through the change in X—in other words, only if the intervention was not done with a fat hand. X is a direct cause of Y if, hypothetically, were all other represented variables held constant, ideal intervention on X would result in a covariation of Y.

That isn't the end of the story. A hypothetical (or actual) intervention on X might remove X from the system altogether, it might force a change on the value of X no matter the other prior influences on X, it might fix a more or less permanent value of X or change X briefly and then let normal influences on X resume, it might not render X independent of its normal causes but instead change the degree of influence of those causes. Brain surgery suggests a further interpretation: An intervention might alter or destroy a particular channel connecting brain areas. Work on graphical causal models in the last two decades has developed a full-fledged mathematical theory of interventions on variables that have a joint probability distribution of a special, but ubiquitous, kind (described later). When the effects of variables is additive, that mathematics trivially extends to interventions on connections, but when effects are interactive, the issue is less clear.

Figure 11.1 shows a particular model that is deterministic. None of the variables represented in the picture have their values determined by values of any other represented variables, but the underlying linear model adds a disturbance term for each variable, and the variables pictured are assumed to be determined uniquely by other variables and their proper disturbance. That necessarily implies constraints on the joint probability distribution of the variables if (unlike figure 11.1) the graph is acyclic— has no closed chains of edges, or edges going both ways between two variables. For any distribution in which the disturbance variables are jointly independent, each variable X will be independent of all other variables conditional on the values of the variables with edges directed into X. That is the Markov property of directed acyclic graphs (DAGs) and probability distributions on the variables that are nodes in such graphs. It does not depend on linearity or on any particular mathematical form for the influences of variables on one another. A somewhat unintuitive purely graphical condition, d-separation, characterizes the conditional independence relations implied by the Markov property for any DAG. The d-separation property extends to cyclic graphs of linear systems, like that shown in figure 11.1.

Linear, polynomial, additive, and logistic regression models; log linear models; path models; structural equation models; and so on are of this kind, with differing families of probability distributions and parameterizations. If the stochastic DAG has a time-repeating graphical unit, and repeating parameter values (e.g., linear coefficients) and corresponding members of different graphical units are treated as the "same" variable at different times, we have the graph of a time series model. Recently, time series models for data sampled noncontinuously have been supplemented with graphical causal models of the "simultaneous" causal processes—those occurring more rapidly than the sampling rate (Dimiralp and Hoover 2003). The causal and statistical relations among variables in systems with feedback are commonly represented by time series, but a long tradition in engineering and in the social sciences represents them as finite cyclic graphs without self-loops.

In measurements of brain function, the correct causal description may require unmeasured common causes, or "latent variables," either to explain the generation of the fMRI signal, or because of misspecification of the specific brain ROIs or omission of relevant regions due to failure in initial identification. Latent factors may be explicitly modeled, as is done in thousands of social science studies, factor analysis, principal components analysis, and elsewhere; or instead, the associations they produce between measured variables may be represented in a way distinct from marking a causal connection between the measured variables. Other graphical representations of probability distributions are available (e.g., chain graphs; see, e.g., Lauritzen 2002), but their causal interpretations are less clear.

What Do Stimuli Do?

Potential causal connections are everywhere. On any day, Hanson could change the population of Rome by flying to Rome, but usually he doesn't. Routine causal connections are also everywhere. On every day, Glymour wakes up and, more or less automatically, brushes his teeth. The brain may, likewise, have multiple nerve paths from one region to others that ordinarily are either not used or used routinely in low-level ways. All serious hypotheses about how brains produce cognition must allow for these background processes or potential processes. A stimulus presented to a subject is an intervention on the subject's brain, with direct or indirect effects indicated by a BOLD response measured in an fMRI signal. There are three pictures of what kind of direct effects a stimulus might have, and they have led to different formalisms.

First, the stimulus may temporarily directly (relative to other ROIs) influence the variables associated with one or another ROI, and indirectly, through connections, stimulate or suppress other clusters of cells.
Second, the stimulus may change the properties of channels connecting ROIs.
Third, it may do both.

A pipeline and reservoir model seems almost apt. One could change the height of one reservoir by adding water, and so by increasing water pressure, increase the flow downstream and the heights of downstream reservoirs; one could open a new channel from one reservoir to another, or increase the opening of a valve on an existing channel. Or one could do both.

The first picture is implicit in the structural equation models (SEM) and time series models proposed by many authors. The stimulus directly changes the values of one or more variables in a directed graphical model, which indirectly changes the values of downstream variables. How downstream variables depend on upstream variables is unchanged in the course of the experiment, although it may be changed from a "rest" condition. In a linear or otherwise parameterized model, the coefficients and disturbances of downstream variables are unchanged in the course of the experiment; more generally, the probability distribution of each variable not directly stimulated, *conditional* on the values of variables with edges directed into it, is unchanged.

The second picture of the effect of stimuli suggests that they alter the rate, or quantity (of something, we don't know just what) per unit time, at or by which upstream variables, or some of them, influence downstream variables.

A third view suggests there are two kinds of stimuli: those affecting the connection channels and those directly affecting some variable values. This is the view taken in so-called dynamical causal models (DCM; Friston et al. 2000), in which uninterpreted state variables attached to each ROI are related by a system of differential equations (in the time). Variable values, some of them, are directly affected by experimentally controlled stimuli. Rate parameters are altered by the experimental environment, such as the experimenter's instructions to the subject, and so on.

The first and third pictures have champions. How different they are is unclear, as we shall see in the next section, where we consider the different inference problems they present, and some they share.

How Are Causal Relations to Be Discovered?

The eventual data for all causal models based on fMRI or other imaging methods are the statistical associations among the time-series variables. These consist of strengths of associations and conditional associations measured in various ways, most familiarly in Gaussian models of the probability distribution by correlations and partial correlations, or the corresponding regression and partial regression coefficients.

In dynamical causal models, the unknowns consist of rate parameters influenced in an unknown way by the experimental setting, and the changes in some variables' states produced by stimuli, and measured indirectly (via a model of the BOLD response with further parameters) by their fMRI signals. Fixed pathways are assumed, but may not all be active. With this cornucopia of parameters and the uncertainty of postulated fixed pathways, how is one to search, systematically and reliably, over their possible values? The standard answer is that for the critical parameters, and the fixed connections, little search is done; in our reading never more than half a dozen alternatives are considered. Each specification of fixed connections determines a directed graph, and conversely, there are four to the (N choose 2) power of the directed graphs on N variables. So either one must assume a lot about the fixed causal connections, or else one can consider only a very small number of variables. With the connections fixed, the result is a model of a kind that econometricians call unidentifiable, meaning that multiple vectors of parameters will produce the same likelihood for the data. The

DCM strategy is to put a prior probability distribution over each parameter (usually, a Gaussian distribution), and estimate a posterior distribution by a heuristic method, expectation maximization (EM). The result is a separate posterior probability associated with each fixed edge in the graph. (Just what it is the probability *of* is unclear to us.)

The EM procedure finds only "local" maxima, which means, first, that it does not actually compute posterior probabilities and, second, that for all one knows there is a different distribution of probabilities for parameter values that fits the data as well as or better than EM estimates. In particular, there are likely to be trade-offs between stimulus effects and context effects, since usually neither is independently measured with respect to the DCM model structure. With larger numbers of possible fixed connections, the uncertainties are, of course, much worse. A variety of other problems exist as well, but these are shared by structural equation models (SEMs), to which we turn next.

Structural equation models or SEMs, as we use the term, include all pseudo-indeterministic models in which the variables are deterministic functions of their parents in a directed graph and of unrecorded, independently distributed disturbance terms. Much of what follows generalizes to models that posit correlated disturbances and also to models of categorical variables that satisfy the Markov property but do not have disturbance terms. A SEM in our usage may be linear or nonlinear, additive or nonadditive, acyclic or cyclic, and have latent common causes or not.

A SEM model for fMRI data is in some ways like a simplified DCM model. Rather than representing context by unobserved parameters to be estimated that influence the rates at which influence is propagated, a SEM is *conditioned* on the context. The parameters in a SEM function relating X to a direct cause Y and to other direct causes of X are components of the partial derivative of X with respect to Y, holding all other variables constant. In the linear case, they represent the change in Y per unit change in X, when all other variables causing Y are held constant.

One way to search for SEM models is to try almost everything: Test every model on a set of variables against the data and select those alternatives with best fit. There are at least two problems. The first is that the distribution family for the variables is generally not known, and may be non-Gaussian. The second is that the number of graphs grows exponentially with the number of variables. The first problem is assuaged by simulation. Our, and others', extensive simulations with combinations of Gaussian and non-Gaussian variables, using Gaussian distribution theory (that is, a variation on the standard asymptotic chi-square test for Gaussian models), have found that exhaustive test procedures, though not error free, do surprisingly well. The computational problems are tractable for up to six variables. The search cannot be strictly exhaustive because some models are unidentifiable, for example, models in which X directly influences Y and, reciprocally, but there are no edges directed into X or Y. In such cases, no maximum likelihood estimate is available. Hanson and collaborators have

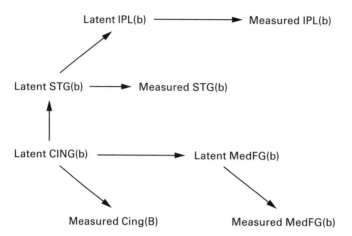

Figure 11.2
Oddball task (left graph), random motion of geometric stimuli (middle graph), and familiar action video ("making coffee," "putting a chair together," etc.). Note shared areas including medial frontal gyrus (MFG), superior temporal gyrus/sulcus (STG), and inferior parietal lobule (IPL). Anterior cingulate cortex (ACC) is specific to oddball task and -random motion task. The t values on each edge indicate the significance of the influence, and p values indicate the frequency of the edge in the top 1% of best fitting graphs. Middle temporal gyrus appears as a node in the familiar action video graph, perhaps involved in "schema" activation—that is, familiar action sequence episodes.

developed a variant voting method using exhaustive search. The method consists of the following steps: (1) Perform region location-clustering and clustering in individuals to maximize brain interactivity interpretation and to produce valid region identification and define NODEs, as discussed earlier. Then designate a common centroid as $\langle x \, y \, z \rangle$ for the NODE. (2) Determine time series per NODE. For fMRI, there are various (nonexhaustive) possibilities: (a) m by m by m smoothed voxels over time (reduced noise, increased signal consistency); (b) eigen-time series: performing Principal Components Analysis on V by V voxel space over time, producing an eigenvector over time for each NODE. (3) Compute covariance matrix over NODE constructed time series. (4) Fit covariance with all graphs and rank using the Akaike Information Criterion (AIC), p, or favorite goodness of fit method. Assuming the AIC distribution (for example) is single peaked and skewed, threshold the distribution at 1%, and use maximum likelihood voting to construct a composite graph representing the "most likely" best graph over the threshold sample.

We provide three examples of this method (see figure 11.2), first using an oddball task, during which subjects were fixating a central point on a display screen and were then asked to press a button if they saw a change in the stimulus ("circle" versus "face"), where the oddball stimulus occurred on 20% of trials. GLM was used to identify *t* peak areas in a visual oddball task, which identified four NODEs (we have subsequently done this with DMC and were able to identify one node as less reliable in cross validation) that then were submitted to the graph search method described earlier. The second paradigm is also a detection task, but one that is inherently more complex (though almost as simple), involving decisions based on category and similarity inclusion. Subjects are asked to watch a video of familiar everyday events ("assembling a chair," "making a bed," etc.), and then press a button when they detect an event change. Subjects readily perform this task and achieve high within-subject reproducibility (>0.9 correlation) and significant between-subject agreement, even though the subjects parse the video at different rates. We used two pre-scripted videos, one low-complexity sequence involving random motion of a geometric stimulus through a geometric set of objects ("geometric" video) and the other a higher-complexity sequence involving a student sitting in a room and studying ("study" video). Note shared areas, including medial frontal gyrus (MFG), superior temporal sulcus (STS), and inferior parietal lobule (IPL). ACC (anterior cingulate cortex) is specific to oddball task and random motion task. The *t* values on each edge indicates the significance of the influence and *p* value indicates the probability of the edge in the top 1% of best fitting graphs. Middle temporal gyrus appears as a node in the familiar action video graph, perhaps involved in "schema" activation—that is, familiar action sequence episodes.

What can be done when there are more variables? There are methods adopted from the social statistics literature, modification indices. The idea is to start with an arbitrary linear model—typically the empty model with a set of nodes and no connections—and then add whatever free parameter representing a directed edge is estimated (by a Lagrangian procedure) to most improve fit after a maximum likelihood estimate of the model with the newly added free parameter, continuing until fit can no longer be improved. Several methods from the machine learning literature are also available, some of which have been used for fMRI data. The oldest search algorithm for DAGs without latent common causes is the PC (for Peter [Spirtes] and Clark [Glymour]) algorithm. The PC algorithm uses a series of conditional independence tests to construct a class of alternative DAGs, all have the same conditional independence implications according to the Markov property—a Markov equivalence class. Some edges may be directed, indicating all DAGs in the Markov equivalence class share that direction for that edge; and some may be undirected, indicating that there are Markov equivalent graphs with different directions for the edge. A more conservative variant of the PC algorithm tends to direct fewer edges but in small- to medium-sized samples makes fewer errors. Another method, the greedy equivalence search (GES) is akin to modification index search, but with important differences. Rather than searching over DAGs, it searches over Markov equivalence classes of DAGs. And rather than scoring based on a fitting function and a maximum likelihood estimate, it adds edges using an approximation of a Bayesian posterior distribution, the Bayes information criterion (BIC). After a

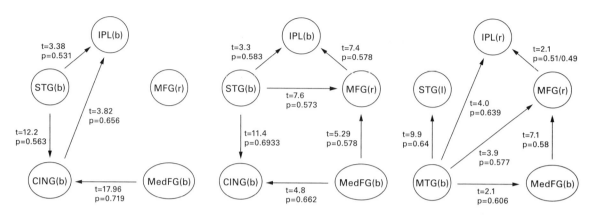

Figure 11.3
Latent structure model consistent with graph in figure 11.1.

forward search until no further improvement is obtained, it carries out a backward search, eliminating edges until improvement stops.

Finally, but not exhaustively, a new class of algorithms search for linear models, the LiNGAM procedures. Roughly, they work this way: Suppose the true model is linear with independent disturbances, at most one of which is Gaussian. The model can then be written equivalently (algebraically and statistically, not causally) so that each measured variable is a function only of disturbance terms—still with unspecified parameters. Independent components analysis then provides an algorithm that specifies each measured variable as a linear function, with specified parameter values, of the disturbance terms. Elimination of "insignificant" independencies and some matrix algebra yields a linear graphical model of the causal relations among the measured variables and estimated values of the linear coefficients for each directed edge. The output is a unique DAG, not a Markov equivalence class. Both the PC procedure and the LiNGAM procedure have been generalized to linear cyclic graphs, the latter more than a decade ago, but one still runs across claims that SEM methods cannot be applied to feedback systems.

What about latent variables? They are the events and processes we are trying to understand or that are only very indirectly measured by fMRI recordings of the BOLD response, but the methods we have just described assume otherwise. Can inferred causal relations among such measured variables be good proxies for causal relations among the neural activities? Not necessarily. For example, the sampling distribution of the measured variables fit by the first model of figure 11.2 could be explained by the latent variable model in figure 11.3 (as well as by several others). Note that there is no direct causal connection in the model between the latent variables for CING(b) and IPL(b). But an association will exist among the corresponding measured variables that is not removed by conditioning on any other measured variables. If the model of figure 11.1 were correct, then for midsize samples, even the exhaustive testing and voting procedure would add an edge between CING(b) and IPL(b). The same is true for all of the other search procedures we have described. The same problem arises for DCM models that actually fit the data.

There are three ways around this problem. One insufficient way is to use a (rather complex) elaboration of the PC algorithm, the fast causal inference (FCI) algorithm, which returns a class of alternative Markov equivalence classes for the measured variables, and specifies when an edge among measured variables is real, when it is due to an unobserved confounder or confounders, and when one cannot tell. The problem is that the procedure tells one nothing about the relations among the unmeasured variables, which is the real aim of inquiry. The same is true of a variant of the LiNGAM algorithm that tolerates latent confounding. A second strategy is to eliminate, in some principled way, edges that form triangles. A third way is to search over latent variable models directly. That involves the procedure known in fMRI work as *deconvolution*. We are only beginning to understand how to do that in such a way that deconvolution is sufficiently accurate to allow search over the latent ("deconvolved") variables. Few algorithmic investigations are more important to the ambition of understanding brain mechanisms from imaging data.

What about time? Functional MRI recordings are time series of records of processes that can begin as much as two seconds or more after the neural events of interest, and last up to eight seconds. How can one resolve time dependencies among neural events with such delayed measures? The DCM procedures estimate parameter values (or at least a probability distribution for them) as a function of time, subject to the liabilities we have discussed earlier. The SEM methods we have discussed in effect ignore time, treating the recordings at various time intervals as independent sample cases, which they often are not. Sometimes it may be best to treat them so nonetheless, but if one wishes to use the time dependencies and understand them, how can that be done? A fashionable method is Granger's, which amounts to positing that X causes Y directly, if the next recording of Y is better predicted (e.g., by least squares regression) by adding preceding values of X to preceding values of all other variables, including Y. The method has two difficulties, aside from the fact, already considered, that the causal process to be understood relates unobserved variables. First, X can Z only by causing Y, which causes Z, but Granger's method will not find the mediation by Y, merely that X causes Y and X causes Z and Y causes Z. (Spurious triangles again!). A remedy is to regress each variable at each time on all other variables, including itself for some number of lags (plausibly one or two lags from fMRI work) and compute the residual values of the variables at each time after subtracting the regression estimates of their values from the recorded values. Then, any of the machine learning algorithms discussed previously can be applied to the residuals (Dimiralp and Hoover 2003).

A second difficulty is that BOLD response delays vary among brain tissues. One solution is to shift the recordings of some variables with respect to others for two to four seconds, and see whether better models are obtained with shifted data. In our experience, shifting one variable at a time does not work well, but shifting all variables in all combinations is computationally impossible except for a small number of variables. A reasonable compromise is to shift all sets of three, or at most four variables (depending on how many there are).

A final problem (for this discussion) is that experiments typically have multiple subjects, and the sets of ROIs extracted from the several subjects may not be identical. Typically, in our experience, unless the ROI generation procedure forces things otherwise, subjects will share some but not all ROIs. That problem can be addressed in exhaustive search by voting procedures, as discussed previously—perhaps weighted by sample sizes when those vary. It can also be solved by iterative search procedures, such as GES, by scoring a model modification separately on each data set and averaging the scores. The same can be done with algorithms such as PC by deciding each combination of conditional independence relations using a function of the p values on each separate data set, although in our preliminary studies this has not worked very well. For DCM, the solution would appear to be to average the posterior probabilities for the parameters over the estimates from the several subjects or to use a hierarchical Bayesian model.

How Can We Evaluate Model Specification Procedures?

One of the most important ways of evaluating model specification procedures, almost never considered in the fMRI literature, is to prove asymptotic correctness of the procedure under explicit general assumptions—which will seldom be strictly true for empirical data. Such proofs exist for the PC algorithm, the FCI algorithm, and their conservative versions, and for the GES algorithm. No proof is available for the LiNGAM procedures, but they should be consistent if the assumptions noted earlier hold and the sampling is identically, independently distributed (i.i.d.). No proof is available for the exhaustive test procedure, but for Gaussian data it is plausible that the procedure converges to a set of statistically indistinguishable models in the large sample limit. No such proof is available for DCM, even assuming that the fixed connections are correctly specified. The modification indices procedure is provably inconsistent, giving the wrong output no matter how large the sample size for simple cases involving as few as three or four variables.

Frequentist statisticians like confidence intervals. It has been shown that no confidence intervals are possible for PC or for similar estimators of causal effects. But they are possible for the conservative version of PC, although no practical procedure is available for computing them.

Another important way to test search procedures is on simulated data, but simulations can be tricky. Misrepresentation of the actual relations between measured variables and unmeasured causal processes of interest can lead to wildly misleading assessments of the accuracy and informativeness of model search procedures, and though models of the BOLD response and the noise in fMRI measurements exist, there are significant uncertainties. So, too, can the omission of backprojections be misleading.

Still another possibility is independent confirmation of methods by more invasive measurements on animals. Such comparisons are unlikely to be available for nonvisual tasks. For the time being, it may be more helpful to compare complex output from searches with previously well-established human processing features; for example, we would expect (in right-handed subjects) that verbal tasks visually presented would first activate the left occipital and then feed forward to left hemisphere areas, and thence to right hemisphere areas. Elsewhere, we report just such results.

Besides verbal tasks, five classes of tasks allow exploration of the diversity of graph structures and how they may recruit similar brain structures. First, we identify a series of tasks that can potentially provide some clues about the validity and usefulness of graph modeling in this domain. For example, one could use simple *motor tasks* involving finger tapping, reaching or grasping for target objects, *oddball/detection tasks*, with geometric and familiar objects (which should preserve graph structure implicated in detection but not in terms of recognition as target changes), *working memory tasks* involving *n*-back tasks varying target classes and similarity, *object recognition tasks*, focusing mainly on face recognition networks, and finally *event perception tasks* involving familiar action sequences that tend to invoke action/social/mirror networks.

Each task can be arranged to consist of the same target experiments where specific objects (e.g., "cups") might be manipulated or identified or recognized or interacted with in some way, thus controlling for task content across similar tasks (e.g., oddball task versus event perception task). We are particularly interested in the types of subnetwork or constituent nodes that appear as common to all such tasks and others that appear to be uniquely associated with a given task or aspect of the task. We discuss specific cognitive function–graph mapping hypotheses further in research focus plans. The identification and decomposition of cognitive tasks that have well-correlated neural circuitry of the kind we consider here is an ongoing research task. Research groups that are just now identifying sets of regions that appear to be constituents of a particular functional account will provide "sensitivity" analysis of graphs produced by the various methods we will be testing. It is possible to develop theories to refine model specification and testing with specific testable hypotheses concerning node presence and edge orientation.

First-order predictions in terms of normative neuroimaging analysis often involve the presence or absence of a node. In terms of graphical analysis, since graphs consist of subgraphs and nodes, we will investigate the stability and reproducibility of graphs by examining node extraction (clustering: Hanson et al. 2007) and validation using classifier methodology to identify cross-validation nodes for clustering verification. In particular, it is critical to develop new methods to

- detect outlier graphs;
- extract models of graphs that may well represent homogeneous subgroup of a given population;
- validate cluster method in "node" detection and determine the nature of individual variability across nodes;validate classifier methods in "node" detection and determine the nature of individual variability across nodes;
- test stability of input to cluster methods based on different classifier methods and GLM;
- test variation in time series distance measures;
- use tasks to construct graphs for contrast and comparison; andtest graph differences across different populations, across sessions and variations.

One can also test the sensitivity of the method as a function of the structural equation method. In terms of validation of this general graph method, it is important to focus on the cumulative cross-validation methods discussed next.

Across task variations there are several possible outcomes. If, as is apparently accepted in present neuroimaging theory, nodes represent factorable functional brain areas, then small variations in a task (target category change in oddball task, or in working memory task) should modulate edges between nodes but not nodes primarily. If, on the other hand, constituent function is distributed over nodes, then even small changes in a task should cause variations in both nodes and edges. To the extent it is possible to validate nodes across subjects, we should be able to detect local changes in graphs versus "catastrophic" changes that alter the complete graph structure as well as the underlying constituents. Logically, one can expect (at least) *four* kinds of outcomes, which are shown in figure 11.4. First, a task manipulation could produce no change (in a cross-validation sense) to the graph, in that the perturbed task graph is statistically identical to the initial task graph.

A second outcome is that the task change is isolated to the edges, while the nodes are statistically stable, suggesting that the underlying constituent is factorable, that is, it could be removed by subtraction in some meaningful sense (assuming additivity).

A third outcome is that the task change adds nodes while leaving the original graph, now effectively a subgraph of the larger structure, implying that the task itself is statistically identifiable by the original graph. (A similar outcome to 3, we term 3a, would be that the graph loses nodes and hence still consists of a smaller subgraph of the original task graph, suggesting a possible contraction of the complexity.)

Graph structure hypotheses as a function
of task significant task manipulation

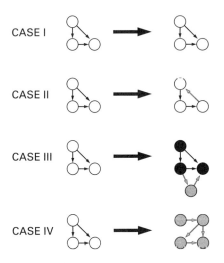

CASE I

CASE II

CASE III

CASE IV

Figure 11.4
Logical cases for outcomes in graphical analysis during perturbation of cognitive tasks.

A fourth outcome is that the task change produces a more radical reorganization that changes all nodes and therefore edge values; essentially the task change produces an entirely new graph. This outcome is obviously the most radical change that might occur from a task variation and, therefore, would represent a type of null hypothesis to test other potential outcomes against. As pointed out in the beginning of this chapter, any graph stability must be established by repeatable node estimation and extraction and between-subject cross-validation. In this way, one can establish a framework to begin looking at task/cognitive function mapping to graph structure (in contrast to the standard practice of producing a single estimated graph as a final output).

A second class of tests involves perturbation manipulations, where a single task, such as object recognition or oddball task, is changed more radically to see what the effects on a previously estimated stable graph might be. For example, one could use an object recognition task (e.g., flanker task) where subjects are asked to determine which of two flanking stimuli match the center target stimulus (say, in the case of three faces). As we vary the similarity of the target face to nonmatching stimuli random objects (cars, flowers, shoes, etc.), we might expect a relatively large change in the graph structure in terms of detected nodes or edges. These types of variations would further test the stability of the graph structure and its sensitivity to potentially large-scale challenges or reorganizations and further help us define the nature of brain interactivity of cognitive function.

Conclusion

We have described some, but not all, of the potential problems in extracting correct causal information from fMRI data, and some possible solutions. This chapter represents our understanding when written, more than a year ago. Since then, we have implemented and applied combinations of the automated search strategies described here to develop independently justifiable models of data on verbal judgments and of data on risk aversion. We have not described still more ambitious possibilities. For example, rather than clustering comparatively small fractions of the total collection of voxels into a few regions of interest, partial graphical causal models could in principle be obtained by running a sufficiently fast algorithm, such as PC, on the entire voxel set of a brain scan. Analysis of the resulting graphical network properties, and their changes with tasks, might identify functional areas and pathways critical for a task or type of task. We believe it is past time for the statistical methodology of search to catch up with the data.

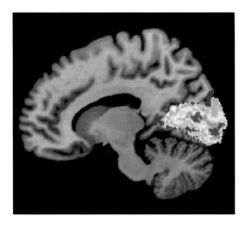

Plate 1 (figure 2.1)

Aligning V1. A sagittal slice of the MNI template brain (x = +12) overlaid with the probability map for the location of V1, determined posthumously from the cytoarchitecture of ten individuals. Color scale shows number of brains in which V1 occupies each position, from blue − 1 subject to red − 10 subjects. From Wohlschlager et al. (2005).

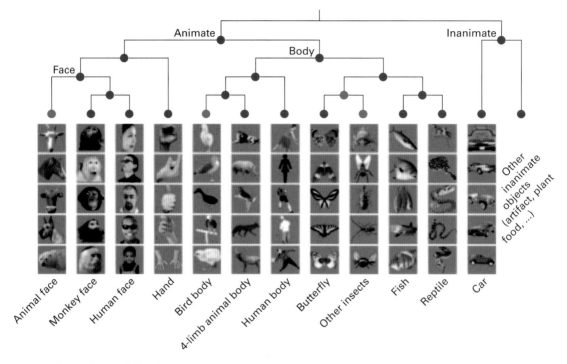

Plate 2 (figure 5.2)

Similarity structure of population responses measured in monkey IT during viewing of a wide variety of images of faces, animals, and objects (from Kiani et al. 2007). Similarity was indexed as $1 - r$, where r is the correlation between the pattern of response strengths across IT neurons. Results are displayed as a dendrogram produced with hierarchical clustering.

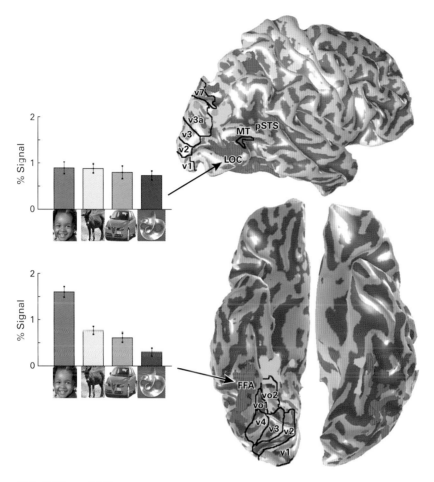

Plate 3 (figure 14.1)

Object-selective regions in the human brain. Object-, face-, and place-selective regions on a partially inflated brain of one representative subject shown from lateral and ventral views. Superposition of three contrasts thresholded at $p < 0.0001$. Red: faces > nonface objects. Green: places > nonface objects. Blue: nonface objects > scrambled. Pink and dark green indicate overlapping regions. Pink: face > objects and objects > scrambled. Dark green: places > objects and objects > scrambled. Boundaries of known visual areas are shown in black on the right hemisphere. LOC includes a constellation of object-selective regions (blue and pink regions) in lateral and ventral occipital cortex. The posterior region adjacent to MT is typically labeled LO and the ventral region is labeled pFUS/OTS. Face-selective regions include the FFA, a face-selective region in the fusiform gyrus; the pSTS, a face-selective region in posterior superior temporal sulcus and a region in LOC (shown here in pink and sometimes referred to as the OFA). MT: motion-selective region in the posterior ITS. Mean percentage signal from LOC (excluding regions that respond more to faces than objects) and FFA averaged across ten subjects relative to a scrambled baseline. Stimuli are indicated by icons and include faces, four-legged mammals, cars, and abstract sculptures. Note that object-selective regions respond to both objects and faces more than scrambled images, but they do not respond more strongly to faces than to objects.

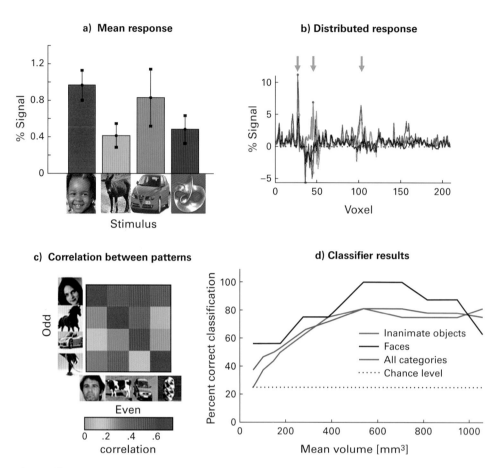

Plate 4 (figure 14.4)

Pattern analysis of distributed fMRI responses. (a) Mean LOC response to different object categories relative to a scrambled baseline, from one subject. Error bars indicate SEM across eight blocks
of a condition. (b) Distributed response across LOC voxels, same data as on the left; x-axis: voxel
number; y-axis: percent signal relative to scrambled. Each category elicits a different pattern of response across the LOC. Arrows indicate some voxels which have strong differential responses to
different stimuli. Adapted from Grill-Spector et al. 2006b. (c) Correlation analysis of patterns of
distributed responses. One way to examine information in the distributed response is to compare
the pattern of responses to the same and different stimuli across split halves of the data. In this
example, the pattern of response from one subject to different faces, animals, cars, and sculptures
was measured. This response was measured separately across odd and even runs that used different
images. The diagonal of the correlation matrix shows the reproducibility of the data across independent measurements. The off diagonal measurements depict the distinctiveness of the patterns.
When the on-diagonal values are higher than the off-diagonal values, it suggests that the distributed activations to different stimuli are both reproducible and distinct. (d) Results of a winner-
take-all classifier on determining which category the subject viewed based on the highest correlation between even and odd runs. Classifier performance is averaged across five subjects from their
standard-resolution LOC data and is shown as a function of the number of voxels selected from
the ROI.

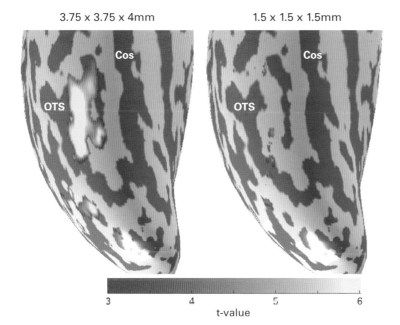

3.75 x 3.75 x 4mm   1.5 x 1.5 x 1.5mm

Cos   Cos

OTS   OTS

3   4   5   6

t-value

Plate 5 (figure 14.5)

Standard- and high-resolution fMRI of face-selective regions in the fusiform gyrus. (a) SR-fMRI (3.75 × 3.75 × 4 mm) and (b) HR-fMRI (1.5 × 1.5 × 1.5 mm) of face-selective activations in the same individual. GLM analysis shows higher activations to faces than to objects, $p < 0.002$, $t = 3$, voxel level, for the same subject at two imaging resolutions. Maps are projected onto the inflated cortical surface, zoomed on the fusiform gyrus. HR-fMRI shows more localized and patchy face-selective activations in the fusiform gyrus than SR-fMRI. Cos, collateral sulcus; OTS, occipito-temporal sulcus.

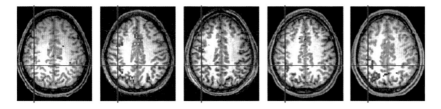

Plate 6 (figure 15.1)

Five individual SPM maps from five subjects performing a computation task compared to a language task. The activity is not always present at the same position in Talairach space. Intensity of activation (threshold: $z = 3$) is also different across subjects.

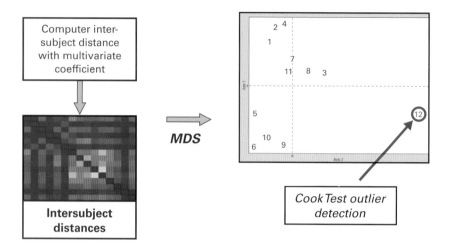

Plate 7 (figure 15.4)

The Distance toolbox principle. It allows for a rapid evaluation of the group functional pattern homogeneity. Models with nonparametric statistics are more sensitive.

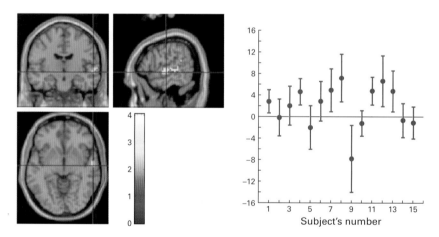

Plate 8 (figure 15.5)

The effect size and intrasubject estimated variability in the temporal lobe responding to language stimulation. In this specific situation, the mixed effect model downweights the measure of the subject with the smallest effect and therefore yields a more sensitive statistic than the random effect model.

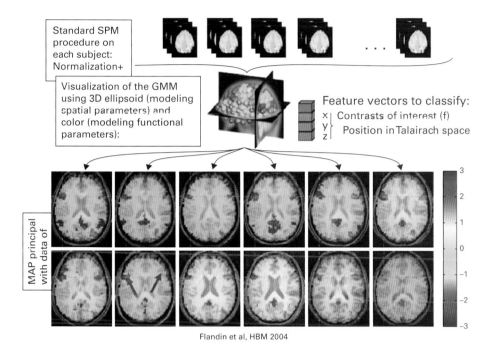

Flandin et al, HBM 2004

Plate 9 (figure 15.6)
Scheme of the Gaussian mixture model parcellation. Notice that the red parcel is not exactly identical across subjects, and may not even be present in outlier subjects (e.g., last subject on bottom row).

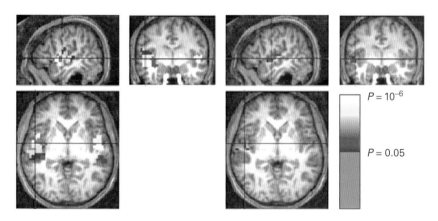

$P = 10^{-6}$

$P = 0.05$

Plate 10 (figure 15.7)
(Left) Random effect analysis using rerandomization and parcellation technique. (Right) Standard analysis. The gain in sensitivity (with controlled risk of error corrected 5%) is due to adaptation of the parcels to individual subject activity.

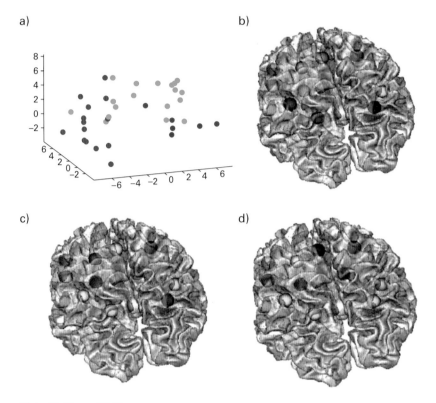

Plate 11 (figure 15.8)

Functional landmarks based on a reproducibility measure. Those landmarks do not have the same intensity of activity across subjects, and the group could be divided into three subgroups (shown with a multidimensional scaling in panel a in blue, green, and red). Panels (b), (c), and (d) show the average intensity of the landmarks for the three groups.

III Design and the Signal

12 Resting-State Brain Connectivity

Bharat Biswall

Systematic, spontaneous low-frequency signal fluctuations (SLFs) have been observed in a number of research laboratories using different imaging modalities and species. These low-frequency signals appear to fluctuate synchronously between functionally related brain regions. Since the discovery of this "resting-state connectivity" (RSC) (Biswal and Hyde 1997), several groups have explored its characteristics in sensori-motor, auditory, visual, and association cortex. RSC differences between Alzheimer's patients, multiple sclerosis (MS) patients, schizophrenics, attention deficit–hyperactivity disordered children and their respective controls have also been characterized. The meaning of these differences, however, remains unclear for a number of reasons.

First, the biophysical basis of SLFs is still poorly understood. On one hand, data obtained in animal models using cytochrome oxidase optical imaging suggest a neural basis for SLF. On the other hand, laser-Doppler flowmetry suggests a vascular basis, specifically a dominant role for red blood cell perfusion in the SLF mechanism. Second, the anatomical basis remains poorly understood. Studies showing increased RSC in MS patients have implicated white matter as the RSC substrate, but the possibility of MS-related vascular changes renders this evidence inconclusive. Moreover, it is unknown whether RSC originates from a single source (e.g., basal ganglia) or from multiple sources (e.g., within local networks). Does RSC vary with characteristics of local vasculature? Little evidence as yet exists to answer these questions. Third, relationships between RSC and functional activity have not been studied in depth. What is the functional relevance of RSC? Some evidence suggests that it represents cellular maintenance of an optimum balance between blood flow and cerebral metabolic rate (a biophysical origin hypothesis). Other evidence suggests that it represents "default mode" of information processing, in which systems are collecting and analyzing internal and external stimuli (a cognitive origin hypothesis). What are the developmental characteristics of RSC? Some work has been done using healthy elderly and healthy children as controls in clinical studies but lifespan data on RSC are practically nonexistent. Finally, little work has yet been done to explore the clinical relevance of RSC. How is RSC affected by disease? Answering this question could contribute to our basic understanding of RSC, but could also establish its clinical relevance in diagnosis. In summary, a basic understanding of the functional and clinical relevance of RSC would help us understand basic properties of brain function and could be clinically useful as well.

In this chapter, we discuss the biophysical mechanisms of SLF and RSC, their anatomic origins, and functional relevance. The studies described here will (a) establish the biophysical basis of SLF and RSC, (b) characterize relationships between SLFs arising at metabolic (neural) and hemodynamic (vascular) levels using multiple imaging modalities in animals and humans, (c) decipher properties of SLFs during perturbed physiological conditions and anesthetic levels, (d) lead to development of processing strategies for analyzing and quantifying RSC within and between brain regions, (e) lead to improved understanding of relationships between RSC and functional activity, and (f) examine how these relationships develop, how they change with age, and how they are affected by childhood- aging-related disease.

Background

Functional Magnetic Resonance Imaging

Functional magnetic resonance imaging (fMRI) (Bandettini et al. 1992; Belliveau et al. 1991) has permitted measurement of local changes in cerebral blood volume, flow, and oxygenation within localized cortical areas of the brain in response to task activation. Neuronal activity leads to local vasodilation, with concomitant increase in blood flow and in the ratio of oxyhemoglobin to deoxyhemoglobin that results in an increase in fMRI signal intensity (Ogawa et al. 1992). Functional MRI is currently being used extensively to characterize and map sensory, motor, and cognitive function in healthy subjects as well as patients. The general approach is to present the subject with a task and look for changes relative to a resting or baseline control state.

In all the studies described here, echoplanar imaging (EPI) was used. We have been able to acquire echoplanar images as rapidly as sixty-four per second in a single slice or from the entire brain at about four per second. The time course of signal intensity in a given voxel typically varies by about 5% about the mean during task activation and 1% during rest. A Fourier transform of a representative resting-state voxel time course shows peaks at the heart and respiratory frequencies. Peaks are also seen at the harmonics of the heart rate and the respiration rate. In addition, low-frequency physiological fluctuations, which are the subject of this proposal, are observed (Biswal et al. 1995).

FMRI has great potential for studying human brain function because of its noninvasiveness, and superior temporal and spatial resolution. In addition to experimental protocols made possible by the absence of ionizing radiation, fMRI has several technical advantages:

• Using a 3T scanner, a spatial resolution of $3.75 \times 3.75 \times 7$ mm in fMRI is obtained with images acquired from the entire brain every second. Higher resolution of $1 \times 1 \times 4$ mm can be obtained by sacrificing coverage or increasing the scan time. Spatial resolution is enhanced with use of higher-field-strength magnets such as 3T because of the increase in signal-to-noise ratio (SNR). For example, the spatial resolution of images (being acquired with a TR of 250 msec and spatial resolution of 1×1 mm) can be traded for a better temporal resolution (images with TR = 50 msec, and spatial resolution of 3.75×3.75 mm).

• The temporal resolution of fMRI is close to a second. Further, by decreasing the area of coverage and using partial k-space, sixty-four images per second can be acquired. This would allow one to sample most of the physiological fluctuations, including the cardiac and the respiration frequency, at a rate faster than the Nyquist rate.

• MRI anatomical images are obtained together with functional imaging data sets, providing excellent registration of functional data sets with high-resolution data sets of brain anatomy.

Spontaneous Low-Frequency Physioloqical Fluctuations

RSC may be defined as significant correlated signal between functionally related brain regions in the absence of any stimulus or task. This correlated signal arises from SLFs. These fluctuations were first observed by Davies and Bronk (1957) in cerebral oxygen availability using polarographic techniques. These low-frequency spontaneous fluctuations have also been observed by several investigators using animal models and a variety of measurement techniques, including laser-Doppler flowmetry (LDF) (Hudetz et al. 1992), fluororeflectometry of NADH and cytochrome aa$_3$ (Vern et al. 1998), and polarographic measurement of brain tissue PO$_2$ with microelectrodes. These fluctuations appear to be independent of cardiac and respiratory fluctuations and hence are termed "spontaneous."

Biophysical Origin Hypotheses of RSC

Testing hypotheses of the role of SLFs has involved attempts to determine their physiological origins. Cooper et al. (1966) hypothesized that these fluctuations represent cellular maintenance of an optimum balance between blood flow and cerebral metabolic rate. Testing this hypothesis has involved manipulating cerebral metabolism with anesthesia. These studies have compared activity during waking and anesthetized states in animals using various techniques including LDF (Hudetz et al. 1992) and fMRI in humans (Biswal et al. 1993; Weisskoff et al. 1993). Signal oscillations in the rodent brain vary with levels of halothane anesthesia, PCO$_2$, and nitric oxide synthase blockade LDF (Hudetz et al. 1992). These results suggest support for the biophysical origin hypothesis that affects the neural vasculature. The neural mechanisms of slow rhythmic fluctuations have not yet been clearly defined, though studies indicate they may be both neuronal and glial in origin (Zonta et al. 2003).

In spectrophotometric studies of the intramitochondrial redox state of enzyme cytochrome aa₃ (CYT) and cerebral blood volume (CBV), continuous slow oscillations and interhemispheric synchrony has been observed between these variables (Vern et al. 1998). The relationship between CYT and CBV oscillations seems to be independent of the physiological state as they have been observed during both awake state and sleep (Vern et al. 1988, 1997b, 1998), anesthesia (Dora and Kovach 1982; Hudetz et al. 1992), and cerebral ischemia (Golanov et al. 1994; Mayevsky and Ziv 1997). Though some studies have indicated the presence of metabolic oscillations in the absence of CBF oscillations (suggesting metabolic oscillations may be primary in origin), there is no concrete evidence for this. On the contrary, flow oscillations can be linked to metabolic oscillations in the presence of evidence that NADH and cytochrome aa₃ oscillations lagged behind CBV oscillations (Vern et al. 1997b, 1998). These results indicate that spontaneous oscillations in the intramitochondrial redox state may be at least in part linked to a rhythmic variation in oxygen consumption of the tissue.

It should be emphasized that the origin of the slow cerebral fluctuations of CBV and CYTox remains to be determined. It is unlikely to be entirely vascular (vasomotion), in view of the complex frequency/time and interhemispheric architecture of these fluctuations in cats and rabbits (Vern et al. 1997b, 1998). A variety of neuronal, glial, and vascular phenomena may contribute to what finally appears as a measurable "fluctuation" (Berridge and Rapp 1979). For instance, glutamate-induced intracellular calcium waves within the glial syncytium may represent an energy-dependent indirect reflection of activity within focal neuronal fields. Such factors would need to be carefully dissected by future efforts. An interesting example of such multifactorial components of the slow fluctuations emerges from the study of CBV and CYTox during the transition from slow-wave sleep to REM sleep in the cat, as discussed in the following sections.

Cognitive Origin Hypotheses of RSC

In contrast to biophysical origin hypotheses, others have proposed cognitive origin hypotheses based on observations that low-frequency signal fluctuations appear to correlate between functionally connected brain areas (e.g., Biswal and Hyde 1997b). Testing these hypotheses has involved observation of resting-state activity between functionally connected regions, and contrasts between RSC and task-induced activity in these regions.

We first demonstrated a significant temporal correlation of SLFs, both within and across hemispheres in primary sensorimotor cortex during rest; 74% of the time series from these voxels correlated significantly (after filtering the fundamental and harmonics of respiration and heart rates) weas only a few voxel time courses ($<3\%$) correlated with those in regions outside of motor cortex. Subsequently, Hampson et al. (2002) demonstrated the presence of RSC in sensory cortices, specifically auditory and visual cortex. In their studies, signal from visual cortex voxels during rest (first scan) was used as a reference and correlated with every other voxel in the brain. A significant number of voxels from the visual cortex passed a threshold of 0.35, but only a few voxels from outside the visual cortex passed the threshold. The researchers have demonstrated similar results in the auditory cortex (Hampson et al. 2004).

Lowe et al. (1997a) extended Biswal and Hyde's (1997) results by showing such correlations over larger regions of sensorimotor cortex (i.e., across multiple slices). Xiong, Fox, and colleagues (1998, 1999) established relationships between motor and association cortex. As in earlier studies, they observed RSC between sensorimotor cortex areas (primary, premotor, secondary somatosensory). Further, however, they observed RSC relationships between these motor areas and association areas, specifically anterior and posterior cingulate cortex, regions known to be involved in attention. Greicius et al. (2004) observed RSC in anterior and posterior cingulate areas. Subsequent observation of activation during a visual attention task indicated similar cingulate activity.

These studies have established the foundation for "resting-state functional connectivity studies" using FMRI (e.g., Biswal et al. 1995; Greicius et al. 2004; Gusnard and Raichle 2001; Hampson et al. 2002; Lowe et al. 1997). Results from these studies form the basis for speculation regarding the functional role of RSC. Bressler (1996) has suggested that such correlated signal fluctuations may represent the functional connection of cortical areas analogous to the phenomenon of "effective connectivity" defined by Friston et al. (1993). Thus, a family of cognitive origin hypotheses (in contrast to biophysical origin hypotheses) has emerged. Gusnard and Raichle (2001), for instance, suggested that such coherence indicates the presence of a "default mode of brain function" in which a default network continuously monitors external (e.g., visual stimuli) and internal (e.g., body functions, emotions) stimuli. Other cognitive origin hypotheses suggest that low-frequency fluctuation is related to ongoing problem-solving and planning (Greicius et al., 2004). Biswal, Hyde, and colleagues (1995) and Xiong, Fox, and colleagues (1998, 1999) observed that analyses of resting-state physiological fluctuations reveal many more functional connections than those revealed by task-induced activation analysis. They hypothesized that task-induced activation maps underestimate the size and number of functionally connected areas and that RSC analysis more fully reveals functional networks.

Comparisons of RSC and Task-Induced Activity

Skudlarski and Gore (1998) compared RSC and signal fluctuations in olfactory cortex during three sustained passive stimuli: a pleasant odor, an unpleasant odor, and no odor. They reported that the presentation of odor altered the strength of correlation in some regions, compared to rest. Biswal and Hyde (1998) studied low-frequency physiological fluctuations in the motor cortex during a sustained six-minute period of bilateral finger tapping. In all four subjects, the frequency and phase of low-frequency fluctuations were similar. The magnitude of the low-frequency fluctuations, however, was significantly enhanced during continuous finger tapping. In addition, RSC maps produced by correlation of low-frequency fluctuations between motor-cortex voxels had an improved coincidence with task-activation maps compared to the RSC. These results suggest that attention to a prolonged task spontaneously fluctuates and that RSC is modulated by attention. These three studies involved a sustained active task, a sustained change in environment, or a sustained task that was repeated twice with different instructions. Numerous other variants and extensions of these ideas are immediately apparent. However, in each case one is comparing differences between small effects. There is a significant challenge to improve experimental methodologies for these kinds of experiments.

We have carried out a study to test the reliability of resting-state functional connectivity maps in fMRI using test-retest analysis. Five resting-state data sets were collected from each subject in addition to bilateral finger tapping to activate the sensorimotor cortex. The reliability of the resting-state data sets was obtained using different measures: (1) *voxel precision:* the ratio of the number of specific activated sensorimotor voxels that passed the threshold in each of the five rest scans to the number that passed the threshold in at least one of the five rest scans; (2) *first-order precision;* and (3) *second-order precision*: the numerator of the above ratio is modified to include voxels that passed the threshold in four out of five rest scans and three out of five rest scan. It was observed in all subjects that all five resting-state functional connectivity maps of sensorimotor cortex had substantial overlap with the corresponding bilateral finger tapping task. It was seen that, though the voxel precision was about 60%, the first-order and second-order precision were about 70%, and 80%, respectively. This suggests that, while variability between the resting-state functional connectivity maps exists, most of it can be accounted by simply taking into account the neighboring voxels.

Voxel time-course intensities from the sensorimotor cortex increased by about 5% during finger tapping, and the same voxel time-courses during rest varied by 1% (Biswal et al. 1996). A significant correlation was obtained between the percent change in signal in an activated voxel from sensorimotor and the percent signal change during rest in the corresponding voxels. Average regression coefficients of about 0.55 were seen. These results show that the percent increase in voxel activation during task is inherently correlated with underlying low-frequency physiological fluctuations.

Finally, Lowe et al. (1997a) sought to examine the role of attention in RSC. They compared correlations during rest and during stimulation in three subjects. Following the rest scan, subjects were presented with sequences of tones and circular symbols.

The sequences of tone and symbol presentation were randomly out of phase with each other. Attention was manipulated by requiring subjects in one condition to press a button when the auditory tone was heard and when the symbol appeared in another condition.

The researchers reasoned that, since all stimuli and responses were identical between the two scans, any change in correlation between motor, visual, and auditory regions across the two scans should be due to the effects of attention on neuronal connectivity. They observed slight increases in intraregional correlations during task performance. Specifically, correlations between visual cortex voxels was increased, compared to rest and to auditory-task performance, while subjects attended to symbols. Similarly, correlations between auditory cortex voxels was increased, compared to rest and to visual-task performance, while subjects attended to tones.

The results of the studies presented here suggest intriguing clues about the relationship between RSC, functional activity, and the role of attention in mediating these relationships. Thus, Gusnard and Raichle (2001), for instance, have argued that the set of brain regions showing correlated activity at rest (the "default" network) continuously monitors external (e.g., visual stimuli) and internal (e.g., body functions, emotions) stimuli. On the basis of similar observations, and apparent hippocampal involvement, Greicius et al. (2004) have argued that RSC may be related to episodic memory retrieval in the service of ongoing problem-solving and planning. Moreover, such activity may be suppressed or "suspended" (Gusnard and Raichle 2001) under conditions of demanding cognitive activity. Such accounts are intriguing because they suggest presumed baseline activity may not be as random as has been nearly universally presumed. Others have argued that RSC represents the tonic activation of networks that are brought "on line" during cognitive task performance. All of these hypotheses suggest that meaningful functional activity may be occurring during rest. Understanding the mechanisms and the functional and clinical relevance of such activity may have profound effects on our understanding of functional neuroimaging results, leading to explanations, for instance, of many poorly understood phenomena including the to-date inexplicable "negative activation" results that have bedeviled neuroimaging research.

Further, understanding RSC activation relationships could lead to plausible accounts for patterns of age-related differences in BOLD activity as well (e.g., Cabeza 2001; Grady et al. 1995; Rympa and D'Esposito 2000; Rypma et al. 2001, 2005), because older adults often show greater activation than younger adults. Cognitive accounts of this phenomenon, such as "age-related compensation," have been unsatisfactory thus far because age-related activation increases have not been consistently related to performance improvements in older adults (e.g., Grady et al. 1995; Rypma et al. 2001). The idea that such age-related activation increases are related to an RSC network that must be inhibited for successful task performance is compelling because older adults are known to have deficits in inhibitory functions at the cellular (i.e., neuronal), structural (i.e., glial), and cognitive (i.e., behavioral) levels (Hasher et al. 1991). Greicius et al. (2004), however, have observed decreased hippocampal involvement in comparisons between older healthy individuals and those with Alzheimer's disease. No studies to date have directly compared RSC between younger and older adults.

Few studies to date, however, have explicitly examined relationships between resting-state connectivity, functional connectivity, and BOLD activity. One aim of the current proposal is to take this step forward. We plan to use such comparisons to investigate RSC-activation relationships, how they develop and change with age, and how they are altered by disease.

Effective-State Connectivity (ESC) Results from Interactions between Brain Regions during Task Performance

ESC may be defined as the influence that one region or system exerts over another during task performance (Buchel 2004; Friston et al. 1993). ESC may be modeled with a number of functions (e.g., linear or quadratic) to characterize the nature of interactions between brain regions (usually specified a priori or on the basis of "level-1," traditional massive univariate analysis). ESC models reflect the hemodynamic change in a given voxel or region as the weighted sum of changes in other regions. More complex structural equation models reflect the relationships between regions by minimizing the least-squared difference between an observed covariance structure and the structure of a theoretical model. The necessary multimodal imaging work has not yet been done to determine the neural substrate of effective connectivity. It is presumed to reflect propagating neurotransmission between brain regions via white matter tracts.

ESC Reveals Functional Activity between Regions Showing RSC

Biswal and his colleagues (1997abcd) have shown that (1) BOLD signal is more sensitive to RSC than flow-based signal implicating a neural basis for RSC and (2) motor regions evincing RSC show increased BOLD activity during finger tap performance. Biswal and Hyde, for instance, studied physiological fluctuations in the motor cortex during rest and during a sustained six-minute period of bilateral finger tapping. They observed that the magnitude of low-frequency physiological fluctuations observed at rest were enhanced during continuous finger tapping. In addition, maps of these motor cortex–based low-frequency fluctuations had significantly greater coincidence with task-activation maps than those in other brain regions. These results suggest that functionally active networks are chronically active at rest. Recently, Xiong et al. (1999) have hypothesized that ESC represents a subset of the RSC network. Analyzing the sensorimotor cortex, they found a number of additional regions, including premotor, to be connected that are not typically connected during bilateral finger tapping.

Task-related patterns of BOLD activity may represent acute activation of the circuits necessary for the task at hand. Such circuitry may be revealed in ESC analysis models advanced by a number of researchers (e.g., Buchel and Friston 2000; Goebel et al. 2003; McIntosh et al. 1996). ESC analyses have revealed interconnections between brain regions known to be active during cognitive task performance. In one working memory (WV) study for instance, McIntosh and colleagues (e.g., 1999) have observed increases in interactions among PFC regions and between Prefrontal Cortex (PFC) and cortico-limbic regions with increasing delay intervals. ESC studies comparing younger and older adults have indicated that older adults show increased ESC during cognitive task performance. Their results indicated that, whereas younger adults showed hippo-campal interactions with ventral PFC, during memory encoding, older adults show hippocampal interactions with both dorsal and ventral, as well as parietal interactions. At present, the meaning of this age- and disease-related increased ESC remains poorly understood. The best evidence suggests that it may reflect either (1) compensatory activity in the service of optimizing memory performance (Grady et al. 1995) or (2) a decreased inhibition of the "default mode," as Greicius et al. (2004) have suggested. Little leverage may be gained on these questions because the results come from different groups of subjects performing different tasks. In the studies proposed here, we compare RSC and ESC within the same subjects performing similar kinds of cognitive tasks.

In recent years interest has been renewed in low-frequency spontaneous fluctuations. Using a variety of neuroimaging methodologies in animals (e.g., LDF, reflectance oximetry, fMRI), studies have reported spontaneous fluctuations in the 4-to-12-cpm range when cerebral perfusion was challenged by systemic and local manipulations. Hypotension, hyperventilation, and cerebral artery occlusion substantially modulate the magnitude of these spontaneous fluctuations. These studies clearly challenge our current understanding of CBF autoregulation and demonstrate the dynamic nature of regional CBF. The work proposed here will contribute to our understanding of the basic neurophysiology of these phenomena and to our basic understanding of brain function.

The literature reviewed earlier indicates that RSC and ESC have been used separately to examine differences between young and old and between healthy old and Alzheimer's disease patient groups. Few studies to date have directly compared RSC and ESC, and no studies have examined the differences between them. Moreover, no studies to date have tied these measures directly to performance in the way we propose to do in the present studies.

Neuropsychological and functional neuroimaging studies indicate that attention is subserved by anatomically overlapping but functionally dissociable networks in the brain (Posner and Petersen 1990). A posterior network that includes the superior parietal lobe and its connections to inferior temporal and lateral premotor regions is important for voluntary detection of target stimuli in space (termed *selective attention*; see Corbetta and Shulman 1998). An anterior network that includes the anterior cingulate and its connections to dorsolateral prefrontal cortex is important for monitoring target detection, and maintaining target- and goal-related information in working memory while resisting interference from competing information (termed *executive control*). The parietal and frontal cortices are anatomically connected directly as well as indirectly via the anterior cingulate gyrus (Goldman-Rakic 1988). The anatomical connectivity facilitates goal-directed behavior that is accomplished by continuous interaction of operations of selective attention and executive control.

Lifespan development appears to reflect disproportionate changes in anterior attentional networks. Cognitive development from childhood into adulthood includes improved executive control of action and attention. These cognitive improvements are subserved by functional anatomical maturation of prefrontal cortex and associated anterior cingulate circuitry (Bunge et al. 2002). Conversely, normal aging is marked by declines in executive control that are related to reductions in inhibitory functions (e.g., Hasher et al. 1991) and functional changes in prefrontal cortex and associated circuitry (Rypma and D'Esposito 2000; Rypma et al. 2004). These findings suggest that the anterior attentional network may be relatively more affected by the deleterious effects of adult aging. These findings suggest that anterior rather than posterior attentional networks are more influenced by neural changes associated with childhood development and aging.

Evidence suggests that, whereas the anterior attentional network is disproportionately affected by diseases of childhood, diseases of aging may affect both anterior and posterior attention networks (e.g., Vaidya et al. 2005; Rombouts and Schelten 2005). Clinically, ADHD is characterized by impulsivity, inattention, and hyperactivity. In the laboratory it is characterized by reductions in performance on anterior attention tasks (e.g., "go/no-go" and "n-back") (Shallice et al. 2002; Vaidya et al. 1999), but relatively preserved performance on visual search tasks (Aman et al. 1998). Alzheimer patients, on the other hand, tend to show deficits in both kinds of tasks (Backman et al. 2005; Drzezga et al. 2005; Rosler et al. 2005).

Analyses that combine ESC and RSC will permit one to observe attentional changes associated with childhood and aging. First, both childhood and aging groups should show greater changes in anterior than in posterior attentional networks compared to their control groups. Second, the anterior attentional network that is weaker in both populations differs in the underlying developmental sequel, specifically immature myelination and pruning in childhood and deteriorating myelination in aging (e.g., Madden et al. 2004; Peters and Sethares 2004). One can expect that relationships between frontal and parietal cortices will be affected in different ways in these two anatomical scenarios. Analysis of RSC-ESC in both healthy and diseased children, healthy young adults, and healthy and diseased elderly will permit us to assess the effects of developing, intact, and deteriorating connections between brain regions and their associated behavioral consequences.

Improved understanding of RSC could benefit diagnosis of age-related disorders across the lifespan. Li et al. have recently demonstrated altered RSC between hippo-campal regions in Alzheimer's disease patients (Li et al. 2000). Across ten Alzheimer patients they observed significantly fewer resting-state correlations between hippo-campal regions than in controls. Moreover, there were minimal differences between these patients and controls in resting-state correlations in visual cortex between these two groups. We have also carried out a study on a diverse group of five patients with Tourette syndrome. The results of these investigations are reported in a paper in *AJNR* (Biswal et al. 1998), which describes motor task-activation studies, and in two abstracts (Biswal et al. 1997c, 1997d) that report on functional connectivity using analysis of physiological fluctuations. Comparisons were made with age- and gender-matched controls. A bilateral finger-tapping paradigm was used for task activation. We believe there is a high likelihood, based on these studies, that analysis of resting-state physio-logical fluctuations will contribute to clinical practice

13   Subtraction and Beyond: The Logic of Experimental Designs for Neuroimaging

Russell A. Poldrack

The goal of functional neuroimaging studies is generally to determine which particular brain regions or systems exhibit altered activity in response to the engagement of particular cognitive, emotional, or sensory processes. In order to determine these mappings between mental and neural processes, experimental designs are employed that attempt to manipulate a particular process and then examine how the manipulations affects brain activity. The goal of this chapter is to characterize the various forms of experimental design that have been used for functional neuroimaging, with a particular eye to how these designs constrain the inferences that can be supported.

When the neuroimaging researcher uses a task manipulation, he or she is (either implicitly or explicitly) assuming that the task can be decomposed into specific processes that can be independently manipulated. If the assumed decomposition is correct, then differences in brain activity can be mapped onto specific mental processes. This assumption of the decomposability of mental processes is shared with cognitive psychologists, who examine the effects of similar task manipulations on such behavioral variables as response times and task errors. Thus, both neuroimaging and cognitive psychology rely critically on the assumption that mental processes can be functionally decomposed; this is a fundamental tenet of cognitive psychology that differentiates it from classical behaviorism. A full discussion of the status of mental decomposition is beyond the scope of the present paper; here I will take the decomposability of mental processes as a given, and refer the interested reader to some previous critiques (e.g., Skinner 1963; Uttal 2000) and rejoinders (e.g., Bechtel 2002b).

The Subtraction Method

The most basic, and still most commonly used, experimental design for neuroimaging is the subtraction method (figure 13.1). At least two conditions are presented, which putatively differ in the presence of a single cognitive process. For example, Petersen et al. (1988) presented subjects with nouns and asked them to either read the word aloud or generate a verb associated with the noun. The subtraction between these

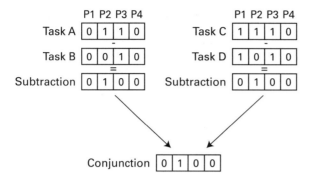

Figure 13.1
The subtraction method.

two conditions was meant to isolate the processes of semantic retrieval, under the assumption that all other processes (e.g., those involved in word recognition, speech production, breathing, etc.) remain constant between the two tasks. This is known as the *pure insertion* (PI) assumption, meaning that a single cognitive process can be inserted without affecting the remainder; this concept was first introduced by Donders (1868/1969) in the context of reaction times (cf. Sternberg 1969). Subtraction remains the most common experimental design in cognitive neuroimaging studies because of its simplicity.

The Core Problem

This simplicity, however, is misleading: The PI assumption is simply not tenable in many situations. In neuroimaging, the PI assumption actually comprises two parallel assumptions, one regarding the insertability of cognitive processes (i.e., the same assumption made in response time studies), and a second regarding the insertability of neural processes. The assumption regarding cognitive insertability can potentially be tested using an approach known as the additive factors logic (Sternberg 1969), in which one manipulates multiple factors in order to test for interactions between putatively separable functions. However, such tests of the PI assumption are only rarely presented in neuroimaging papers. In addition, the additive factors approach requires the strong assumption that transfer of information between processing stages occurs in a set of serial and discrete steps. The strongly interactive and recurrent nature of neural processing and prevalence of feedback connections between regions suggests that this assumption is incorrect. In addition, there is specific evidence for partial information transfer between stages of processing occurring in different brain regions from single-unit recordings (Bichot et al. 2001) and human electrophysiology (Miller and Hackley 1992). These violations of the discrete stage assumption make it impossible to determine using additive factors logic whether different systems are additive or interactive (McClelland 1979).

As Friston et al. (1996) have pointed out, it is perfectly possible that a design could satisfy the PI assumption at the cognitive level yet fail to satisfy it at the neural level, and failure at either of these levels compromises any inferences based on the subtraction. In fact, the highly interactive and nonlinear nature of neural processing makes it very likely that this assumption will fail. Jennings et al. (1997) provided evidence of just such a failure. Subjects in their study performed judgments regarding semantics (deciding whether the object was a living thing) or letters (deciding whether the word had an "a"), under three different response conditions (spoken response, silent response, or mouse movement). Behavioral data revealed no interaction between task and response type for memory encoding (i.e., memory performance was similarly affected by the task across different response types), but there was a substantial interaction in the neural response as measured by positron emission tomography (PET): A much larger difference existed between encoding tasks in the left inferior prefrontal cortex under mouse response conditions than under mental response conditions, with spoken response falling in between. These data suggest that, even if the assumptions of the additive factors logic are tenable, demonstrating additivity at the level of behavior may not be sufficient to ensure the PI assumption of the subtractive method. If the PI assumption fails, then there is simply no way to determine what cognitive processes are reflected in the activation observed in the subtraction experiment.

The Need for Task Analysis

A further problem with subtraction designs lies in how task comparisons are designed. A number of authors have noted (Poeppel 1996; Sartori & Umilta 2000; Sergent et al. 1992) that cognitive subtraction requires a formal task analysis to determine which particular cognitive process is being isolated by a subtraction. Such an analysis lays out the processes involved in performing the task, which is equivalent to a theory of how the task is performed.

Unfortunately, such task analyses are very rarely presented in neuroimaging papers. Whereas formal theories from cognitive psychology could often provide substantial guidance as to the design of such tasks, it is uncommon for neuroimaging studies to take meaningful guidance from such theories. Rather, the task comparisons in many studies are based on intuitive judgments regarding the cognitive processes engaged by a particular task.

As an example, Poldrack et al. (1999) set out to isolate semantic and phonological processing in separate task comparisons. To do this, we presented subjects with four tasks: abstract/concrete judgments, syllable-counting judgments (with either words or pseudowords), and uppercase/lowercase judgments. The comparison of most interest was that between abstract/concrete judgments and syllable-counting judgments, which was meant to isolate processes specific to semantic retrieval (positive differences) or phonological manipulation (negative differences). However, no formal task analysis was presented to motivate these tasks (indeed, they were adopted because they had been previously used by other experimenters, who also did not present formal task analyses).

An assessment of these tasks with regard to psycholinguistic theories of phonological or semantic retrieval reveals a number of difficulties in interpreting the findings. First, syllable-counting judgments with written materials actually require a number of processes that might fall under the umbrella of "phonological processing": retrieval and/or assembly of phonological output forms, syllabification, metalinguistic counting of the syllable units, and working memory for phonological and metalinguistic information. Likewise, the semantic task may involve lexical semantic access, resolution of lexical ambiguity, retrieval of specific semantic cues in service of the decision, and working memory for this semantic and metalinguistic information. Thus, activation for subtractions between these tasks could reflect any of a number of theoretically distinct processes that differ between them. Together, these points suggest that the conclusions deriving from many imaging studies using subtraction designs may provide a relatively coarse mapping of cognitive processes to brain function; to the degree that one wishes to map cognitive processes to brain regions as specifically as possible, this is problematic.

A Defense of Subtraction

In opposition to arguments against subtraction, Petersen et al. (1998) argued that

[C]onfusion results from the lack of appreciation for the distinction between "cognitive subtraction" as an experimental design and interpretive strategy, and image subtraction as an analysis methodology. As seen above, cognitive subtraction can be used to design and interpret an imaging study, and imaging subtraction can be used to mirror the cognitive strategy. However, image subtraction does not make the assumption of pure insertion: experimental designs, analysis choices, and interpretive strategies do. Image subtraction is performed in part to mirror experimental design strategy, but more importantly it is done to reveal the differences in the hemodynamic signal between two conditions by subtracting the large amplitude complex anatomical background present in hemodynamic images. (p. 854)

It is certainly true that the computation of a subtraction between images does not require any assumptions about the underlying processes; however, most cognitive neuroscientists are not interested in creating subtraction images for the sake of making pretty pictures. Rather, they do this with the goal of mapping the observed subtraction results onto the mental processes that were manipulated in the study. This argument thus fails to salvage the subtraction approach.

Petersen et al. (1998) also argued that the assumption of pure insertion can be tested if the appropriate control conditions are performed. They focused on a particular kind of violation of pure insertion, wherein a process is engaged during the baseline task but not in the experimental task (e.g., daydreaming during a resting baseline). In order to assess the assumption of pure insertion, they compared activation during both a baseline task (word reading) and an experimental task (verb generation) with a resting baseline. Most regions showed a pattern that they took to confirm the PI assumption, with no difference between word reading and rest but a significant activation for verb generation versus reading; however, at least one region (in the posterior insula) showed activation for word reading versus rest but deactivation for word reading versus verb generation. This approach is interesting and does provide some added confidence in the results of a subtraction analysis, but it cannot unequivocally save the PI assumption. In particular, it makes a fairly strong assumption that it is possible to find some kind of ultimate neutral baseline against which to compare all other tasks (in this case, rest). However, there is a growing realization that all baseline conditions for fMRI are arbitrary, and in particular that resting is associated with engagement of specific mental processes (Binder et al. 1999; Stark and Squire 2001).

Confounds and Subtraction

One of the most common problems with subtraction designs is the presence of behavioral confounds between conditions. In nearly every case where two tasks are compared in a subtraction design, the task of interest is more difficult (as defined by longer reaction times or lower accuracy) than the baseline task. Given that the duration of neural firing is directly related to the resulting BOLD signal, this results in a difficulty for interpretation: Does the difference in activation result from the differential engagement of a particular process, or from engagement of that process for different durations? This distinction is often taken to be rather esoteric in the neuroimaging field, but it is actually fundamental. For example, imagine a study that compared social versus nonsocial judgments about faces, in which the latter are performed more quickly than the former. A difference in activation is observed in a particular brain region, and this difference is attributed to social processes. However, it is equally possible that the region showing the difference in activation is actually related to motor programming, and that the more protracted response process in the social task results in more activation in the region. A number of studies using subtraction have dealt with this issue by using multiple baseline tasks that vary in their difficulty (e.g., Demb et al. 1995); this approach provides greater confidence that the resulting differences in activation are not driven by confounds.

The Subtraction Approach: What Can We Infer?

The foregoing arguments provide strong reasons to distrust subtraction as a means of mapping cognitive processes onto neural activity. However, the approach remains quite prevalent in many parts of the functional imaging literature. It is striking that many subtraction studies find a common set of brain regions that are activated regardless of the specific task (Duncan and Owen 2000), as well as a set of regions that are commonly deactivated relative to a baseline task (known as *task-independent decreases*: e.g., Gusnard and Raichle 2001). One interpretation of this set of findings is that they reflect the previously mentioned effort/executive control confounds, which are nearly always present in subtraction studies. Without the use of multiple baselines that vary in difficulty, it is nearly impossible to determine the specificity of activation in a subtraction design. Based on these concerns, it appears that simple subtraction designs are unable to establish reliable links between cognitive processes and neural structures.

Alternatives to Subtraction

In order to sidestep the problems inherent in simple subtraction designs, a number of other fMRI design approaches have been developed (for other discussions of these approaches, see Aguirre and D'Esposito 1999; Friston et al. 1997). Most of these methods do appear to avoid some of the criticisms of subtraction methods. However, closer examination reveals that they are subject either to many of the same fundamental assumptions as the subtraction approach or to different but equally stringent assumptions regarding the relationship between task manipulations and the underlying cognitive processes.

Conjunction Analysis

Price and Friston (1997) recommended an approach called *cognitive conjunction*, which they suggested could circumvent the assumption of pure insertion. In the conjunction approach, subjects are presented with at least two task subtractions, wherein only one putative cognitive process is shared between the different subtractions. For example, one might examine phonological processing by conjoining two task comparisons: rhyme generation versus word naming (which isolates phonological processing operations) and syllable counting versus silent reading (which isolates a large number of word recognition processes along with phonological processing). In the original version of this analysis (Price and Friston 1997), a significant conjunction required that each of the different subtractions showed activation and that there were no significant differences between the subtractions. Price and Friston (1997) argued that this version of conjunction analysis does not require the PI assumption, because regions showing differences across subtractions are by definition excluded.

In contrast, the subtraction approach explicitly assumes a lack of interaction, and thus will be invalid in the presence of such interactions. In more recent versions (Friston et al. 1999), this approach was changed so that the conjunction simply finds regions that are commonly active at a particular threshold, without regard to differences across subtractions; this version abandons the goal of discounting regions show-

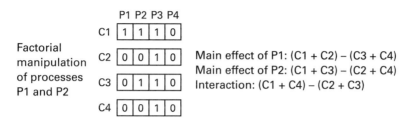

Figure 13.2
Factorial design.

ing interactions, and thus is no more immune to the effects of interactions than standard subtraction analyses (cf. Caplan and Moo 2004).

Another requirement the conjunction approach shares with the subtraction approach is the need for a detailed task analysis to determine which components are subtracted in each comparison. In particular, conjunction analysis requires that the conjoined subtractions have only a single process is common. Take the previous example of phonological processing: It is quite difficult to ensure that phonological processing is the only common process between these two subtractions. For example, both rhyme generation versus naming and syllable counting versus rest comparisons involve differential working memory demands, as well as differences in overall task difficulty that could differently engage task monitoring and effort mechanisms. Another problem Caplan and Moo (2004) have pointed out is that subjects may implicitly process stimuli in ways that the task does not require; for example, if a subject is asked to simply name a word, he or she may also automatically retrieve semantic knowledge about that word. These problems suggest that conjunction analysis may not generally overcome the fundamental limitations of the underlying subtractions. Compared with simple subtraction, however, it does offer some degree of additional confidence in putative mappings of cognitive processes to brain activity.

Factorial Designs

Factorial designs involve the simultaneous manipulation of multiple experimental factors (figure 13.2). In such a design, the data are analyzed using an analysis of variance approach, which allows measurement of both main effects (equivalent to subtractions) and interactions that occur when the effect of one factor is modulated by the level of another manipulated variable. For example, Gläscher et al. (2004) examined the interaction between facial identity and facial expression, to test whether the fusiform gyrus and amygdala showed different patterns of interaction between these factors. Activity in the amygdala showed one pattern of interaction, wherein activity was greater when consistently fearful expressions were seen across a number of faces, compared to all other combinations of identity and affect. The fusiform gyrus showed a different

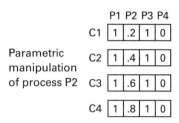

Figure 13.3
Parametric design.

pattern of interaction, such that constant images (where the identity and emotion were held constant) showed less activity than any of the other conditions, which were all equal.

These results show how factorial designs can be used to identify the ways in which specific factors interact. Rather than globally assuming pure insertion, it is possible to directly test whether the effects of one cognitive manipulation are modulated by other factors. The finding of such interactions provides additional insights into the mapping of cognitive processes to neural systems, by showing whether putatively distinct cognitive processes may converge or interact at the neural level. However, factorial designs still require the PI assumption, because each particular factor is assumed to isolate a specific cognitive process (cf. Aguirre and D'Esposito 1999); tests of the additivity of processes are possible for the manipulated processes, but PI must be assumed for all other processes. In the foregoing example, for instance, interpreting the results requires the assumption that manipulations of facial expression do not cause changes in other factors, such as attentional arousal.

Parametric Designs

Parametric designs involve the manipulation of a particular task parameter across multiple levels rather than comparison between different tasks (see figure 13.3). This strategy has been used extensively in studies of the visual system, in which there are well-known relations between psychophysical parameters (e.g., stimulus contrast) and neural activity (e.g., Wandell 1999). Similarly, studies of working memory have used a task paradigm known as n-*back*, in which subjects are presented with a stream of stimuli (such as letters) and asked determine whether the present stimulus matches the one presented N trials back. The value of N is manipulated, with 1-back being relatively easy, 2-back more difficult, and more than 3-back being impossible for many subjects; a 0-back condition is often implemented by asking the subject to match each stimulus to a predefined target. Studies using this task have shown parametric increases in activation as N increases (e.g., Braver et al. 1997). With sufficient levels of the parameter, parametric designs also allow the estimation of nonlinear effects; for example, some parametric studies of the *n*-back task have shown an inverted-U function relating activation to working memory demands (e.g., Callicott et al. 1999). The inability of simple subtraction designs to find such nonlinear effects may underlie the conflicting results that are often seen in studies comparing patient (e.g., schizophrenia) and control groups; patients could show either greater or lesser activation than controls (or no difference), depending on where in the function the two groups fall.

Because they involve the modulation of a single process rather than its presence or absence, parametric designs theoretically avoid the pure insertion assumption. However, they replace it with what might be called the "pure modulation" assumption— the assumption that the manipulation affects only the degree to which the process is engaged and not the engagement/disengagement of any other processes. This assumption may fail in cases where changes in the parameter cause the task to be performed differently, or drive the engagement of additional processes. For example, if working memory load is increased parametrically to a level beyond the subject's capacity, then additional processes will be engaged at the point where memory fails (e.g., processes related to frustration or error detection). Parametric designs also require a task decomposition to understand exactly what process the task is parametrically manipulating. For example, increased working memory load increases the load on processes involved in memory maintenance, but may also increase the need for monitoring processes. One particular concern is that parametric manipulations are often correlated with task difficulty and response time.

Priming/Adaptation Designs

Another class of designs, referred to as either repetition priming (e.g., Demb et al. 1995; Squire et al. 1992) or fMRI adaptation (Grill-Spector and Malach 2001; Grill-Spector et al. 1999) designs, take advantage of the fact that net activity in task-relevant regions often decreases when items are repeated in a task. In priming designs, regions showing repetition-related decreases in activity are inferred to process those stimulus properties that are repeated. Because the comparison is between two instances of exactly the same task, there is no need for the PI assumption. However, priming/adaptation designs require the assumption that the cognitive processes engaged during performance change only quantitatively and not qualitatively, similarly to the pure modulation assumption for parametric designs. Given that some theories have proposed that repetition priming involves a change in processes rather than diminution in a single process (e.g., Logan 1990), this issue is of potential concern. In addition, this approach requires a task analysis to understand the cognitive processes that are changed by repetition, in order to associate these processes with the regions of neural change. It should also be noted that repetition is almost invariably associated with decreased reaction time, and thus it is necessary to rule out whether observed decreases in activation reflect the consequences rather than the causes of the repetition effect.

It has been argued that adaptation fMRI designs can provide better resolution of neural representations than direct comparisons between conditions (Grill-Spector and Malach 2001; Grill-Spector et al. 1999). In this approach, a stimulus is repeatedly presented, thus putatively inducing adaptation in those neurons that respond selectively to that stimulus. Some feature of the stimulus is then changed (e.g., size of an object). Regions showing release from adaptation are inferred to code for the particular feature that was changed, because neurons that are invariant to the altered feature should treat the stimulus exactly like the previous repetition and thus not show a release from adaptation. The adaptation method may be more powerful than simple categorical comparison of different stimulus types, because it equates everything except the processing history of the stimulus, and thus avoids some of the potential confounds inherent in comparing different items (cf. Henson 2005. However, recent work on the nature of the BOLD signal (e.g., Logothetis, 2003) suggests that interpreting these changes in terms of the local representation in the regions showing adaptation might be invalid. More likely, they reflect representations in upstream regions (where the changes in spike rate actually occur). Furthermore, evidence from single-unit recording suggests that stimulus selectivity inferred from adaptation responses may differ from the selectivity of the neuron's response to novel stimuli (Sawamura et al. 2006).

Blocked versus Event-Related Designs and Behaviorally Driven Comparisons

Somewhat orthogonal to the experimental design distinctions outlined in the preceding section is the distinction between blocked and event-related fMRI designs. In a blocked design, subjects perform the tasks of interest for alternating blocks of time (generally lasting about 16 to 40 seconds), and the statistical model treats the entire block as a single entity (e.g., modeling the task design using a boxcar function). In an event-related design, trials of various types or tasks are presented in a pseudorandom order, with periods of rest or visual fixation interspersed between trials (Buckner et al. 1996; Wagner et al. 1998), and trials are modeled individually. Event-related designs have been embraced because they may be more psychologically realistic than blocked designs by making events less predictable. For example, in a study of recognition memory designed to compare activity evoked by old versus new stimuli, the presentation of long, predictable blocks of old or new stimuli may result in undesirable strategic effects. Event-related designs are also useful because they allow trials to be sorted based on the subject's behavior. For example, Brewer et al. (1998) presented subjects with pictures to study, and then tested their later memory for those pictures. The trial-by-trial fMRI data acquired during memory encoding were sorted depending on whether the subject subsequently remembered or forgot each item, which revealed several regions whose activity predicted later memory. This approach is very useful because it relies on actual behavior rather than the putative effects of a task manipulation.

Despite the power of event-related designs, there are cautions that must be appreciated. First, the use of behaviorally defined comparisons, rather than task comparisons, does not eliminate the need for a decomposition of the cognitive processes revealed by the comparison. The finding that behavioral differences are associated with differences in brain activity is not particularly enlightening, unless it provides insights into how the cognitive processes underlying that behavioral difference are implemented in the brain. For example, studies of memory retrieval have compared activity on different classes of trials sorted by behavioral outcomes, such as successfully remembered items ("hits") versus forgotten items ("misses") (e.g., Eldridge et al. 2000). When activity is found in particular regions in relation to memory outcomes in particular brain areas (e.g., hippocampus), it has been associated with particular aspects of mnemonic experience. This conclusion may be well founded, particularly given everything else that is known about the role of the hippocampus in memory, but such differences could also reflect other cognitive processes (e.g., processes related more generally to success on a task). It is thus necessary to decompose behaviorally driven comparisons in the same way as task-driven comparisons.

Second, it is sometimes incorrectly assumed that event-related fMRI does not require the same subtraction assumptions as blocked designs. This illusion may stem from the fact that event-related fMRI allows one to estimate the hemodynamic response evoked by a particular trial condition; what is sometimes overlooked is the fact that this response is estimated against a particular baseline, generally a "null event" such as visual fixation or resting state. In this sense, inferences from event-related fMRI are no different from those based on blocked designs with regard to the logical nature of the comparisons.

Conclusions

This chapter has outlined the primary methods used for experimental designs in neuroimaging. In response to the well-known problems of the subtraction method, a number of approaches have been proposed. However, none of these approaches eliminates the need for an understanding of how the task manipulation relates to the underlying cognitive processes, because in each case interpretation of the results relies on knowing exactly what processes have been modulated. Although the parametric and priming approaches do not require the PI assumption, they instead require a "pure modulation" assumption that may be equally tenuous. Event-related fMRI designs do not alleviate the need for any of these assumptions. Furthermore, in any fMRI design, an understanding of how neural activity relates to cognitive processes requires that the task be decomposed into particular processes, in essence requiring a theory of how the task is performed.

The less charitable reader might be tempted at this point to ask why the appropriate response to the foregoing review is not to give up on fMRI as a means of understanding the relation between cognitive and neural processes. Before addressing this specifically in the context of fMRI, one should first note that the project of cognitive psychology suffers from many of the same conceptual difficulties regarding the mapping of cognitive processes onto data (which, in the case of cognitive psychology, comprises data regarding behavior rather than brain imaging data). Not surprisingly, the harshest criticisms of neuroimaging have come from theorists who more fundamentally reject the decomposition of cognitive processes, either behaviorists (Uttal 2000) or dynamic systems theorists (van Orden and Papp 1997). Thus, giving up on fMRI for these reasons would entail a more general abandonment of the goal of a mechanistic theory of mental processes.

Regarding fMRI more specifically, there are glimmers of hope amid the sea of futile subtractions. One source of optimism comes from a number of recent meta-analyses of neuroimaging data (e.g., Nee et al. 2007; Owen et al. 2005; Turkeltaub et al. 2002; Wager and Smith 2003). These analyses have demonstrated a strong degree of consistency in associations between classes of task manipulations and activation patterns. These findings can be viewed as a "conceptual conjunction analysis," showing that specific regions are consistently associated with particular brain regions even when other factors are varied across studies. The finding of consistency does not salvage the pure insertion assumption, but it does suggest that whatever processes are being mapped in subtraction studies are reliably associated with particular brain structures.

More important than consistency is specificity, wherein particular patterns of brain activity are selectively associated with particular cognitive manipulations. Meta-analyses have shown some degree of specificity. However, particularly in higher-order association cortices, any particular region may be associated with a number of cognitive manipulations, though there do seem to be broader-scale functional gradients across cortical regions. For example, more anterior regions in prefrontal cortex appear to code for higher-order relations compared to more posterior regions (cf. Koechlin et al. 2003). Further work will be necessary to determine to what degree this lack of specificity reflects problems with the current cognitive ontology versus true distribution of function across the cortex (Poldrack 2006). If highly specific patterns of brain activity related to specific cognitive manipulations can be identified, then this would blunt (though not eliminate) some concerns about the possible problems with subtraction, by suggesting that whatever processes are being isolated by convergent subtractions are neurobiologically coherent.

Another source of optimism comes from the integration of computational modeling with functional neuroimaging. To the degree that a computational model reflects an explicit theory of the processes underlying a task, it provides a more principled way to relate brain activity to specific cognitive functions. There is a wide range of approaches to integrating computational modeling and neuroimaging, but most involve the use of computational models to create model-based regressors that are then used for analysis of fMRI data. For example, Brown and Braver (2005) compared the predictions of two different computational models to determine whether activity in the anterior cingulate was better explained by conflict detection or error likelihood prediction. Other approaches have used model comparisons to determine whether separate brain systems may be characterized by different computational functions. For example, Hampton et al. (2006) used two computational models that varied in their degree of structure (a simple reinforcement learning model and a more complex Markov model), and found that different brain systems showed patterns of activity that correlated with each of the different computational processes. Such analyses still involve comparing imaging conditions, but the comparisons are based on quantitative outputs from a computational model rather than qualitative manipulations of task or stimulus conditions. Although they do not eliminate the need for assumptions regarding the relationship between cognitive and neural processes (such as the pure modulation assumption of parametric designs), they do provide more confidence that brain activity is being mapped to processes that play a specific cognitive role by virtue of performing a particular computation.

Acknowledgments

Preparation of this chapter was supported by grants from the National Science Foundation (DMI-0433693) and National Institutes of Health (P20 RR020750 to R. Bilder). Thanks to Martin Bunzl and Marisa Geoghegan for helpful comments on a earlier draft.

14 Advancements in fMRI Methods: What Can They Inform about the Functional Organization of the Human Ventral Stream?

Kalanit Grill-Spector

Object recognition is an amazing human feat. Humans effortlessly recognize objects within a fraction of a second. Recognition is largely invariant to changes in the appearance of objects due to the variability in viewing conditions, which can change objects' location, size, viewpoint, illumination, occlusion, and other characteristics. However, the underlying neural representations and computations that enable recognition are still mysterious.

Neuroimaging techniques (especially functional magnetic resonance imaging, or fMRI) offer an opportunity to investigate neural mechanisms underlying object recognition. Functional MRI studies have revealed a constellation of object-selective regions in lateral and ventral occipitotemporal cortex (lateral occipital complex, or LOC; see Malach et al. 1995) that respond more strongly to objects than to noise patterns, textures, and scrambled objects (figure 14.1, plate 3), and face-selective regions that respond more strongly to faces than to nonface objects (figure 14.1), the most studied of which is the fusiform face area (FFA) (Kanwisher et al. 1997b).

Activation in these regions correlates with subjects' recognition performance (figure 14.2). When stimuli are ambiguous or presented close to the perceptual threshold, activity in face- and object-selective cortex correlates with subjects' recognition of faces (Grill-Spector et al. 2006a; Hasson et al. 2001; Moutoussis and Zeki 2002; Tong et al. 1998) and objects (Grill-Spector et al. 2000). Further, prolonged experience with objects (Gauthier et al. 1999, 2000) and faces (Golarai et al. 2007) modifies these representations.

These studies provide fundamental knowledge about which brain regions are involved in object and face recognition. However, many questions about the nature of the underlying neural representations remain: (1) How do these representations provide for invariant recognition without losing the acuity to distinguish between similar items that share the same parts and configuration? (2) What mechanisms underlie rapid categorization? (3) Are the same representations used for between-category (e.g., distinguishing between a car and a boat) and within-category discrimination (e.g., distinguishing between a sailboat and a motorboat)? (4) Are representations of faces

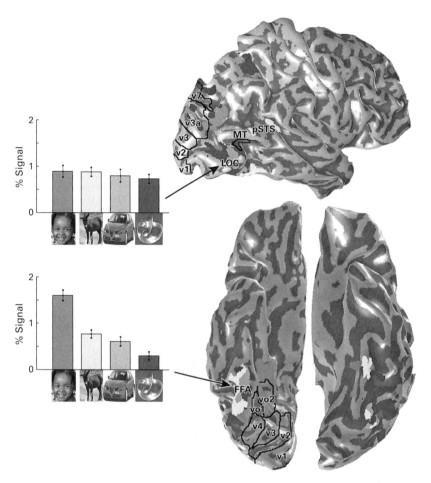

Figure 14.1 (plate 3)

Object-selective regions in the human brain. Object-, face-, and place-selective regions on a partially inflated brain of one representative subject shown from lateral and ventral views. Superposition of three contrasts thresholded at $p < 0.0001$. Red: faces > nonface objects. Green: places > nonface objects. Blue: nonface objects > scrambled. Pink and dark green indicate overlapping regions. Pink: face > objects and objects > scrambled. Dark green: places > objects and objects > scrambled. Boundaries of known visual areas are shown in black on the right hemisphere. LOC includes a constellation of object-selective regions (blue and pink regions) in lateral and ventral occipital cortex. The posterior region adjacent to MT is typically labeled LO and the ventral region is labeled pFUS/OTS. Face-selective regions include the FFA, a face-selective region in the fusiform gyrus; the pSTS, a face-selective region in posterior superior temporal sulcus and a region in LOC (shown here in pink and sometimes referred to as the OFA). MT: motion-selective region in the posterior ITS. Mean percentage signal from LOC (excluding regions that respond more to faces than objects) and FFA averaged across ten subjects relative to a scrambled baseline. Stimuli are indicated by icons and include faces, four-legged mammals, cars, and abstract sculptures. Note that object-selective regions respond to both objects and faces more than scrambled images, but they do not respond more strongly to faces than to objects.

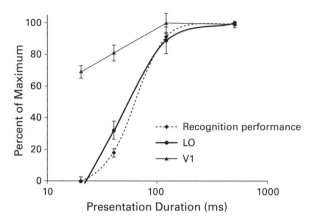

Figure 14.2

Relationship between LOC activation and recognition performance; BOLD signal and recognition performance as a function of image exposure. During scanning, subjects viewed gray level images of faces, animals, common objects (e.g., cars, boats, etc), which were followed by random scrambled image masks. Subjects were asked to name pictures covertly at the basic level (e.g., face, dog, car, boat, etc). In different blocks, images appeared for a different duration (20, 40, 120, or 500 ms) followed by a mask completing a 500 ms trial (480, 460, 380, or 0 ms mask duration). Immediately after fMRI scans (but while in the scanner), subjects saw the same images at the same duration, and participated in a behavioral experiment in which recognition performance was recorded. Recognition performance (dashed black) is correlated with LO activation (red) but not with V1 activation (blue). Adapted from Grill-Spector et al. 2000.

(or objects of expertise) fundamentally different from standard object representations, and if so, how do they differ? (5) How do experience and development shape these representations?

In addressing these questions, the inherent limitations of standard-resolution fMRI (SR-fMRI) pose significant challenges. SR-fMRI measures the pooled neural responses across a voxel or many voxels that constitute a brain region. Since a cubic millimeter of cortex contains approximately 10,000 to 50,000 neurons, fMRI signals from regions that extend ~250 to 5,000 mm^3 (which is typical in standard fMRI) reflect the activity from tens to a few hundred million neurons. Given results from electrophysiology studies, it is highly likely that such measurements pool across diverse neural populations that process different aspects of objects.

Evidence from electrophysiology suggests that a fine-grain neural organization (in the order of a few millimeters) may be particularly relevant for understanding the neural representations of faces and objects. Single unit recordings from monkey infero-temporal (IT) cortex suggest that neurons with similar properties (e.g., similar shape preference, see Fujita et al. 1992; or face preference, see Tsao et al. 2006) are physically clustered. Tanaka and colleagues have suggested that IT cortex contains a columnar structure, which is organized perpendicular to the cortical surface. These columns are about 400 microns in diameter and contain clusters of neurons tuned to similar features of objects (Fujita et al. 1992). The basic columnar structure is prevalent throughout the visual cortex and is thought to be a basic computational unit. In monkey visual cortex, columns are 50 to 500 μm in diameter, and in humans they are thought to be twice as large. Histological measurements in postmortem brains of human ocular dominance columns in V1 (Horton et al. 1990) reveal that they are about 1 mm in diameter in contrast to 400 to 500 μm in diameter in the macaque brain. If the columnar structure is prevalent in humans as in monkeys, it suggests that higher-level visual cortex— such as object- and face-selective cortex may also have a fine-grain structure (on the scale of 0.5 millimeter to a few millimeters).

Here we review recent methodological advances in fMRI that elucidate the neural representations underlying recognition. These include the method of fMRI-adaptation (fMRI-A), multivoxel pattern analysis (MVPA), and high-resolution fMRI (HR-fMRI). Each of these approaches examines the underlying representations in a different way: fMRI-A relies on adaptation of neural populations within a voxel by repeated stimulus presentations. MVPA capitalizes on small but systematic modulations across voxels, and HR-fMRI images cortex directly at a substantially higher resolution. As we discuss these methods we will highlight how these methods have advanced theories of object recognition.

fMRI Adaptation

Repeated presentation of objects or faces typically leads to a reduced fMRI response in object and face-selective cortex, or fMRI adaptation (fMRI-A) (Grill-Spector et al. 1999). This reduction is stimulus specific. Adaptation is maximal for the repetition of an identical stimulus, but is less (and may disappear) for transformed versions of the same item (e.g., the same object presented in different locations; Grill-Spector et al. 1999). fMRI-adaptation is a robust phenomenon that is present even when repetitions of the same object occur after many intervening stimuli (Sayres and Grill-Spector 2006) and across various time scales ranging from seconds to days (Sayres and Grill-Spector 2006; van Turennout et al. 2000). It is hypothesized that this reduced response measured by fMRI is related to the stimulus-specific decrements in the firing rates of IT neurons to repeated objects. However, the exact relationship between neural adaptation and fMRI-A is not understood (Grill-Spector et al. 2006a).

fMRI-A allows tagging of specific neuronal populations within a voxel by adapting them with a repeated stimulus and then examining the sensitivity of the representation to different factors, by testing which factors lead to a recovery from adaptation. For example, SR-fMRI of lateral occipital cortex shows a similar level of response to dif-

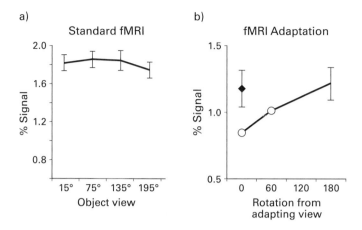

Figure 14.3

fMRI adaptation. (a) Standard fMRI of LO responses to different animal views relative to a scrambled baseline. Error bars reflect SEM across seven subjects. (b) Short-lagged fMRI adaptation experiment: Recovery from adaptation in LO as a function of object rotation. Diamond: unadapted response (different animals at the same view). Open circle: significant adaptation, $p < 0.05$ as compared to the response to different images. There is monotonic recovery from adaptation as the object is shown in a new view, which is rotated further away than the adapting view. Signal is measured relative to a blank baseline. Error bars indicate SEM across same seven subjects as (a). Adapted from Andresen, Vinberg and Grill-Spector 2009.

ferent views of the same object (figure 14.3a). This may reflect either a homogeneous population of neurons that responds equally across object views, or a heterogeneous population of neurons within a voxel, each tuned to a specific view. Using fMRI-A, these possibilities can be distinguished. Recovery from adaptation indicates that LO is sensitive to object viewpoint (figure 14.3b). A lack of recovery from adaptation would have indicated view invariance.

fMRI-A has been used to examine theories of view-invariant object recognition. Some theories of object recognition posit that objects are represented by a set of relatively simple, view-invariant features and their spatial relationship (Biederman 1987; Biederman and Gerhardstein 1993). Other theories suggest that object representations are view-dependent and invariant recognition is accomplished by interpolation across several object views (Bulthoff and Edelman 1992; Bulthoff et al. 1995; Edelman and Bulthoff 1992; Hayward and Tarr 2000; Poggio and Edelman 1990; Tarr and Bulthoff 1995). fMRI-A experiments have provided support for view-dependent cortical representations in LOC (Grill-Spector et al. 1999; Vuilleumier et al. 2002), by showing that there is a recovery from adaptation when rotated views of the adapted object are shown. Further fMRI-A studies demonstrated a hierarchy of representations in LOC, where more posterior regions recover from adaptation (and therefore are sensitive) to changes in object size, position, illumination, and view, and more anterior regions along the occipitotemporal sulcus and fusiform gyrus remain adapted when object position and size are changed, but recover from adaptation when object viewpoint and illumination are changed (Grill-Spector et al. 1999). In addition, there is evidence for hemispheric differences: The right fusiform gyrus recovers from adaptation when the same object is shown in a different view from the adapting view, whereas the left fusiform gyrus remains adapted (Vuilleumier et al. 2002). Recent experiments using parametric measurements of recovery from adaptation (Andresen, Vinberg, and Grill-Spector 2009) provide more precise measurements of the degree of sensitivity across the ventral stream to different object transformation and constrain theories of object recognition by providing quantitative measurements of sensitivity to object transformations. Overall, fMRI-A studies suggest that any comprehensive theory of invariant object recognition should include a hierarchy of processing stages involving intermediate stages containing view-dependent representations and higher stages containing more abstract representations.

Another area of intensive research is the neural representations underlying face identification (e.g., identifying "Albert Einstein"). This research has focused on characterizing the response properties of face-selective regions in the fusiform gyrus (FFA), because of findings that activity in this region correlates with face identification performance (George et al. 1999; Grill-Spector et al. 2004). Several recent studies have used fMRI-A to characterize the representation of faces in the FFA. However, to date these studies have not provided a consistent model of the neural basis of face identification.

Several studies have used fMRI-A and a morphing algorithm in which one identity is gradually transformed to another identity, to examine which level of morphing produces a recovery from adaptation due to identity changes. Rotshtein and colleagues (Rotshtein et al. 2005) have shown that the FFA recovers from adaptation when the perceived identity of a face changes (e.g., Marilyn Monroe versus Margaret Thatcher), but remains adapted when the same level of physical changes does not change the perceived identity. Results of this study suggest that the FFA may contain neurons that represent specific individuals, that is, neurons are sharply tuned to either "Marilyn" or "Maggie." However, two other recent studies (Gilaie-Dotan and Malach 2007; Jiang et al. 2006) reported a monotonic recovery from fMRI-A with the level of the morph. In these studies, degrees of morphing that were not strong enough to be perceived as a different face nonetheless caused recovery from adaptation in the FFA. These studies provide evidence for a different model of face identity representation based on a population code. According to this model neurons code stored face exemplars, their response is proportional to the similarity between the input face and the stored exemplars, and a particular face is represented by the distributed response across this neural population. The source of the disparate results may be the use of familiar faces (in which identity boundaries may be more salient) in the Rotshtein study and unfamiliar faces in the studies of Jiang and Gilaie-Dotan.

Although the method of fMRI-A is widespread and has provided important knowledge about representations in the human ventral stream, its weakness is that it is an indirect measure of neural selectivity and its underlying neural mechanisms are not fully understood (Grill-Spector et al. 2006a). Further, recent physiological investigations of the neural mechanisms of fMRI-A suggest that cross-adaptation in IT neurons across stimuli may not be predicted simply by the number of spikes the stimuli produce, as stimuli that drive a cell similarly may not produce cross-adaptation (Sawamura et al. 2006). Future experiments examining the relationship between neural adaptation and fMRI-A (Grill-Spector 2006; Grill-Spector et al. 2006a) will improve understanding of the underlying neural mechanisms and will be important for the interpretation of fMRI-A results.

Multivoxel Pattern Analyses

Many studies reported regions in the brain specialized for processing unique object categories such as faces, places, body parts, animals, tools, and letter strings. These findings of regions specialized for particular stimuli are highly reproducible, and built on previous neuropsychological evidence that lesions in the human ventral stream can lead to specific deficits in object and face recognition.

The presence of category-preferring regions poses a theoretical problem: Is there a special region in the brain that codes for every category humans recognize? Kanwisher and colleagues propose that the brain contains a few domain-specific modules, specialized for processing faces, places, and body parts, whereas other objects are processed and recognized by a general-purpose object recognition system (e.g., the LOC). According to this model, activation of domain-specific modules is tightly linked to recognition of these specialized categories and items from these categories. Another model, posited by Haxby and colleagues (Haxby et al. 2001), suggests that a single system recognizes both faces and nonface objects. According to this model, objects and faces are represented by highly distributed and overlapping patterns of brain activity across the ventral stream, and this distributed activity codes object category. This model builds on connectionist models, which showed that a distributed code provides a greater representational capacity and thus allows for the representation of a large number of objects and categories.

Proponents of each of the preceding models have provided evidence for their view by employing pattern analyses (MVPA). MVPA differ from region of interest (ROI) analyses used in SR-fMRI in that they examine the distributed pattern of response across voxels instead of measuring the average response across a region, which is typical in many fMRI studies (figure 14.4, plate 4). To support their model of distributed object

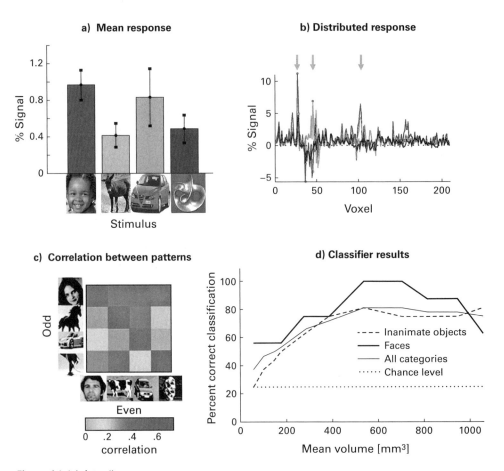

a) Mean response

b) Distributed response

c) Correlation between patterns

d) Classifier results

Figure 14.4 (plate 4)

Pattern analysis of distributed fMRI responses. (a) Mean LOC response to different object categories relative to a scrambled baseline, from one subject. Error bars indicate SEM across eight blocks
of a condition. (b) Distributed response across LOC voxels, same data as on the left; x-axis: voxel
number; y-axis: percent signal relative to scrambled. Each category elicits a different pattern of response across the LOC. Arrows indicate some voxels which have strong differential responses to
different stimuli. Adapted from Grill-Spector et al. 2006b. (c) Correlation analysis of patterns of
distributed responses. One way to examine information in the distributed response is to compare
the pattern of responses to the same and different stimuli across split halves of the data. In this
example, the pattern of response from one subject to different faces, animals, cars, and sculptures
was measured. This response was measured separately across odd and even runs that used different
images. The diagonal of the correlation matrix shows the reproducibility of the data across independent measurements. The off diagonal measurements depict the distinctiveness of the patterns.
When the on-diagonal values are higher than the off-diagonal values, it suggests that the distributed activations to different stimuli are both reproducible and distinct. (d) Results of a winner-
take-all classifier on determining which category the subject viewed based on the highest correlation between even and odd runs. Classifier performance is averaged across five subjects from their
standard-resolution LOC data and is shown as a function of the number of voxels selected from
the ROI.

representations, Haxby and colleagues performed MVPA of the distributed responses across face- and object-selective cortex (Haxby et al. 2001). They showed that the distributed response across the ventral stream to particular object categories is reproducible, and different categories produce distinct activation patterns. It is therefore possible to decode from the distributed response pattern which category subjects viewed. Subsequent studies showed that the distributed response for a certain category is consistent across sessions (Cox and Savoy 2003), and extends to other exemplars of a category and objects presented in a different format (line drawings versus photographs; see Spiridon and Kanwisher 2002).

It has also been argued that pattern analyses of distributed responses achieve subvoxel resolution (Haynes et al. 2005; Kamitani and Tong 2005). In this kind of analysis, the mean response from each voxel in an ROI is entered into a vector, which then represents the distributed response, as opposed to using the average response from the entire ROI. In a recent paper, Tong and Kamitani demonstrated that orientation sensitivity in V1 could be measured by MVPA (Kamitani and Tong 2005). They showed that individual voxels have a small but reliable orientation bias and the orientation of a visually presented grating could be decoded from the distributed responses across all V1 voxels.

Nevertheless, since the MVPA method is new, its theoretical foundations and limitations should also be considered. For example, MVPA relies on small but systematic modulations of responses across voxels. If these modulations are not reliable, then results of MVPA may not show information found in fMRI-A data. Another problem is that MVPA relies on sampling biases in fMRI, that is, how fMRI voxels combine across neural populations that have a spatial structure at a finer scale, such as orientation columns. If these sampling biases are not present, MVPA may fail, even when there is information at a smaller spatial scale. Another caveat is that, while MVPAs reveal what information is present in the distributed response, they do not show whether the brain uses the entire distributed activity during object recognition, or just information present in localized regions (but see Williams et al. 2007).

High-Resolution fMRI

More recently, researchers have used high-resolution fMRI (HR-fMRI) to directly image the fine-grained structure in object- and face-selective cortex. SR-fMRI uses voxels ranging between $3 \times 3 \times 3$ mm and $3.75 \times 3.75 \times 5$ mm to provide coverage of the entire brain. HR-fMRI uses voxels between $1 \times 1 \times 1$ mm and $2 \times 2 \times 2$ mm across parts of the brain, providing less coverage but a substantial increase in the imaging resolution by a factor of 27 to 70 (figure 14.5, plate 5). One of the goals of HR-fMRI is to image cortex at a higher level of spatial precision and distinguish heterogeneous responses that may be averaged with SR-fMRI. We believe that understanding the spatial scale of

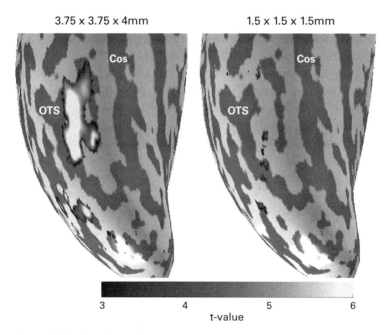

Figure 14.5 (plate 5)

Standard- and high-resolution fMRI of face-selective regions in the fusiform gyrus. (a) SR-fMRI (3.75 × 3.75 × 4 mm) and (b) HR-fMRI (1.5 × 1.5 × 1.5 mm) of face-selective activations in the same individual. GLM analysis shows higher activations to faces than to objects, $p < 0.002$, $t = 3$, voxel level, for the same subject at two imaging resolutions. Maps are projected onto the inflated cortical surface, zoomed on the fusiform gyrus. HR-fMRI shows more localized and patchy face-selective activations in the fusiform gyrus than SR-fMRI. Cos, collateral sulcus; OTS, occipito-temporal sulcus.

the representation matters. For example, examination of face-selective responses with HR-fMRI shows that there are several smaller clusters in the fusiform gyrus that respond to faces more than objects, in contrast to a larger and more diffuse region that shows higher responses to faces than objects with SR-fMRI (Grill-Spector et al. 2006b; see figure 14.5). Indeed, experiments using HR-fMRI have revealed that in the fusiform gyrus, body part–selective voxels are adjacent to (but distinct from) face-selective voxels (Schwarzlose et al. 2005) and a multimodal region in the superior temporal sulcus contains mixtures of unimodal voxels (Beauchamp et al. 2004).

HR-fMRI improves the signal because it images more localized cortical responses and there is less partial voluming (less mixing between different types of tissues, such as gray matter and white matter). The hope is that with HR-fMRI brain measurements will be closer to the scale of cortical representations. For example, if there are columns tuned to objects or object features, as suggested by electrophysiology experiments, perhaps HR-fMRI can be used to directly image these representations. Whether or not this will happen is an empirical question and depends on several factors including the following:

1. The size of the point spread function of the BOLD signal (How spatially diffuse is the BOLD signal relative to the localized neural response?). Current estimates of the point spread function of the BOLD signal using gradient echo (EPI) sequences are on the order of 2 mm (Shmuel et al. 2007). However, recent results suggest that when spin-echo sequences at high magnetic fields (7T) are used, the point spread function is small enough to enable robust measurement of orientation columns in human V1 (Yacoub et al. 2007).

2. The spatial scale of the underlying representations: Are there clusters of neurons that code for features, objects, or categories? If so, what are the dimensions of these clusters?

3. The cortical distance between neural clusters tuned to similar properties. Clusters may be less than 1 mm in size, but if the distance between clusters of similar properties is of the order of a few millimeters, it may be possible to resolve them with HR-fMRI.

4. The signal-to-noise ratio (SNR) of HR-fMRI. SNR is thought to decrease with voxel size because the signal decreases while the noise does not. Further, HR-fMRI may be particularly sensitive to fMRI-related noise factors such as subject motion. However, it is not entirely clear by how much the SNR decreases with smaller voxels because HR-fMRI produces lesser partial (sampling across diverse tissues) and measures across more homogeneous neural populations which may increase the fMRI signal. The SNR may be further improved by using higher field scanners and by advancements in fMRI protocols and coil designs.

Summary

Recent advancements in imaging methods and analysis approaches provide fundamental constraints for cognitive theories of recognition and offer important insights about the nature of cortical representations of faces and objects. We believe that studying these representations at the appropriate scale is important. We addressed the limitations of SR-fMRI for understanding the neural bases of object recognition: (1) SR-fMRI may not be the appropriate resolution for investigating the underlying representations. We suggested methods for approaching a resolution that may be more appropriate for studying object and face representations. (2) Methods that examine the mean response across a region may overlook important components of the representation because the information present in the distributed response may be different from that present in the average response. We believe future directions that utilize multiple advancements such as a combination of fMRI-A, HR-fMRI, and MVPA will be the most fruitful for progress in understanding the neural representation of objects and faces and providing empirical constraints for cognitive theories.

Acknowledgment

This research has been supported by NIH R21 EY016199-01 and Whitehall Foundation 2005-05-111-RES grants to KGS.

15   Intersubject Variability in fMRI Data: Causes, Consequences, and Related Analysis Strategies

Jean-Baptiste Poline, Bertrand Thirion, Alexis Roche, and Sébastien Meriaux

Functional Brain Imaging and Standard Procedures for Analyzing fMRI Data

Functional brain imaging has generated many hopes for further understanding the neural mechanisms that sustain our cognitive or sensorimotor processes, or the dysfunctions that lead to neurological and psychiatric diseases. The field has emerged with imaging tools such as positron emission tomography (PET) and single photon emission computed tomography (SPECT), but magnetic resonance imaging (MRI) has revolutionized the field because of its wide availability in general hospitals, its lack of known effect on health, and its technical potential in terms of temporal and spatial resolution. Compared to well-established electrical techniques developed since 1930, the spatial resolution and the signal-to-noise ratio (SNR) are major advantages of functional MRI (fMRI). Functional MRI has therefore become a major tool for investigating brain activity, despite well-known limitations such as the need to interpret the signal measured and the difficulty of obtaining absolute quantification. Nevertheless, the potential of fMRI, associated with anatomical MRI (including diffusion imaging) or other techniques, is immense in basic and applied science, generating an increasing number of research work and publications over the past ten years. This fast growth has not occurred without fundamental questions regarding how we structure our data analysis and what framework is required for interpreting the data of several subjects.

For decades, experimental psychology studies have relied on the reaction times in psychological tests, on the one hand, and on neuropsychology and patient deficits in relation to brain tumor resection, on the other hand, to form models of functions. Brain imaging, and fMRI in particular (Ogawa 1990), has brought a class of new potentials and challenges for which psychologists are not necessarily prepared, such as the amount of data to be analyzed, the specificities of imaging data, and the related statistical issues such as multiple comparison problems, data reduction, accounting and interpretation of dynamic aspect of the signal, and most of all, how to summarize, describe, and interpret the results from several subjects in group analyses or group comparisons. One aspect of this is the observed interindividual variability in fMRI, its origin and causes, and the strategies needed to model it. While this variability is a major difficulty when attempting to pool data from several subjects, it is also the source of information for understanding brain functions with respect to other subjects' data such as behavioral or genetic measurements.

The goal of this chapter is therefore to review some fundamental issues linked to intersubject variability and point to better methods of reporting observations across individuals. We first describe the usual course of action when analyzing multiple-subject data in fMRI. We show the limitations of the current hypotheses proposed in the standard analysis framework. We then consider some intersubject variations described in the psychological literature and consider how they might or might not be linked to imaging anatomical or functional variations. Finally, we depict some analysis strategies that should help us better consider the issues in fMRI analyses or study these variations in relation to other sources of variability.

What We Need to Know about the Data and Standard Analyses Procedures

As described previously, the origin of the data is hemodynamic. Following an increase of synaptic and spiking activity, neurons require more energy conveyed through the blood in the form of oxygen and glucose (Raichle et al. 2001). Through a mechanism not fully known, the result is first an increase of oxygen extraction followed by an increase of blood flow that overcompensates the loss of oxyhemoglobin.

The blood oxygen level–dependent (BOLD) contrast can be measured with MRI because the oxyhemoglobin is diamagnetic whereas the deoxyhemoglobin is paramagnetic, such that the MR signal increases with the ratio oxyhemoglobin over deoxyhemoglobin. The timing of this brain measure is relatively slow and peaks around 4 to 6 s after a short stimulation and returns to baseline in about 20 to 25 s. Hemodynamic responses are the subject of many research, with the long-term goal of extracting from the response shape quantitative information on neural activity. It is interesting to note that even if the absolute timing may be considered as poor, the differential timing between two conditions can be precise to the order of 100 ms. The BOLD contrast does not show much anatomical details, and is sensitive to artifacts caused by magnetic field variation around air-tissue interfaces, inducing loss of signal or volume deformation in these areas.

Usually, an fMRI data set is composed, per subject, of several runs of a few hundred three-dimensional scans typically acquired every 2 or 3 s. Before statistical analysis proper is performed, a few essential preprocessing steps are necessary: intrasubject realignment in space (subjects' movements inside the scanner are rarely negligible and are an important source of false detection or loss of signal) and time (each slice is acquired at a different time and the data are usually temporally interpolated to impose a unique timing for all voxels of one brain volume), correction for distortions due to the echo planar imaging characteristics (the technique that measures the BOLD signal), and alignment between functional and anatomical images. These steps are not appropriately dealt with because the corrections have so far been considered independently while they, in fact, depend on each other. In a first approximation, however, it is assumed that the intrasubject data are corrected and can be used for further analyses.

Second, subject activation patterns are constructed. This is most often done with the use of a linear model, which includes a series of variables to model the expected variation of the signal with time. This step is crucial, as the selected model is largely arbitrary. The model usually includes time courses that should account for the variation due to the experimental conditions, but also to scanner drift, movement effects, physiological signals measured within the scanner such as respiratory and cardiac signals, and any experimental factor that varies with time and is thought to have an impact on the measured BOLD signal. This step is generally performed heuristically by experimentalists who will try several models and choose one on the basis of the obtained results. This clearly introduces a bias in the reported findings. Also, the model itself is identical across voxels or brain regions (only the parameters of the model vary), even though hemodynamic properties or a priori information may vary greatly across brain regions. A better approach would be to select the model used at each voxel (or region of interest), but this would be computationally expensive and add a great complexity in the analysis.

Third, data from several subjects have to be pooled and tested for an effect. This is the most crucial and controversial step of fMRI analysis. Two schools of thought have been developed and present different arguments: the *Talairach atlas–statistical parametric maps (TA-SPM)* and the *individual functional localizer approach (IFLA)*. These approaches are also known as *voxel-based* versus *individual region of interest–based*. In the TA-SPM approach, the subject brain images are warped in a common space by spatially deforming the anatomy to match a template (most often this is the brain template constructed at the Montreal Neurological Institute, MNI-305) that should match a brain atlas such as the Talairach atlas (Talairach and Tournoux 1988), designed originally for the subcortical structures. If the match is generally found to be good in those structures (putamen, thalamus, etc.) at the resolution of functional images, matching of smaller anatomical structures or cortical features is much more problematic. The difficulty lies at several levels, the most fundamental being that there is no clear correspondence between the many cortical structures across individuals, which in itself is a subject of active research (Mangin et al. 2004; Rivière et al. 2002). While it is not too difficult for a neuroanatomist to label the main cortical sulci and gyri, it is not possible to define unambiguously an isomorphism between two normal brains, and clearly the problem is even more severe in case of pathology. At a less fundamental level, the results of the stereotactic normalization rely on the choice of an anatomical atlas that is not unique across laboratories or even studies, and on a normalization procedure that has to be parametrized. A more elaborate approach that is also based on deformation but takes the cortical anatomy into account has been developed by Fischl and colleagues (1999a). In this work, the deformation is done on the cortical surface and the match is driven by the depth of the main sulci. The procedure has been shown to better register functional information in the visual cortex, providing higher SNR when averaging functional images recorded during a primary visual experiment. Nevertheless, the method still relies on matching structures between which a unique transformation is not necessarily defined. It also involves practical problems such as defining a template surface, and in addition the technique is not robust, with distortions between the functional and the anatomical images (see, e.g., Grova et al. 2007, for a dedicated interpolation method to account for those possible small distortions).

In the IFLA, subjects are matched in a completely different manner. The underlying idea of IFLA is that a given robust paradigm will yield increased activity in the same functional regions across subjects. This was advocated first in the visual system by the work of Sereno and others (Sereno et al. 1995), who defined the visual cortex retinotopic regions V1,V2, V3, and so on, subject per subject, with a "functional localizer." The averaging or summarizing across subjects is then based "solely" on the defined functional regions, whereas these may not have the same size, exact matching of anatomical boundaries, or even the same topology.

In practice, individual regions of interest (ROIs) are defined when their positions are approximately in the same position as defined by the Talairach coordinate system (and therefore require a preliminary stereotactic normalization), or at least are within the same anatomical macrostructures (cortical lobes), so that only small spatial variations are allowed. Implicitly, the macroscopic anatomical structures are acknowledged as constraints for the functional organization. (We discuss this issue later in the text.) This approach has been pursued for several years, for instance, by Kanwisher and colleagues (see, e.g., Grill-Spector et al. 2004; Yovel and Kanwisher 2004), for whom defining subject–per-subject functional regions is a prerequisite to further functional investigation in the defined region, and who in a sense were using functional imaging almost like electrophysiologists might have studied the response of a neuron to a condition of interest after selecting it on the basis of a more standard condition. Their work led to the use of standard procedures to define robustly the parahippocampal area, the fusiform face area (FFA), and several other regions.

The approach is not without technical or more fundamental difficulties that have been pointed out by its detractors (Friston et al. 2006). First, the SNR will vary across subjects, such that the definition of the region based on a threshold on an SNR map may have to be adapted across subjects. There is no clear or easy way to do so, as the between-subject difference of the activated region size may be due to true variations but also to scanning specificities (amount of subject movement, scanner signal to noise, etc.). Second, the approach could limit the interpretation of the data to a single region that may badly represent the network sustaining the task. Third, the experimental condition that defines the fROI may itself not be very representative of the cognitive process under study. Having a unique set of experimental conditions to study brain modules may prove too constraining. Nevertheless, the approach does provide the experimentalist with a solution to the fundamental question of how to relate the different subjects' functional information that may show better reproducibility. This is crucial to the field, as we will develop further later. An excellent review of the localization issue in neuroimaging can be found in Brett et al. 2002.

In summary, current approaches (see also Ashburner et al. 2004; Worsley et al. 2002) do not offer an appropriate general solution because there is no clear definition of a referential or spatial coordinate system based on either anatomical or functional features. One of the goals of brain imaging should indeed be to define this referential that would allow the study of stable (reproducible) landmarks of brain functional organization across individuals or groups of individuals. This can be seen as a prediction problem: what minimal set of anatomical or functional features need to be defined such that the position of activity in a subject who has not yet been scanned can be predicted, and with what level of certainty and precision? Once this localization system has been defined, to what extent can we relate subjects' functional pattern variations in amplitude or position to variations of individual psychophysical or genetic features?

In the following, we discuss the origin of the functional variability, and propose some strategies to account for this variability.

What Is the Origin of Functional Variability?

In this section, we review various sources of the observed functional variability across subjects with fMRI and classify them according to their different nature.

Are Functional Patterns Different across Subjects?

First, we show an example demonstrating that functional patterns observed across subjects are not easily superimposed in the standard coordinate system, whatever the cause for this misregistration. Figure 15.1 (plate 6) presents the functional patterns of several subjects scanned during a computation task after coregistration to the MNI template using the most common software (SPM5). Although the differences may be due partly to the thresholding procedure, partial view of the data, one can see differences in signal amplitude and localization at a local level (small spatial mismatch of the order of a few voxels), but also the same network may not be involved in this task across subjects. Variability results, first, from all factors that are specific to the time of the scanning, such as state of the scanner or its equipment or state of the subjects. For instance, a subject may have a more or less rapid cardiac rate, which will influence the BOLD signal, or have more or less head movement during the scanning. These factors are generally of little interest. The limitation of stereotactic normalization

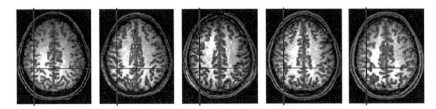

Figure 15.1 (plate 6)
Five individual SPM maps from five subjects performing a computation task compared to a language task. The activity is not always present at the same position in Talairach space. Intensity of activation (threshold: $z = 3$) is also different across subjects.

would typically induce variations in the position of the brain signal at a local level (about 1 cm). The crucial observation is that the variability across subjects is much greater than the intrasubject variability (see Wei et al. 2004), and this is a robust observation that has been made a number of times in the neuroimaging literature. It occurs despite the learning or habituation effects inherent to intrasubject reproducibility studies.

The more interesting variability arises from the intersubject variability. Clearly, this variability is demonstrated through many studies that first classify subjects on the basis of specific abilities, behavioral or psychological tests, and endogenous characteristics such as age, sex, or pathologies, and then compare the functional patterns of activity between the groups. Group size varies from ten individuals to large cohorts of fifty or sixty individuals in some cases, but many groups include between twelve and fifteen subjects. Additionally, correlation studies linking subject characteristics (age, psycho-physics scores, etc.) with BOLD activity are numerous and avoid the difficult issue of selecting a reference group for comparison, very much as so-called parametric experimental designs vary a parameter during scanning to find the BOLD variation as a function of this parameter (also avoiding the choice of a "control" condition). Phenomenological observations such as "subject's memory score correlates with magnitude of activity in the insula" may tell us something of how memory is implanted in neural circuitry.

The link between the results of these studies and the underlying anatomical variability is also generally unclear in the literature. One could design a case where the variation in the underlying structure position, not appropriately corrected by spatial normalization, would yield a variation in intensity for a given position. One could thus observe only positive and negative correlations that were due to the displacement of the activity within a region or of the underlying anatomical structure with the regressed parameter. For instance, if the anatomical structure of the subjects in one group is located 5 to 10 mm away from the anatomical structure of the subjects in a control group, one would observe a spurious difference when comparing the functional brain activities of the two groups. Functional imaging has likely not paid enough attention to these issues so far since those anatomical differences are not easy to detect and characterize.

Because of the very large number of variables or parameters that, in principle, could classify subjects, it is obvious that even after grouping on the variable of interest a large variation would remain within groups. This variability has not often been studied, mainly for methodological reasons: A large number of subjects is needed to study this variability. This remaining intersubject variability should have a dramatic impact on group study sensitivity but may also affect group studies specificity. In a recent study, Thirion and colleagues (Thirion et al. 2007a) analyzed a large database of more than eighty subjects. Using several different groups of fifteen subjects or fewer, they showed that current analyses performed with this number of subjects are poorly reproduced and recommend using at least twenty subjects. With twelve to fifteen subjects, it is generally not possible to detect the presence of several subpopulations within the group. The classification of subjects in groups with similar functional patterns has rarely been attempted, simply because such investigations require a very large number of subjects, leading to high cost. It is likely, however, that the intersubject variability mostly considered as noise so far will be the subject of investigations and eventually be explained. This may require new generation of web-based tools and analysis methods for accessing and using previous neuroimaging results in current analyses.

Anatomical Variability: Cytoarchitectonics, Sulcogyral, and Other Anatomical Structures
Cytoarchitectonics, first studied by Brodmann in 1909, has been recently revisited by Zilles and collaborators (Zilles et al. 2004). Their work demonstrates that the intersubject variability of cytoarchitectonic areas may be important. For instance, it is reported that the size of the early visual area can vary greatly, possibly up to a factor of 2 in some extreme cases. While this variation may be linked to functional ability, systematic studies of such correspondences are still rare and extremely difficult to perform on a (large) cohort, because cytoarchitectonics can be assessed only postmortem. The progress of MRI resolution and diffusion imaging may provide such information in the future.

The link between cytoarchitectony and sulcogyral anatomy is also a subject of further research. The main sulci formed early in the development are very likely good frontiers for cytoarchitectonic areas as demonstrated in Fischl et al. 2007, but smaller structures may or may not be linked with functional modules or variations of cytoarchitectony. Studies of sulcogyral anatomical variability across subjects (Rivière et al. 2002) demonstrate that the variability is important even for normal subjects, and the euclidean distance between two structures labeled as identical can be of the order of a centimeter. These authors also show that small structures may or may not be present.

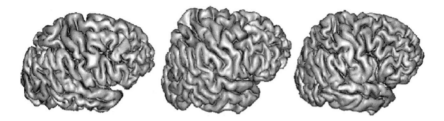

Figure 15.2
The cortical lateral surface of three normal subjects. It is clear from this picture that the sulcal structure cannot be matched voxel to voxel across subjects.

In figure 15.2, three brain cortical surfaces are represented (see BrainVisa, www .brainvisa.info). It is clear from this figure that the correspondence is extremely difficult to perform in some areas (for instance, at the position of the colored circles). To find the correspondence, one has to define the reproducible structure across individuals, and therefore the criteria on which these measures of reproducibility can be based. It is interesting that almost the same issues are the subject of research in comparative anatomy. Across species, criteria for homology are defined as follows for the nervous system:

• similarity of position in "natural coordinates," not cartesian coordinates (position in a network, in a chain of elements);
• similarity of specific criteria (e.g., same cytoarchitectonics, same proportion of neurotransmitter receptors); and
• continuity of the criteria in close by species in the evolution tree (this criterion is important to differentiate homology and homoplasy).

Other anatomical structures such as white matter fiber tracks are only at the early stages of investigation with diffusion MRI. It is possible, and in our opinion very likely, that important variations will be found across subjects for small tracks. Future research should investigate the link between these variations and functional variability found in fMRI or other imaging techniques.

Intersubject Variations Observed in Psychology
In psychology, intersubject variability, its status, its meaning to, and how it impacts on or participates in current theories is not fully resolved. The question is how one could combine the observation of stable differences between individuals with the search for a general law, for which intersubject variability would be treated as an error term. This error is the quantity that will be used to show differences between groups of subjects, and this framework leads to the analysis of variance often used in classical psychology.

On the other hand, "differential psychology" searches for stable variations between individuals, using correlation methods to demonstrate that behavior variations are due to individual differences. Interestingly, differential psychology was born with the work on intelligence of Galton, who invented the correlation coefficient to show that intelligence had an hereditary component, using parents–children cohorts, an enterprise that was inspired by the evolution theory. But differential psychology and classical psychology have not yet been unified into a single framework, despite the work of many (e.g., Lautrey 2002; Reuchlin 1999). Individual differences are considered using two models. First, the variations are not fundamental, but simple modifications of the parameters of a single model. In other words, subjects use the same information processing but with different time constants or speed for the various operations. The second possibility is that the differences correspond to different cognitive strategies, leading to different observed patterns with fMRI. It has been shown, for instance, that to memorize words, some subjects use subvocal repetition, others memorize the words first letters, others use the words meaning (Logie et al. 1996). Depending on the ability to mentally rotate figures (Eme and Marquer 1999), for example, a cognitive task can be resolved differently.

Another well-known domain in which individual differences are particularly striking is the representation of language, which depends strongly on both gender and laterality, but atypical language representations are found frequently in the general population (see Crivello et al. 1995, in which a right-handed subject showed a right inferior frontal gyrus activity in a comprehension task).

Though these differences are well known in psychology and brain imaging, it is generally not practical to have submit a subject to many long psychological tests to make sure he or she can be safely grouped for the cognitive process under study before being scanned. Furthermore, the interaction between possible categorizations of subjects may be important and unknown in many cases, making the grouping extremely hard to detect. While groups with or without specific abilities/pathologies can be formed and their functional patterns compared, undetected subgroups may exist. If the groups are selected using strong behavioral or demographic constraints, it must be remembered that the results of the study will only stand for those specific subject populations. It should also be noted that, in general, finding differences in the fMRI patterns between groups does not necessarily imply that these differences reflect the neural cause for the group partition.

Brain Imaging: A Promising Phenotype for Genetic?

Genetic information and brain imaging already have a common significant history, through the study of either genetic pathologies, large samples, or family links such as siblings or homozygous (MZ) or heterozygous (TZ) twins. In a recent review of the relationship between anatomical brain structures and genetic information, Leonard and colleagues (2006) argued that brain structures could be a plausible intermediate phenotype between "genome" and "cognome," the cognitive phenotype. They reviewed the variations in cortical size, asymmetry, and sulcogyral shape with the variation of genetic proximity, and how these variations can predict differences in the subject's ability to perform a verbal task or demonstrate computation skills. It was demonstrated that the labeling of the cortical structures, as performed in Rivière et al. 2002, is a promising avenue for such studies.

The relation between *functional* brain imaging pattern and genetics has recently attracted renewed attention (Hariri et al. 2002; see also the work of Weinberger and colleagues, e.g., Winterer et al. 2005). For instance, Hariri and collaborators studied the 5HTT-LPR: a variable number of tandem repeats polymorphism in the promotor region of the serotonin transporter gene. People have either two short (*ss*, 20%), one short and one long (*sl*, 50%), or two long alleles (*ll*, 30%). The *l* (long) allele is linked to higher concentration of 5HTT mRNA and greater 5-HT reuptake (as shown in cultured human lymphoblast cell lines). In vivo SPECT imaging also shows differences in 5HTT binding levels. The *s* (short) allele appears to be dominant. The level of serotonin transporter translates into differences in anxiety levels and cognitive capacities. The authors show that groups sorted as a function of their genotype differ in the functional activity of structures such as the amygdala: individuals with one or more 5HTT-LPR short alleles show an increased amygdala response to threat-related stimuli. Though these types of results are still rare, it is expected that the construction of large databases mixing anatomical and functional brain imaging, psychophysics, and genetic data will, in the near future, better relate subjects' brain imaging phenotypes and genotypes. This obviously involves important ethical issues that are only partly common to any genetic study.

In *Genes, Brain, and Cognition: A Roadmap for the Cognitive Scientist* (2006), Ramus and others review the issues of the genetic influence on cognition, and the neuroimaging intermediate phenotype. It is argued that if many cortical areas are prewired, their final tuning or functions are largely the effect of environmental factors.

Genetic information or phenotype closely related to genetics such as functional genomic data offer a vast spectrum of possible characteristics for subject classification. For instance, recent DNA chips can provide one million single nucleotide polymorphisms (SNP) per subject, and the latest very high throughput platforms an even greater amount of data. Studying the relation between brain anatomy and function using the current imaging tools with this tremendous amount of genetic or epigenetic information is certainly a challenge for the future. The endophenotype provided by neuroimaging may explain more of the intersubject variability than the current behavioral phenotypes used in genetic studies. Eventually, this wealth of information may be used in more individualized therapies for patients.

Consequences: Lack of Reproducibility of fMRI Group Analyses and Some Strategies to Increase Reproducibility

An important consequence of the many sources of variation that can affect functional pattern is, in our view, the lack of reproducibility in brain imaging. This lack of reproducibility is difficult to quantify. It strongly depends on the brain system being studies and the strength of the observed signal. Clearly, the primary visual system generates very strong and reproducible signals in the primary visual areas, simple motor tasks define a network of regions that are clearly seen in standard protocols, the signal of a single sentence can be detected in the superior temporal gyrus, and parahippocampal place area (PPA) or fusiform face area (FFA) are well reproduced. But experimental psychologists are often concerned with weaker signals and less reproducible patterns. One crucial factor is that the number of subjects involved in a particular study is often around twelve to fifteen (Murphy and Garavan 2004). With such small numbers, the influence on the average result of only a few subjects (and sometimes only one) can be very significant. Nevertheless, scanning is costly, long and tedious and rarely involve large groups, making the study of potential group inhomogeneity more difficult. A second crucial factor is the large amount of imaging data (around 40,000 intracranial voxels in a BOLD image). This prevents simple categorization and implies data reduction techniques that may impose interpretation constraints.

As previously mentioned, the study by Thirion et al. on a large database of more than eighty subjects using a unique functional protocol is one of the first to systematically quantify the potential lack of reproducibility for group analysis, using various testing procedures and two reproducibility measures. To summarize, cluster level tests are more reproducible than local maxima tests, mixed effect models accounting for intrasubject variance also provide more reliable results, and more important, the number of subjects should be around twenty-five for a good reproducibility. This study also makes it clear that the lack of reproducibility has much to do with the lack of sensitivity of studies with small numbers of subjects. This is an important point because papers often base their interpretation of the data not only on the results found at a given statistical threshold but also on the negative results, as it is easy to forget that lack of significant results does not imply no signal. This, of course, does not mean that one should lower the statistical threshold that would increase the risk of false-positive findings.

Furthermore, analyses techniques are not standardized, nor are they easy to compare and reproduce. A recent experiment in which a single data set was made available for analysis to all on the Internet demonstrates that analysis techniques are also a significant source of variation in the reported results in the literature. The "Functional Imaging Analysis Contest," presented at the 2005 Human Brain Mapping in Toronto, involved most of the main producers of data analysis software and methods (SPM, FSL,

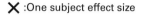

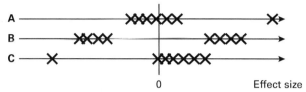

A: positive outlier; weak risk of false positive
B: two groups: the average is a bad summary
C: negative outlier: risk of false negative

Figure 15.3
Three cases for nonhomogeneous groups. Subjects' activity intensity (effect size) is represented by red crosses.

BrainVoyager, AFNI, and many others). Though all methods found very strong activity in primary auditory cortex, other reported results varied significantly with the analysis method used (Poline et al. 2006). It is worth noting that the reproducibility issue has been pioneered in particular by Genovese et al. (1997), Strother et al.(2002), Laconte et al. (2003), and Liou et al. (2003).

Analysis Strategies to Better Deal with Intersubject Variability

We present here some techniques and strategies that partly address the issues exposed in the preceding sections. First, we show how group homogeneity can be assessed in the framework of the standard coordinate system with the use of global intersubject distances, and discuss the use of robust statistics, diagnostic tools, and model selection techniques. Second, we extend these ideas in the spatial domain and describe techniques that should correct for small variability in the Talairach space, the so-called parcellation techniques. Last, we briefly describe new approaches based on reproducibility measures, together with the use of a large database to investigate the relation between variations of functional patterns and variability of the subjects' psychophysics scores.

Group Analysis in Inhomogeneous Populations
Group analyses that can be performed from standard software packages such as SPM, FSL, AFNI, and others test for the differential effect of one experimental condition versus another by averaging BOLD signal across subjects at each voxel, and comparing each such average with the corresponding across-subject variance. Figure 15.3 shows a number of cases where this test may badly represent the group activity. All these cases

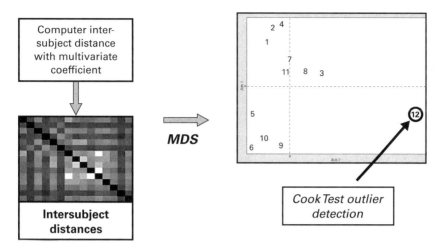

Figure 15.4 (plate 7)

The Distance toolbox principle. It allows for a rapid evaluation of the group functional pattern homogeneity. Models with nonparametric statistics are more sensitive.

are examples of "nonhomogeneity" because either the underlying distribution of subject is indeed not unimodal or the sampling of a unimodal distribution has yielded extreme values. Kherif and colleagues (Kherif et al. 2004) showed that pairwise global distances between individual functional patterns can be computed and the resulting distance matrix represented in a two-dimensional subspace to help spot potential outliers or groupings. A test for the influence of a particular subject over the average (the Cook test) can then be used to label subjects as potential outliers in the sense that their distance from other subjects is abnormally high (under multivariate normal distributional assumptions). We illustrate the method's principle in figure 15.4 (plate 7). Mériaux and colleagues (2006) developed a software to allow neuroscientists to perform outlier diagnosis ("Distance," downloadable as an SPM toolbox) and demonstrated that outliers occur relatively frequently in fMRI studies by analyzing more than twenty fMRI data sets. They showed that more than a third of the data sets and contrasts studied presented outliers and potential grouping effects. The potential causes for these have yet to be established and are study-dependent.

This work can be complemented by a voxel per voxel analysis, as developed in the diagnostic toolbox by Luo and Nichols (2003). Compared to the global pattern approach, this enables to detect individual brain regions that show inconsistent signal with respect to the other subjects, even if the general pattern does not demonstrate strong differences across subjects. However, this approach, being univariate, has a multiple comparison problem that may require further investigations.

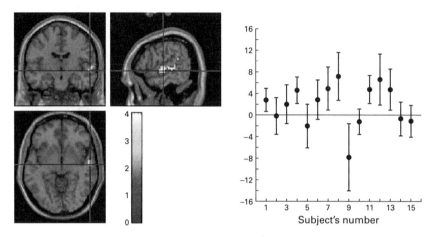

Figure 15.5 (plate 8)

The effect size and intrasubject estimated variability in the temporal lobe responding to language stimulation. In this specific situation, the mixed effect model downweights the measure of the subject with the smallest effect and therefore yields a more sensitive statistic than the random effect model.

Mériaux and colleagues therefore considered the use of robust and nonparametric statistics to better account for potential subject random or nonrandom dispersion (see also Wager et al. 2005; Woolrich 2008). Outlier diagnosis provides a valuable tool to assess group homogeneity. However, outliers detected from a joint analysis of all subjects' data cannot be dropped from the ensuing statistical test without breaking the fundamental assumption that the subjects are sampled independently. Robust statistics coupled with nonparametric resampling techniques such as permutation or bootstrap tests offer a valid statistical framework for group analysis in inhomogeneous populations. Standard statistics are fragile with respect to normality hypotheses when too few subjects are included, and the use of robust statistics such as the Wilcoxon signed rank, the sign test, or the empirical likelihood ratio may result in significantly enhanced detection power compared to the conventional t-statistic (Roche et al. 2007). A closely related idea is to use mixed-effect models, which explicitly incorporate the intrasubject variance in the inter subject variability model (intra subject variance may be due to thermal instability, respiratory signals, spikes, poor movement correction, etc). Mériaux, Roche, and collaborators (2006) also considered, and showed that this often increases sensitivity as well since subjects' signal will be downweighted according to the reliability of their measurements. Figure 15.5 (plate 8) shows an example of a group analysis in which the subject with the lowest effect size also has the highest intrasubject variance. In such a situation, mixed effect models associated with a nonparametric test would typically yield improved detection power.

Parcellation Technique to Account for Small Spatial Misregistration

It should be noted first that reports of brain imaging results are most often presented as a list of the positions in the standard space (Talairach space) in millimeter units. The results summary tables are formed with the local maxima of smoothed images. This means that the voxel resolution, although apparent in result tables, is lost and local maxima in fact represent a certain volume of activity. The data are generally smoothed by a spatial filter of 10 to 12 mm (full width at half maximum) such that a peak of activity represents a brain region on the order of the centimeter in the three directions of space. In other words, description of the results is performed at the voxel level, but the underlying biological phenomenon is thought to be at a regional level and therefore is the analysis. Indeed, the description and the communication of the results are done at the level of a functional region. The smoothing operation does help by allowing for some overlap between activities that are not located in the same place across subjects, but it is blind to the actual form of the signal, and indeed the amount of smoothing to be performed is rather arbitrary.

We are in search of a method that can account for signal difference in terms of spatial extent, localization, intensity, and possibly allowing for zero activity in some subjects. Flandin et al. (2002a, 2002b, 2003) proposed to use a mixture of Gaussian low to model both the location (through the spatial coordinates x, y, z) and the intensity of one or several contrasts of interest (say f1, f2, ... fn). Having chosen a number of classes corresponding to the usual resolution of group analyses (e.g., 500), it is possible to fit the parameters of the Gaussians through maximization of the likelihood of the model and expectation maximization procedure, including all subjects' activation maps in the data. The result of the algorithm is, for each class, a set of parameters describing the average position and average activation for each contrast. Grouping the voxels by their closest center of class, one can visualize that not all subjects will have the same number of voxels in the class, allowing some subjects to more extended activity than others. Some subjects may not even be represented in a class. Figure 15.6 (plate 9) shows the result of such an algorithm on an fMRI data set comprising twelve subjects. The number of classes (also denoted intersubject parcels) can be chosen for a study using either Bayesian information criteria (since a model distribution of the data is constructed) or cross-validation (Thyreau et al. 2006). This data reduction scheme should also allow for testing a region by condition interaction (Jernigan et al. 2003). Simon et al. (2004) use a similar strategy but with only functional information and a predefined (small) number of classes.

Recently, Thirion and collaborators (2005) developed the concept further. They considered a technique to constrain (soft constraint) every subject to be represented in all parcels, a desirable feature. The inference is then performed through randomization tests. It can be seen on figure 15.7 (plate 10) that the detection may prove to be much more sensitive than usual analysis techniques. This is because the algorithm adapts to

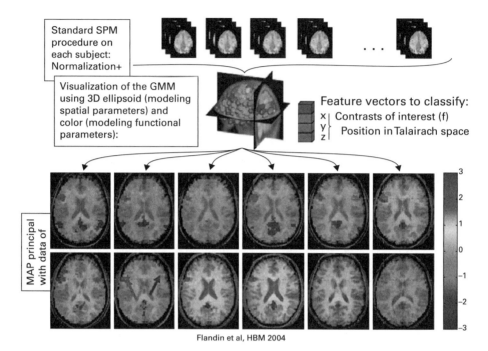

Flandin et al, HBM 2004

Figure 15.6 (plate 9)

Scheme of the Gaussian mixture model parcellation. Notice that the red parcel is not exactly identical across subjects, and may not even be present in outlier subjects (e.g., last subject on bottom row).

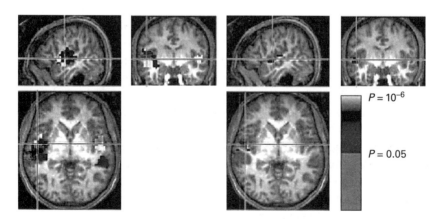

Figure 15.7 (plate 10)

(Left) Random effect analysis using rerandomization and parcellation technique. (Right) Standard analysis. The gain in sensitivity (with controlled risk of error corrected 5%) is due to adaptation of the parcels to individual subject activity.

individual signals, but is constrained enough so as not to produce high statistics under the null hypothesis. (See Thirion et al. 2005 for further details.) The increased sensitivity is a desirable feature, but more importantly these techniques provide *a subject per subject information on the intensity, extent, and position of the activation signal*. These individual parameters can then be related to the subject's behavioral, demographic, or genetic data and yield more robust results than voxel-based analyses.

Analyses Based on Reproducibility Measures and Large Databases

New techniques for group analysis may follow the work of Thirion et al. (2007a), who developed a method that searches for regions showing a high degree of reproducibility across subjects. The technique makes an important conceptual shift from the current detection strategy. It is based on a leave–one-out cross-validation scheme. Potentially interesting regions are selected on the basis of standard group analysis with one subject removed. The left-out subject is then searched for local maxima in a region close to the group activity, and if activity is found in the vicinity, the area is marked as a potential functional landmark. The operation is repeated for all subjects and landmarks showing a reproducibility of more than a given threshold are retained for further analysis. It therefore implements a top-down strategy, using (partial) group results to find individual activity, as opposed to techniques that rely solely on a bottom-up strategy (finding individual results first, then averaging). The advantages of the approach are numerous: It allows a (small) variation of the subject position activity, it can deal appropriately with cases in which only a significant number of subjects responded, and it yields a sparse representation of the networks involved in different contrasts. (See figure 15.8 and plate 11 for an example for which the landmarks activity could be clustered into three groups of subjects with different functional patterns.) The technique was further refined by Thirion et al. (2006b), who used belief propagation networks to associate activated regions that are found in the same relative position across subjects.

As noted above, studying individual neuroimaging variations in relation to other data may require a large number of subjects. Indeed, if the full multivariate distribution of activity were to be estimated, the number of individuals would have to be extremely large because the number of neuroimaging variables is high (around 40,000 at the voxel level for fMRI, but still several hundreds if this is to be reduced at the scale of brain regions). Whole genome association studies face a similar challenge, and they resort to increasingly larger groups of subjects (from several thousands to tens of thousands). Acquiring this amount of neuroimaging data is usually not feasible.

Nevertheless, large neuroimaging cohorts are being acquired in order to better investigate the interactions of larger number of imaging, behavioral, or biological variables. Cohorts of anatomical data or fMRI resting state are easier to collect because they do not require the selection of a number of experimental tasks. For instance, Kiel and collaborators, scanned a large population of schizophrenic patients ($n = 100$).

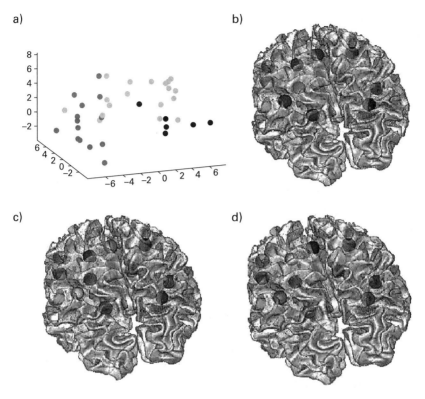

Figure 15.8 (plate 11)
Functional landmarks based on a reproducibility measure. Those landmarks do not have the same intensity of activity across subjects, and the group could be divided into three subgroups (shown with a multidimensional scaling in panel a in blue, green, and red). Panels (b), (c), and (d) show the average intensity of the landmarks for the three groups.

A large cohort of normal subjects is still under construction in Orsay/Neurospin (see Pinel et al. 2007 that should allow the investigation of results reproducibility, and the association of these data with genetic and behavioral data should also provide an extremely useful resource for studying the links between genetic, behavioral, and neuroimaging data.

In the near future, these databases should store not only data, but also models of the data such as multivariate distributions, and evolve from a data repository into a data investigation system. Those models can be refined when new data are entered and while providing a priori for analyses on independent datasets. If completed with statistical query systems, these databases would in fact be converted into expert systems to which neuroscientific questions could be addressed.

Conclusion

We believe that the conjunction of two nonindependent problems has hampered functional brain imaging research: first, the localization problem (Brett et al. 2002) and, second, the lack of reproducibility of group analysis results caused by both intersubject variability and the small number of subjects included in group analyses. These two issues should be better dealt with using coherent intersubject anatomical information, larger sample size and reproducibility measures, respectively. How to and at which scale these coherent structures should be defined is a research question that may be best addressed with the use of predictive models. In the future, we hope that the accumulation and annotation of data will permit a better statistical modeling of interindividual variations and eventually better models of brain function and structure.

The problems described in this chapter are general to brain imaging, not only to detection/localization, and should eventually impact other research areas such as connectivity analyses. It is likely that effective connectivity studies still lack robustness with respect to the number of regions included in the study (the regions form the nodes of the graph) or the definition of these regions. Those approaches should also benefit from reproducibility approaches and better anatomical information integration.

Acknowledgments

We would like to thank P. J. Toussaint for great help in correcting this manuscript. J.B.P. was partly supported by the IMAGEN project, which receives research funding from the European Community's Sixth Framework Programme (LSHM-CT-2007-037286). This manuscript reflects only the author's views and the Community is not liable for any use that may be made of the information contained therein.

IV   The Underdetermination of Theory by Data

16 Neuroimaging and Inferential Distance: The Perils of Pictures

Adina L. Roskies

Cognitive neuroscience has made tremendous gains since the time of its baptism in a taxi in the late 1970s (Gazzaniga et al. 2002). Numerous technical and technological inventions have made those gains possible. Perhaps the most visible of these inventions are new brain imaging techniques, such as functional magnetic resonance imaging (fMRI). Functional MRI, along with a few other imaging techniques, has enabled us to probe brain activity in normal, behaving humans, providing us with novel information about the functional organization of human cognition. Results of fMRI studies are often represented in grayscale images of the brain, overlaid with colored regions denoting areas of activity. Although these images are now omnipresent in the cognitive neuroscience literature as well as the popular press, only recently has any explicit attention has been paid to the epistemic status of neuroimages themselves, either actual or apparent. What is the relation between fMRI data and the conclusions of cognitive neuroimaging experiments? How are neuroimages perceived and interpreted? How should they be? Answers to these questions have implications for the role neuroimaging results play in the scientific process, and for how neuroimages are received and interpreted beyond the scientific community.

Neuroimages are epistemically compelling: They invite us to believe. The phenomenology of the pull of credibility is introspectively undeniable, and its effects recently confirmed by empirical studies. For example, McCabe and Castel found that poor arguments are rated as better when accompanied by neuroimages as opposed to bar graphs or no figures at all (McCabe and Castel 2008). Weisberg and colleagues explored a related issue, finding that the scientific explanations are judged to be improved when accompanied by neuroscientific data, even when that data are irrelevant to the point at issue. They found that both naïve subjects and those with some college-level neuroscience or psychology training rate scientific explanations as better when they include explanatorily irrelevant reference to neuroscience data, such as neuroimages (Weisberg et al. 2008).

Reassuringly, this biasing effect is not seen in experts. Although their study did not focus explicitly on neuroimaging data, Weisberg et al.'s results support the notion that information from neuroimaging adds to the apparent epistemic weight of scientific reasoning, even when it fails to be epistemically relevant. Another study showed that neuroimages can affect mock juror's legal decisions (Gurley and Marcus 2008), but whether the effects were evidence of bias or proper weighing of evidence is impossible to say. At this juncture, it is clear that neuroimages affect epistemic assessment, and that sometimes they do so by introducing confusion and bias, but separating cases in which neuroimages mislead from cases where their evidential value is properly assessed is challenging. Further studies that focus on neuroimages are needed to properly characterize the sources and extent of the prejudicial impact of neuroimages.

Weisberg et al.'s data might indicate that the biasing effect is a worry only for nonexperts, but to conclude that the epistemic status of images is not an issue for experts would be premature. I suggest that the epistemic status of neuroimages is difficult to assess, even for experts, because of inferential difficulties that arise prior to, and even independently of, the construction of images. Thus, interpretive problems arise in the inferential chain not only because of the images themselves, but because of the nature of imaging. Our epistemic limitations in this area are quite real. Although these do not undermine the value of imaging, their impact is easy to overlook. None of the studies undertaken so far has tried to determine whether or how epistemic limitations affect experts' assessment of the epistemic status of imaging data. As studies show, the proper appreciation of the epistemic status of neuroimages is even more problematic for the layperson. One possible explanation for the epistemic effects in nonexperts is a mismatch between what I have called the *actual inferential distance* and the *apparent inferential distance* between neuroimages and that which they are meant to represent (Roskies 2008).

Inferential Distance

A central question in the philosophy of science regards how we should understand the epistemic status of scientific conclusions. Intuitively, some conclusions are more warranted than others, because of the quality of evidence, the support the evidence can provide for a particular claim, the availability of alternative explanations, and the epistemic status of assumptions that play a role in the reasoning that leads us to the claim in question. There has been little agreement about how to unpack the notion of epistemic status. One might attempt to quantify the amount or degree of error to which a conclusion may be subject on the basis of error potentially introduced by the technical and inferential steps relied on in the course of an experiment. Error analysis has been used in this regard.

Alternatively, one might look to the range of states of affairs compatible with a conclusion based on observations, and thus the degree to which a scientific claim is equivocal. Information-theoretic approaches such as this have been championed by some

(Dretske 1981). Bayesian epistemology assesses the degree of confirmation or confidence we ought to have in our conclusion, based on the degree of confidence we have in the steps involved in reaching it. One might also consider relevant the probability that a scientific statement will have to be jettisoned or revised if assumptions it is based on are overturned.[1] Each of these notions is logically independent of the others, although, in fact, they are often highly correlated. Regardless of which measure one prefers, or whether ultimately what matters is some combination of several of them, determining actual epistemic status will involve a characterization of the inferential steps that mediate between observations and the phenomena they purport to provide information about. This characterization will include both the nature of the steps, and their relative certainty, as measured in one or a combination of the above ways. I'll call this characterization *inferential distance*.

My goals in this chapter are modest. There is no univocal way of characterizing inferential distance, or even the number and nature of inferential steps, as the logical positivists found to their dismay. Thus, I use the term primarily metaphorically, to gesture toward whatever epistemic dimensions best characterize the relation of scientific hypotheses to observations. My aim is to describe in rough terms the relation between the conclusions of cognitive neuroimaging studies, as represented by the neuroimage, and the data on which they are based. In so doing, I will point out some of the assumptions and theories that ground the inferential steps operative in actual scientific practice, as well as the limitations that must attend our interpretations.[2] In the absence of a means of quantifying inferential distance, we can view it as a comparative measure: Our conclusions cannot be more secure than the assumptions on which they rely. Future studies may provide more concrete measures of neuroimaging's epistemic status.

There can be a gap between a measure of how epistemically grounded a conclusion is, as based on actual methods and reasoning, and its perceived epistemic status, for instance, as apprehended by the layperson. I use "actual inferential distance" to refer to the inferences explicitly employed in a scientific practice, while "apparent inferential distance" indicates a more subjective measure characterizing the confidence people place in a conclusion on the basis of evidence.[3] In addition to characterizing the inferential distance of neuroimaging, this chapter explores the hypothesis that the actual and apparent (or perceived) inferential distance of neuroimages differ, and that this difference can largely be attributed to the misperception (or misconception) of neuroimages as photographs. I surmise that the difference is the source of the biasing effect of neuroimages for naïve consumers. When actual and apparent inferential distances come apart, people are prone to assign an unwarranted epistemic status to claims. Neuroimaging seems to be a case in which this mismatch is pronounced. On the one hand, the phenomena that neuroimaging studies investigate are inferentially far removed from the images produced; on the other hand, the image format is familiar and accessible. Like photographs, brain images seem be simple and straightforward:

They appear to wear their content on their sleeves. A consequence is that images are liable to be mistakenly apprehended as inferentially proximate.

The scientific content of this chapter will not be new to neuroscientists who employ imaging to investigate cognitive function, though it may be a jolt to be reminded of the epistemic compromises we make, awareness of which we often relegate to the back-burners of consciousness when actually doing the hard work of science. I hope the science discussed will be enlightening to those less familiar with the scientific under-pinnings of functional neuroimaging. The complexities of the technology and inter-pretational difficulties are points of fertile discussion and sometimes fervent debate in the field, and I make no attempt to weigh in on them here. However, these foci of de-bate may be good indicators of points at which the inferential distance of steps in the reasoning process is greatest. The main advances here consist in situating these issues in the context of a discussion of the epistemic role that images play, and in contrasting that role with what is plausibly and popularly taken to be an analogous technique.

This approach to the epistemic issues may be valuable in several ways. First, it be-hooves us to periodically reconsider the inferential distance of our techniques, in order to properly interpret and assess our data. Second, it is of interest to investigate whether a gap exists between the actual and the apparent inferential distance in the science itself, and whether and how that might affect scientific practice. Third, the discussion may be relevant for understanding the public consumption of neuroimages, and its potential social, political, and neuroethical implications. Finally, thinking of things in these ways may have particular importance for public discourse, and may help inform scientists about how to better convey their results to the public through the popular media.

Inferential Distance of Neuroimages

Inferential distance is a relational measure, so in explicating inferential distance we need to specify the relata. The inferential relata for any scientific program are interest-relative, as dictated by the scientific project. The goal of cognitive neuroscience is to map functional components of mind to neural structures. Long before imaging the brain was conceivable, William James identified the task of integrating mind and brain research:

A science of the mind must reduce ... complexities (of behavior) to their elements. A science of the brain must point out the functions of its elements. A science of the relations of mind and brain must show how the elementary ingredients of the former correspond to the elementary functions of the latter. (James 1890, 28)

Cognitive neuroimaging studies seek to fulfill these demands by enabling us to mea-sure the neural activity underlying cognitive and/or behavioral tasks in brain images constructed from MR data. Observables in these neuroimaging experiments are thus measures of subject behavior (including, for example, button pushes, reaction times, errors), and the MR signal collected during task performance. What we'd like to infer from these data are, on the one hand, behaviorally relevant component processes (the "elements of behavior") and, on the other, the patterns of neural activity that cause the MR signal (the "elementary functions" of the brain). The foregoing suggests we conceive of the process of imaging as consisting of two largely separable projects, what I will call the causal stream and the functional stream. The relevant relata for specifying the inferential distance of the causal stream are thus neural activity and the MR image, and for the functional stream they are the behavioral-cognitive elements and the MR image.[4]

The causal stream concerns the relation between the neural activity and the MR image. This stream requires the understanding of two different relations: the relation between neural activity and raw data, and the relation between raw data and image. The inferential distance of the causal part of neuroimaging can be thought of as the additive distance of these two measures. The functional stream is important for interpreting the functional relevance of neuroimaging data: In order to link neuroimaging data to cognition and behavior, an understanding of experimental design and its underlying assumptions are important. The complexity of the neuroimaging process makes it impossible to go into full detail about either stream in a short chapter. Here, I can indicate roughly what inferential steps are involved.

The Causal Stream

Neural Activity to Raw Data

Neuroimaging is so often characterized as a tool for measuring brain activity that people are frequently surprised that the magnetic resonance signal is insensitive to the electrical signals generated by neurons. The blood oxygenation level–dependent (BOLD) signal, which is by far the most widely used paradigm for functional neuroimaging, is not a direct measure of neural firing, or any immediate causal consequence of neuronal activity.[5] Instead, the MR signal is a measure of a quantity that changes as a downstream consequence of neural activity, and bears to it a complex relation. Sometimes the BOLD signal is described as measuring changes in blood flow that correlate with changes in neural activity. Even this is inaccurate, for BOLD imaging is also relatively insensitive to blood flow. As its name suggests, the BOLD MR signal depends on the blood oxygenation level. It is a direct measurement of the dephasing of spins of water molecules in blood, caused by local changes in magnetic susceptibility. The magnetic susceptibility of water (in this case, water in the blood) is affected by the local concentration of deoxygenated hemoglobin. Increased levels of deoxyhemoglobin reduces the BOLD signal; reduced concentrations increase it. Neural activity is linked to susceptibility changes in the following way: It increases local metabolic demands, and these are compensated for by an increase in local blood flow and capillary volume. Although active neurons consume oxygen, and thus increase the amount of deoxy-hemoglobin in the blood, the increased supply of oxygenated blood outstrips the oxygen consumed, resulting in a net increase in the concentration of oxygenated hemoglobin and a concomitant increase in the MR signal. Thus, a constellation of factors, some with opposing effects, are altered in the wake of neural activity.

The correlation between neural activity and increased MR signal is empirically well confirmed (Logothetis 2003; Logothetis and Pfeuffer 2004; Logothetis and Wandell 2004), but the quantitative relationship between changes in magnetic susceptibility and neural activity is not well understood. The underlying physiological mechanisms and their quantitative relationships remain phenomena of scientific inquiry. Our confidence in our ability to relate changes in the fMRI signal to neural activity depends on empirical generalization and corroboration by other methods that more directly measure metabolic demands and blood flow (Buxton 2002; Mukamel et al. 2005; Shmuel et al. 2006).

When considering the steps that allow us to draw conclusions about neural activity from imaging data, it becomes evident that a large number of neural states could conceivably give rise to the same signal, and furthermore, we currently lack means of ruling out many of those possibilities as improbable.[6] For example, with so many factors contributing to susceptibility effects, it is likely that the same net magnetic susceptibility changes can result from different combinations of changes in blood flow, volume, and oxygen extraction. If these correspond to different macroscopic activity patterns, then the signal is univocal with respect to this class of activity patterns. Moreover, the spatial and temporal resolution of the technique is such that the information it provides is orders of magnitude coarser than the neural firings we suppose are at the appropriate grain for understanding many aspects of cognition and behavior.

In addition, when making claims for the functional relevance of changes in activity, it is important to bear in mind that evidence suggests neuroimaging data reflects local synaptic activity, irrespective of whether it is excitatory or inhibitory. Thus, although the functional implications of these two types of synaptic transmission are quite different, the MR signal does not allow us to distinguish them. Moreover, the MR signal may reflect subthreshold neural activity and modulatory inputs from distant areas in addition to neural firing. It is not clear whether it could distinguish other physiologically relevant parameters, such as large changes in the firing rate of a few neurons, small changes in the firing rates of many neurons, or changes in neuronal synchrony in the absence of changes in mean firing rates. Finally, because the MR signal is not a direct measure of neural activity, the signal may be temporally and even spatially out of register with the activity changes that are ultimately the phenomenon of interest. For example, the vascular response to neural activity occurs with a delay of several seconds, and has a time course significantly broader than that of the neural activity it reflects. Although this might appear to be a problem, studies have found that the hemo-dynamic response is relatively stereotypical, so the temporal factors that distinguish the blood flow from the neural signals can be well accounted for during statistical modeling (Friston et al. 1995; Kruggel and Yves von Cramon 1999). In addition, both the geometry of the vasculature and the particular pulse sequences used in generating the MR data can sometimes lead to artifacts in which signal increases appear to come from regions at some remove from the active neural tissue.

All these possible sources of the MR signal illustrate the inferential distance between the signal and the scientific conclusions we draw from it; to bridge the gap, we have to make a variety of assumptions about the temporal and spatial relationships between blood flow changes and neural activity. To the extent that we can expect these issues to manifest equally across conditions, their influence will be effectively negated with direct contrast analyses. While experimental findings corroborate these assumptions in some paradigms, we must assume that the relations that have been established hold in diverse brain areas and independent of task.

Thus, fMRI doesn't directly measure neural activity, but rather reflects the net effect of other physiological factors that are causally related in a rather complex way to downstream consequences of neural activity. From this signal, neural activity is inferred to have increased or decreased. Inferences are grounded by a rough theoretical conception of the physiological changes that are influenced by activity and that themselves influence the MR signal; the rough theory is anchored at points by empirical results from other types of studies that more directly measure the relationship of blood flow, glucose and oxygen metabolism, and neural activity (Raichle and Mintun 2006). Although the general relationship is well established, the inferences that are justified by our current knowledge are rather coarse. Many neuroimagers who are more interested in cognition than in physiology take this relationship for granted; this is often warranted, but it is worth bearing in mind that unanswered questions about this most basic foundation of neuroimaging remain. Fine-grained inferences about local neural activity are much less warranted.

Raw Data to Image

There are a number of unknowns when it comes to inferring conclusions about brain activity based on the MR signal. However, it is not the raw signal that is typically analyzed to make claims about neural activity, but rather pooled and processed data from multiple trials, and often multiple subjects. This pooling is necessary, for the signal-to-noise ratio for neuroimaging is quite low. BOLD signals typically range about 0.5 and 2% above baseline, and there are numerous sources of noise, both biological and technical. To achieve significance and minimize effects of random noise, data from multiple scans is averaged. These averaging processes alter the inferential distance of the techniques in ways that are unclear, for while they enhance the signal–to-noise ratio, they also introduce additional factors that must be considered when interpreting the images. The pooled data are then analyzed and finally represented as an image. In constructing such a representation, certain conventional choices are made that can dramatically affect the visual appearance of the image. The very same visual image could represent any of a group of data sets, and the very same data set could be used to generate a variety of images. This multivocality also is a factor in determining the robustness of inferences based on neuroimages. These steps in converting raw data to an image are discussed further in the following text.

Of increasing concern to neuroimagers are the consequences of averaging or pooling data for inferential robustness. In most studies, multiple scans are averaged across persons. Averaging data across subjects introduces particular complexities. For example, there is considerable variation in individual brain structure as well as in structure-function relationships. Variation in structure is addressed by warping the individual data in order to register the brains in a common space, but we lack independent means for assessing the adequacy of the warping algorithms (Crivello et al. 2002; Gispert et al. 2003; Kruggel and Yves von Cramon 1999). Although warping may adequately address complexities introduced because of anatomical variability, functional-anatomical variability remains an issue.

At least some studies have shown highly variable patterns of brain activation in certain tasks (Miller et al. 2002). Dispersion in the location of functionally active areas can reduce the statistical significance of the data and/or produce resultant images that show activated regions that don't correspond to any actual functionally delineated brain region. Moreover, it is difficult to determine whether variability observed reflects true functional-anatomical differences, or different cognitive strategies. Because we often lack an independent handle on how tasks are performed, it is often impossible to distinguish between differences in functional anatomy and strategic differences as sources of variability.

Finally, the extent of variability itself is not well characterized, which makes inferences from group data to the individual subject, and to particular events, exceedingly problematic. Attempts to use fMRI for many practical purposes, such as lie-detection or making predictions about individual behavior, ought to be viewed with extreme skepticism. Better ways of assessing these factors will be critical in moving the field forward.

Even in single-subject studies, in which scans are averaged within-subject, satisfactory signal-to-noise still requires many trials. Thus, the final image data reflects not a brain event, but the aggregate of many. There are questions about whether and how people's strategies in tasks change over time (in many cases we know they do), the degree to which different trials are relevantly alike and in which ways they differ, and a host of potential confounds such as priming effects or habituation. Neuroimagers tend to be apprised of these issues, and often employ various behavioral measures to control for these factors, but all these factors contribute to inferential distance.

The low signal-to-noise ratio of the BOLD technique makes it impossible to simply read off results from a scan (even an averaged one), as one might read the presence of a protein off a Western blot, or a fracture off an x-ray. Instead, a number of methods are employed to extract significant results, including smoothing and a variety of statistical tests. Technical debates about proper statistical and data analysis abound in the literature, ranging from questions about how to correct for multiple comparisons to whether analysis should be hypothesis driven or whether brute-force statistics suffice. This chapter does not take on these technical questions, but notes their prevalence in order to underscore the point that, to the extent that there is disagreement about the proper way to analyze the data, we can presume that different background assumptions are called into play, and the different analytical approaches may affect the actual inferential distance of an imaging study. This supposition is confirmed by the fact that different ways of processing the data may affect results. For example, which voxels are identified as statistically significant can be affected by experimenters' choices, such as whether or not the raw data are spatially filtered. To the extent that we know the same raw data can produce different results depending on reasonable choices made about processing, we know there is not a one-to-one correspondence between data and image. This is true of any form of data reduction, but it emphasizes the need to know what analysis procedures are used in determining the results of a study and the importance of understanding their effects. For example, it would be of interest to know how much leeway there is in experimenter choice of various analysis parameters without radically affecting conclusions.

A number of features of imaging make inferences about brain activation from imaging data less secure than one might initially think, regardless of whether the data are represented as an image. The robustness of inferences about the causal stream is compromised by the preliminary nature of the theoretical grounding linking the BOLD signal to neural activity, and the nature of the information gained makes inferences about brain activity at the level of small groups of neurons tenuous. In addition, the signal–to-noise ratio necessitates averaging and creates difficult statistical issues, generating new interpretive problems at a variety of levels. We now turn to consider the other part of functional neuroimaging that allows us to link the image data to cognitive function.

The Functional Stream

Neuroimaging has been criticized as "the new phrenology." This is inapt: Despite the popularity of phrenological cartoons showing brain areas for loyalty, humor, or remembering where one put one's car keys, it has long been recognized that complex cognitive functions are not atomistically located in the brain. For instance, relatively early in the development of functional neuroimaging techniques, Petersen and Fiez wrote:

Elementary operations, defined on the basis of information processing analyses of task performance, are localized in different regions of the brain. Because many such elementary operations are involved in any cognitive task, a set of distributed functional areas must be orchestrated in the performance of even simple cognitive tasks.... A functional area of the brain is not a task area: there is no "tennis forehand area" to be discovered. Likewise, no area of the brain is devoted to a very complex function; "attention" or "language" is not localized in a particular Brodmann area or lobe. Any task or "function" utilizes a complex and distributed set of brain areas. (Petersen and Fiez 1993, p. 513)

The goal in neuroimaging is to assign function or processes to brain regions. How to identify those functions in the first place is a crucial question, critically dependent on work in cognitive psychology. Just how localized the identification must be is a matter of contention; new techniques suggest that attention to widely distributed patterns of activity is necessary to characterize neural representations and processes. Since all forms of interpreting images involves data reduction, one's starting assumptions can affect what aspects of the data are regarded as significant; strong localizationists may consider more of the data as below-threshold than those who focus more on pattern analysis. Ultimately, which way is best will depend on an as-yet-unarticulated theory of brain function. Regardless of how these issues play out, it is impossible to properly interpret data from neuroimaging without understanding task analysis and experimental design.

MR provides information about the global levels of magnetic susceptibility in blood and tissue, so images corresponding to unanalyzed data show signal throughout the brain. The bulk of metabolic activity and blood flow is devoted to supporting ongoing, non-task-related brain function. Raw MR images look quite unlike the grayscale images with colorful splotches that grace the pages of popular magazines and scientific journals, and little can be discerned from visual inspection of the images resulting from scans during performance of different tasks. In fact, only a small fraction of what is recorded by neuroimaging corresponds to task-related changes (Raichle and Mintun 2006). But then how do neuroimages provide information about the functional architecture of cognition? A number of methods have been developed to help identify regions involved in different tasks. These involve comparing MR data across different task conditions. Whether one uses standard subtractive techniques or more recent event-related designs, having a functional decomposition of a task is essential to good experimental design as well as interpretation.

A functional decomposition is a working theory of what sorts of processes are involved in task performance. In subtraction, one typically tries to identify task components by subtracting from the data collected during performance of a task of interest the data from another task involving many of the same components, ideally save one. Thus, one might believe that a memory task involves seeing a stimulus, holding it in working memory, seeing a second stimulus, judging whether the two are the same, and pressing one button if they are and another if they are not. To try to isolate the region(s) involved in working memory, one would then want to design a similar task in which the subject sees another stimulus but is not prompted to remember it, sees a second stimulus, makes a judgment not involving memory, and presses one of two buttons dependent on the judgment. If all worked according to plan, subtracting the scan from the nonmemory condition from the one generated by the task of interest, one would isolate the brain region(s) involved in holding something in working memory. This is an ideal characterization; despite widespread misunderstanding (Uttal 2001; Van Orden and Paap 1997), it is not necessary to isolate a single task component to learn something about cognition. Nonetheless, the interpretability of the data will depend on understanding the way in which complex tasks functionally coincide and ways in which they diverge in their demands.

A consequence of relying on these methods is that experimental design and outcome are heavily dependent on one's theoretical commitments to functional architecture. If, for example, one was mistaken in one's theory of the task components, one would misidentify the function of the region(s) resulting from a subtraction. For instance, with respect to the preceding example, if there were more task components in the first scan unmatched by corresponding tasks in the contrast, more regions would result from the subtraction than the ones actually subserving memory; if more were involved in the contrast task, deactivations would result; if the task analysis were largely mistaken, function could not properly be identified (though one could still conclude that the differences in performance of the two tasks involved the regions resulting from the subtraction). Some of these ambiguities can be addressed by obtaining adequate baseline data.

Similarly, when analyzing results of event-related designs, one must identify the types of events and the temporal profile of their occurrence during a sequence of task executions. This identification of event types and their time courses is essential to the workings of the general linear model (GLM) that tries to maximize the amount of signal fluctuations accounted for by fitting the data with different event-type time courses. Here, too, misidentification of event type or the appropriate occurrences can lead to errors in functional attribution. Pattern classification techniques often take deviations of signal from the mean and correlate them with particular stimuli or task types, providing information about large-scale patterns of brain activity that characterize particular task types or individual representational contents, often with surprisingly good predictive value (Haynes 2008; Mitchell et al. 2008; Soon et al. 2008). However, insofar as these techniques can provide insight into the computational basis of cognitive processing, some sort of functional model must underlie the analysis (see, for example, Mitchell et al. 2008).

There is much to be said about the issues surrounding functional decomposition. Many worry that our hypothesized functional decompositions reflect a naïve and inaccurate understanding of the cognitive processes underlying the performance of complex tasks, and worry that such inaccuracies would invalidate neuroimaging (Van Orden and Paap 1997). If, indeed, our understanding of tasks was massively in error and remained so, imaging would prove to be a problematic technique for investigating cognitive function. However, ontology is rarely if ever handed to us on a silver platter in any science, yet we generally maintain some confidence that science can provide us better and more accurate ways of looking at the world. For instance, the triumphs of physics and chemistry are the discoveries of basic concepts/entities such as electrons, kinetic energy, and x-rays, and a look at their histories reveals numerous erroneous posits. Much of the work ahead for neuroscience is in conceptualizing the proper ontology for understanding brain function, but neuroscience is not on worse footing than any other science. Moreover, neuroimaging should not be seen as working in a vacuum. It should and does draw on various other disciplines for theoretical insight and empirical corroboration. Data and theories from cognitive psychology provide a theoretical background with which to work, and results from anatomy, comparative neurobiology, and neuropsychology can also help constrain theories of brain function. Functional triangulation and corroboration from other brain-imaging studies are also essential to the development and refinement of our psychological theories about functional decomposition (Bechtel 2002a; Roskies and Petersen 2001), and computational models can be used to test hypotheses. Those models that effectively predict relations between representational content and patterns of brain activity can lend credence to certain functional hypotheses. Thus, though some are apt to see the glass half empty, those more optimistic about the scientific endeavor are inclined to point to the practical success of scientific bootstrapping in order to see the glass as half full. Any way you look at the glass, however, it is shot through with theoretical commitments. One cannot discern its contents purely by visual inspection.

What is the relevance of this discussion for the issue of inferential distance? It seems that the inferential distance for functional attributions is going to be a function of how well established various functional components of tasks are. In task analysis, identifying sensory and motor components is relatively straightforward, but identifying more cognitive components is more speculative. Their plausibility is tested by experimental manipulations designed to target a specific functional component, for example, by changing task load or creating interference. Understanding the functional or computational components of various cognitive tasks is a primary focus of cognitive psychology, and has also been addressed by other fields such as computer science and linguistics. Just how well established a particular component is will vary, and judgments about its nature will depend on the evidence in its favor, the availability of alternative accounts, and its ability to unify different task accounts. In the case of neuroimaging, the direction of explanation need not be entirely from the side of cognitive psychology. We can also rely on convergent evidence from the neurosciences to help inform our functional decompositions. Neurophysiology in nonhuman animals and lesion studies and other noninvasive techniques in humans can provide independent confirmation for our hypotheses, increasing our confidence in our functional specifications. In general, however, the farther things get from the sensory and motor peripheries, the more speculative will be the inferences that support functional attribution to brain areas.

Of the two streams discussed, the functional and the causal, the functional stream is more inferentially problematic. The causal stream involves assumptions for which our evidence is incomplete or inconclusive at many places, but this can forseeably be remedied with further work, and our current assumptions are likely to be close to correct. The assumptions that are invoked in the functional stream are more global and more difficult to independently verify, and at some level they involve the entire conceptual framework on which neuroimaging is based. Especially in the absence of an overarching theory of cognitive function, or careful physiological corroboration at lower levels, conclusions about function should be viewed as provisional. Neuroimagers, like those in any other science, tend to work within the paradigms established for their field, but it is essential to recognize that our current functional ontology is on epistemically shaky ground. As mentioned before, this is a problem all the natural sciences face— nature does not come with a manual delineating her joints. While this by no means invalidates the technique or undermines the inferences about functional anatomy it enables, a proper appreciation of the epistemic status of neuroimages requires acknowledging these dependencies.

Neuroimaging as Photography

In everyday life, and in science, vision is one of our most important faculties for gaining knowledge about our world. Vision seems effortless and "direct": The phenomenology of vision is that we just *see things as the objects they are, or see that something is the case*.[7] Moreover, we usually think that what we see justifies us in our beliefs. A vast amount of knowledge of the world that we have does come from visual observation; that we consider vision of primary importance in establishing veridical beliefs about the world is evident in common phrases like "seeing is believing," and "I saw it with my own eyes," and even in the import of eyewitness testimony in court cases. Sometimes what we see is mediated by images, as in photographs or film. Through photographs we can see things with which we are not spatially or temporally collocated (Meskin and Cohen 2006). For some time, photographs have been thought to be evidentially privileged: they are, in most cases, what we would see were we there. Photographic images have been typically granted an epistemic status almost as privileged as vision itself (but see Farid 2006), and because of the potential failures of memory, it is in some cases even more privileged.

Photography is a relatively direct means of representation. Photographs of scenes or objects represent the scene or object through a causal process: An image visually resembling a scene is produced on a film by the light reflected or emitted by the objects in the scene. In our experience of looking at photographs, we see in them the objects or scenes they are of. Although seeing a photograph as a representation of a scene involves an inference, the inference is generally automatic, and mediated by implicit background knowledge and judgments of visual similarity. In most cases, relatively little explicit theoretical apparatus needs to be deployed to understand the content of a photograph; in this sense they are inferentially close. Perhaps partly by virtue of this inferential proximity, photographs play important evidential roles in our society, and philosophers have explored their status as evidence (Cohen and Meskin 2004; Walton 1984). Cohen and Meskin, for instance, state:

[P]hotographs seem to have a distinctive epistemic status as compared with other sorts of pictures. Unlike [the aforementioned examples of] non-photographic depictions, photographs typically provide evidence specially about what they depict. Most significantly, the epistemically special character of photographs is revealed by this fact: we are inclined to trust them in a way that we are not inclined to trust even the most accurate of drawings and paintings. (p 513)

A number of features have been adduced to explain their importance as evidence. Here I discuss three that appear prominently in some form in the literature: mimesis, counterfactual dependence, and theory-independence. In addition, I claim that photographs are revelatory: They display their contents.

Briefly, a representation is mimetic if it instantiates a represented property by means of the same property (Kulvicki 2006). Photographs are visually mimetic in various respects, for many of the visual properties of the objects and scenes that are photographed are instantiated in the photograph, such as their colors, visual texture, patterns of shading, and perspective-relative spatial relations and outlines shapes. It is in part because of their mimetic properties that some philosophers think we literally "see through" photographs to the objects they are of (Walton 1984), or that we see in them their objects (Wollheim 1987). Cohen and Meskin argue that photographs are distinguished in the way they preserve visual information about their subjects, while discarding information relating the perceiver to the subject (Cohen and Meskin 2004).

Counterfactual dependence refers to the fact that the content of photographs depends systematically on the scene photographed. If the scene were different, the photograph would be different (modulo differences not visible from the perspective of the camera). This counterfactual dependence is ensured by the mechanical methods of photography (Cohen and Meskin 2004). The epistemic value of photographs is related to this counterfactual dependence and our background beliefs about photographs as a type. This isn't the case with other types of depiction such as painting. Moreover, because of our background beliefs, the way in which the photograph depends on the scene photographed is intuitively clear, usually enabling us easily to make inferences from the photograph about the nature of what was photographed.

Our intuitive abilities to interpret photographs obviate the need for explicit theories to interpret them. In this sense, photographs are theory-independent. In addition, photographs have a characteristic that Walton has termed belief-independence (Cohen and Meskin 2004; Walton 1984). Photographs are belief-independent in that the beliefs of the photographer do not influence the content of the photograph by disrupting or diverting the causal process by which it carries information about its subject[8]; the photographer's beliefs also need not be invoked in order to interpret the photograph. Both these qualities I subsume this under the rubric of theory-independence. Theory-independence is related to a psychologically salient feature of photographs: They are revelatory, that is, they wear their contents on their faces. The qualities described here are by no means uniformly endorsed, and they may hold to greater or lesser degrees for particular photographs. In general, however, these features contribute to the evidential status of photographs.[9]

Visualization is an important tool for gaining and conveying scientific understanding. Images provide ways of representing manifold information at once, and we apprehend some relationships better when they are represented visually than when verbally described. However, the familiarity we have with the visual images we are best acquainted with—photographic images—and the epistemic status we accord them do not always easily translate to images in science.

Exploring the Photograph Analogy

Superficially, neuroimages are like photographs. They are generated by machines that produce representations about events in the mind and brain that may mistakenly be thought of as brain cameras. The representations they produce are images, typically brightly colored, that appear to represent a real object (a brain or brain slice) and some of its visual characteristics; the colored contours delineate regions of neural activity.[10] My contention is that people tend to appreciate neuroimages as if they were photographs of brain activity (Roskies 2007). It is plausible that our familiarity with photography and with the use of photographic images in science and the automatic way in which we interpret photographs dispose us to impart to other images that bear superficial resemblance to photographs similar evidential characteristics.

The characteristics of mimesis, counterfactual dependence, and theory-independence that have been invoked to explain why photographs have historically served as a reliable and psychologically compelling form of evidence may illuminate the perceived epistemic status of imaging. Although brain images may be thought to be mechanically derived direct measures of a state of affairs just as photographs are, we can realize here relevant departures from the features thought to ground the inferential proximity of photographs. Consider the relation of counterfactual dependence. While neuroimaging is counterfactually dependent on the blood oxygenation characteristics of the brain, accounting for its suitability as a scientific tool, the previous discussion elaborated some ways in which we lack a clear understanding of precisely what the dependence relation is between signal and neural activity. Because it is likely that many kinds or patterns of activity can result in the same fMRI signal, our ability to infer relevant characteristics of the activity is limited. This is much less true for photography, where the counterfactual relation is relatively transparent and the possibilities are generally intuitive and well delineated.[11] In addition, the foregoing discussion emphasizes the extent to which the interpretation of the functional relevance of the MR signal is theory-dependent. Certain theoretical relations must hold between the MR signal and neural activity interpreting the signal as reflecting activity to be warranted. The limits of our interpretation are governed by the nature of these relations.

The mismatch between the actual and apparent inferential proximity of neuroimages may be further illuminated by considering the sorts of transformations in format data undergo in neuroimaging. In photography, negatives and prints are both isomorphic to a two-dimensional projection of their subjects. In contrast, data from functional neuroimaging experiments are not originally in the format of an image, but rather of data structures that encode numerical values of phase- and frequency-dependent signal intensity collected in an abstract framework called "k-space." Visual representations of data in k-space bear no visual resemblance to images of brains. These data are transformed to spatial values of signal intensity with a Fourier transform, resulting in an image that looks roughly brainlike. This analytical transformation doesn't alter the information encoded in the data, and thus may be taken not to introduce any inferential distance, in that it introduces no error or range of possible causes. However, the radical transformations in format indicate the indirectness of the technique relative to photography. The fact that these transformations are completely invisible to the consumer of the image implies that neuroimages are not revelatory and illustrates the inaptness of imposing an epistemic framework paradigmatic of photography. The mandatory use of statistics also illustrates the differences between neuroimaging and photography with respect to the nature of the counterfactual dependence relation. It suggests as well that images are not revelatory, in that the choices made are not visible in or recoverable from the image itself, and thus the proper interpretation cannot be discerned on the basis of the image alone.

Much of the inferential distance of neuroimages is due to the necessity of dealing with low signal to noise, and the resulting introduction of variable information from combining scans within and across subjects. It is interesting that, regardless of the particular methods one uses, what results from averaging is a brain image, but not an image of a brain. Brain images are best thought of as generalizations, not particulars. In this respect, brain images are more akin to scientific diagrams or schematics than to photographs (Perini 2005). Although generality is not a feature unique to scientific images, it is foreign to photography. Photographs are always of particulars. They thus support existential inferences: From a photograph of a scene with a dog in it, one can conclude that a dog was there. This does not hold true for neuroimages, for there may be no particular that corresponds with the generalization; for instance, no single subject may display the pattern of activation shown by the group data. In this way, too, they are unlike photographs.

As noted, conventions of image construction also affect brain images. Brain images typically indicate activation levels or statistical significance by overlaying colored areas on a grayscale structural image. The representation of the analyzed data relies on a number of conventional choices that can affect both the final informational content of the image and its visual appearance.[12] Thresholding, for example, reduces the informational content of the image and displays only information that reaches or exceeds the threshold chosen by the experimenter. Other methods discard activated areas that fail to contain a minimal number of statistically significant contiguous voxels. These methods produce images that typically look cleaner than ones that merely compute statistical significance, and the impression of cleanness may affect people's apprehension of the image and their appraisal of its epistemic status. Color manipulations may also have psychological impact. Some experimenters use color gradations to indicate relative levels of activity, while others use color gradations to indicate relative levels of statistical significance. The very same visual image can thus represent quite different, albeit related, contents. Again, the nature of these contents is not revelatory, for it is not discernible from the image alone. Finally, even the choice of color scheme, which is purely conventional and does not affect the information content of the image, can affect the way an image looks to an observer. Blues are cool colors, while reds are hot, and thus often blues are used to represent deactivations and reds activations. It is an empirical question whether purely arbitrary color assignments or other conventional decisions have any psychological effects on how such images are apprehended or interpreted, by both the layperson and the expert. Some work is currently being conducted on these issues.

The fact that some conventional decisions affect the visual appearance of the image without changing its content implies that images are not mimetic in the way photographs are. That neuroimaging is not mimetic is underscored when we recognize that the properties they are meant to represent, location and level of neural activity, are not visual properties, though they can be visually represented. Understanding what is represented requires a knowledge of the choices made in analysis and image construction, and is therefore theory-dependent and nonrevelatory. In considering the causal stream, then, we have seen ways in which imaging differs from photography in terms of mimesis, counterfactual dependence, theory-independence, and revelation.

Some features of the functional stream also affect apparent inferential distance. For example, in neuroimaging the data generated always depend on the chosen tasks, and subtle differences in task can matter to the resulting image.[13] With subtractive designs, the data displayed in the image are contrastive, and it is impossible to read off the image itself what the tasks are that contribute to its content. In particular, the baseline or contrast task is effectively invisible, contributing to what isn't seen or what is seen as deactivation. The image that results from an experiment, therefore, is heavily dependent on both the task of interest and what contrast task is chosen, yet naïve consumers of functional images often overlook the contrast tasks as irrelevant. Because the images don't explicitly carry the information about what the relevant tasks are for interpreting the image, they are not revelatory. Moreover, the layperson might view the image as a confirmation of the experimenter's hypothesis without realizing how critically the interpretation depends on the experimenter's hypothesized functional decomposition. Thus, the content of a neuroimage is highly dependent on the tasks used in its generation, and an understanding of those tasks is theory-laden. Again, when comparing the functional stream to our characterization of photography, we see that neuroimaging fails to share many features of photographs that make them inferentially proximate. In contrast to photography, interpreting the functional significance of neuroimages is highly theory-dependent.

Cognitive function itself is not represented in images, so trivially images are not mimetic with respect to their functional significance. Since neural activity has no relevant visual properties, the conventions of the brain image are representational translations of certain nonvisual aspects of properties related to neural activity, namely, magnetic properties of the water of the brain. All imaging experiments rely on the consumer to correlate functional descriptions with imaging results. In general, scientists tend to be more aware of the importance of other information presented alongside neuroimages, such as figure legends and long discursive accounts of experimental design and methods that are part of every scientific paper. This information is necessary to properly interpret imaging results. However, rarely is adequate information presented in the popular venues in which neuroimages appear, and their visually arresting qualities and seemingly revelatory nature make detailed information seem redundant or unnecessary. Often, it seems, a short caption will do. The foregoing discussion is meant to underline how misleading this can be.

The Illusions of Inferential Proximity

Superficially, neuroimages share many qualities with other types of image that we interpret unproblematically. Both photography and imaging are useful evidential techniques because of their counterfactual dependence on relevant aspects of their objects of investigation.

Neuroimaging is especially scientifically valuable because it is one of the few techniques that provides evidence about brain activity in awake behaving humans. Here I have discussed the actual inferential distance of neuroimages, and highlighted ways in which the inferences made in analyzing and interpreting neuroimages may be less robust than they appear. For example, the counterfactual dependencies in neuroimaging are often mediated by provisional or incomplete theories, and many details are still poorly understood. In addition, methods necessitated by the low signal to noise inherent in the technique increase the inferential distance in ways we have yet to fully understand.

For the layperson, these interpretive problems are compounded. I have suggested that there is an illusion of inferential proximity to neuroimages that is likely to result from people's tendency to view neuroimages as if they were photographs of brain activity. In a variety of ways, however, neuroimaging is unlike photography. For example, the generation and interpretation of neuroimages is highly theory-dependent, and the ways in which neuroimaging differs from photography are not generally apparent in the images themselves—the images are not revelatory with respect to the considerable degree of background information needed to understand how to interpret neuroimages. Thus, the illusion of inferential proximity: Neuroimages are inferentially distant from brain activity, yet they appear not to be. The layperson is prone to see the data represented in an image as a direct view of parts of the brain that "light up" or turn on when some task is performed, and is generally completely unaware of the inferential distance between image and biological phenomenon. This situation is exacerbated by the popular media, which represents results simplistically and rarely discusses actual procedure or methodological challenges in their reports (Racine et al. 2006). The inferential distance between image and neural activity makes their use in public discourse especially fraught and risky.

Neuroimaging is in its early days, and though there has been remarkable progress and there is remarkable promise, we must be diligent in reminding ourselves of the tenuousness of many of our inferences and the continued need for caution in interpreting the data from neuroimaging studies.

Acknowledgment

This work was supported in part by a grant from the Australian Research Council. Thanks to Mark Colyvan, Richard Joyce, Neil Levy, and C. C. Wood for helpful comments on earlier drafts, and to the editors for their suggestions. The main ideas for this chapter appeared previously in Roskies, A. L. (2008). Neuroimaging and inferential distance. *Neuroethics* 1: 19–30.

Notes

1. Thanks to Paul Griffiths for this suggestion.

2. Though ideally a discussion of actual inferential distance would provide an objective metric by which to characterize inferential distance, such a task looks impossible in the absence of an inductive logic. In addition, since the task of breaking down a complex inference into logical atoms is underdetermined, there is no way of uniquely identifying inferential steps in a sequence of reasoning. Thus, actual inferential distance cannot be determined by simply counting or classifying inferential steps according to a clear taxonomy of inferential kinds. However, that does not mean that inferential distance cannot be characterized at all.

3. In this context, one might view actual inferential distance as providing some sort of normative epistemic measure, and apparent inferential distance as providing a descriptive measure.

4. This is actually a simplification, for in many cases the relevant relatum is not the MR image, but the MR data. To the extent that the data are preprocessed and indicate values (average intensity levels, statistical significance, etc.), I will speak of them as if they are characteristics of the image, even if they are never so displayed. It remains an empirical question to what extent the scientific conclusions of scientists are affected by their visual inspection of images, and to what extent they are based purely on numerical values. The answers will likely vary on a case to case basis.

5. For the purposes of this chapter, I focus on BOLD echoplanar imaging, which dominates the cognitive neuroimaging literature. Those familiar with MR imaging will recognize that I have said nothing about this or other pulse sequences. Pulse sequences can be tailored to make the MR image more or less sensitive to different factors. This imparts MR imaging with a great degree of flexibility. Details about inferential distance will depend on what sorts of imaging parameters are chosen. A discussion of this is beyond the scope of this chapter, but relevant details can be found in Buxton (2002).

6. This highlights the fact that inferential distance is a measure that can change given our state of knowledge. The more refined or well confirmed our theories on which inferences are based, the less distance there is.

7. Although there is philosophical debate regarding whether visual perception is direct or mediated, the phenomenology of vision is of direct and unmediated access to the world.

8. Of course the photographer's beliefs may affect what and how he or she chooses to photograph, but once the physical parameters of the photograph are established, the outcome is independent of belief or theory.

9. Although not much attention has been devoted to it in philosophy, the digital age has led to a change in status of the actual inferential distance of photography. As more effective techniques of digitally manipulating photographs have been developed, photography's evidential characteristics have been compromised. The rise of digital forensics reflects this change (Farid 2006). Insofar as this is so, photography's evidential status should wane, although the psychological evidence

reflecting such a change may lag well behind. This suggests that more attention to the contrast between actual and apparent inferential distance may be relevant in photography as well as in neuroimaging. For the time being, however, I will speak of photography as if it indeed were as inferentially proximate as most of the literature suggests. Moreover, if people's intuitive judgments about photography's epistemic status should change as a result of the increased ease of photographic manipulation, and the hypothesis presented here is correct, those changes should be reflected in the future apprehension of the epistemic status of neuroimaging.

10. One might here construe photography widely. Perhaps we may think neuroimages are more like weather maps, but I contend that people think of weather maps as if they were photographs of atmospheric conditions as well.

11. Again, these distinctions are quantitative; in some cases, even traditional photography can mislead (for example, photographs of the Ames Room). The arguments here are meant to reflect more of a difference in degree than in kind.

12. The same is true for photography, but the effects on interpretation seem less dramatic than for imaging, perhaps because of the familiarity with the choices and their counterfactual dependencies. For example, we almost never interpret a black-and-white photograph as being of a grayscale world.

13. Indeed, even differences as subtle as the word frequency of lexical stimuli have been shown to have noticeable effects on imaging outcomes.

17 Brains and Minds: On the Usefulness of Localization Data to Cognitive Psychology

Richard Loosemore and Trevor Harley

In the early 1990s, one of us wrote a textbook about the cognitive psychology of language; in this book there was hardly a mention of the brain (Harley 1995). There was a great deal of neuropsychology, but it was cognitive neuropsychology; indeed, the book discussed (and tacitly adopted) the position of ultracognitive neuropsychology, which maintains that although we can learn a great deal about how the mind works from looking at the effects of brain damage, we cannot learn very much about the mind from looking at the brain.

How times have changed! The third edition of the same book is full of reports of studies of brain imaging in one form or another (Harley 2008). Furthermore, if you look through a journal such as *Science* or *Nature*, you will find that most articles on psychology contain or refer to imaging. And what now passes as psychology in the popular press is mostly reports on brain imaging studies. The brain is back in cognitive psychology. But is this change for the better? Are we really learning anything new or important about psychology (the science of mental behavior), or rather about the science of the substrate on which the mind is based?

One of us has previously argued (Harley 2004a, b) that psychologists are becoming obsessed with brain imaging, and that this obsession shows no signs of abating; indeed, imaging is now taking over the world. Harley argued that imaging the localization of function of components of anything—parts of cars, computers, or brains—can be described at four levels:

1. The "tokenism" level. In the way that a glossy magazine might print a picture of a luxury kitchen because it looks good, sometimes brain images seem to be included just because they are available, and look good. There's no denying that they do look impressive, but what they add to the science of the paper in *these* cases is either unclear or obviously nothing. We admit that imaging devices are fun to use, are expensive, and require big grant money for their care and feeding, and no doubt all of these characteristics add to their popularity.

2. The "absolute location" level. A car engine is in the middle of the engine compartment. This level of description, of course, assumes that we can identify the engine, or

else we are reduced to saying "there is a big box in the middle of the car." The results of knowing just where things are is not really that interesting, for psychologists at least.

3. The "relative location" level. For example, the little fan is above the CPU. This level is more interesting, because it might tell us how things are connected together, but is subject to a new assumption, proximity. This assumption states that adjacent regions of a complex machine do related tasks. While plausible some of the time, this assumption is clearly often wrong (e.g., although proximity between fan and CPU is essential, the fan doesn't carry out computations, it just keeps the CPU cool). Similarly, we cannot assume that just because regions of the brain are near each other, they do similar things. An extension of the proximity assumption is the wiring assumption—if we can spot tracts of fibers, or brain regions mediating between two areas, then they must be working on related tasks.

4. The "functional" level. For example, the engine drives the axles, which in turn drive the wheels. Car manuals provide clear diagrams showing where the components are, what each does, and how they cohere to create a machine that fulfils a particular function. The diagrams explain why components with particular functions are in the places that they are. The trouble here is that you already need to know mostly what each component does before you can begin to make sense of it. In addition, the absolute location of components is rarely critical to the workings of the system; what is more important is the pattern of connectivity.

In an ideal world, brain studies would always be situated at level 4, the functional level. Many of the published reports do indeed make claims that seem to place them near the top of this hierarchy, but in the analysis we present here, we are going to push back on these claims and ask whether the apparent level is the same as the level actually achieved. If we analyze these studies carefully, might we find that those that superficially appear to be at level 3 or 4 are really only at level 2 or 1? We have long suspected that even those brain imaging studies that appear to give us valuable information might actually be suffering from subtle ambiguities or confusions that could invalidate their conclusions.

What we propose to do now, then, is deepen this "levels" analysis by putting six recent brain imaging studies under the microscope.

Before we describe the specific method of analysis to be used on these six studies, here are some of the general background questions we hope to answer:

• Is "where-it-happens" information of any use to present-day psychology? A modern automotive engineer, for example, might find it useful to know that a heavy battery was located in the rear of a car, because that might imply the car was a hybrid; but how useful would this information have been 150 years ago, when internal combustion was barely imagined? At some point in time, when we have an adequate model at the higher levels of analysis, this kind of information undoubtedly becomes useful, but is it useful today?

▪ Are the specific claims about neural localization internally and theoretically coherent? For example, it would be incoherent if a localization study claimed to have found a particular mechanism, but the putative mechanism could do the job it is supposed to be doing only if every one of the brain's neurons was directly connected to all of the others: Since we know that neurons are not totally connected, we know the mechanism cannot be right, and so claims about its location would be incoherent.

▪ Do the localization claims refer to components of the mind that are clearly defined? We would not be interested in an fMRI study that located the id and superego, for example, unless the author could say exactly what the id and superego are supposed to be, how they work, and why we should believe that there are such things.

▪ Are the inferences researchers make theory-laden? Do they depend on acceptance of a particular functional theory of how the mind works? For example, it would make no sense for someone to establish the location of "consciousness" if later developments in our theory of cognition show that consciousness is not a physical place at all, but a process involving many scattered components.

▪ Are today's studies, which give us only crude localization data (both spatially and temporally), just a prelude to later research that will pin down location and function precisely? Or is crude localization all that we can ever expect from brain imaging technology?

Over the last year or so we have kept track of the reports of psychology and imaging we have come across in the popular press. We have made no attempt to be exhaustive, or to make the sample random or representative in any way, so we make no claims to methodological rigor about what is presented in the press; we just wanted to generate a sample of what the popular press finds interesting about psychology and the brain. We certainly have no intention of denigrating these studies just by picking them, or because they have been widely reported in the press. (Indeed, we believe that it is important for scientists to publicize their work, and to explain science to a wider audience.)

Of course, it could be that our sample is biased toward where-it-happens studies because the press is obsessed just with where things are in the brain, rather than any more detailed level of explanation. We don't believe this for a moment: We have yet to come across an article titled "Hippocampus near amygdala shock horror!" No, the press is interested in behavior, explanations of behavior, and unexpected connections between types of behavior—just the things they should be interested in. Nevertheless, the press has clearly bought the "where it is, is important in explaining how and why" argument.

In each of the studies, our main focus will be on what the article claims to tell us about location, and how that information relates to the background theories in cognitive science. Do we feel better informed after reading that such-and-such a function happens in, near, or connected to a particular brain structure, and if (to anticipate a little) it turns out that we do not feel satisfied, can we be more specific about the source of our dissatisfaction?

Using a Theoretical Framework as a Tool

One persistent feeling we get, when reading the brain imaging literature, is that stated conclusions often seem reasonable if psychological mechanisms are interpreted in a relatively simple or simplistic way, but these same conclusions could easily become unreasonable if the mechanisms are interpreted in other ways, or if they are implemented in a less-than-obvious manner. Brain imaging conclusions, in other words, often seem theory-dependent and vulnerable to any future winds of change that might blow through cognitive science.

In order to test this intuition about theory-dependence, we are going to adopt a rather unusual strategy. In this chapter, we sketch the beginnings of a new, unified framework that describes the overall architecture of the human cognitive system, and we use this framework to ask how well the conclusions of our target brain imaging studies would hold up if this framework should one day become the standard, functional-level model of how the brain works.

The framework has some unusual features, and it is these features in particular that we believe could do some damage to the conclusions some imaging studies have arrived at.

We should be clear about what we are trying to achieve in proposing this new framework. We are not really trying to suggest that we have come up with a new interpretation of each of our target studies, which should then be taken as a challenge to be overcome by new, more cleverly designed imaging studies. Of course, we would be happy if our proposals were taken in this light, because this kind of interaction between theory and experiment is the mark of a healthy scientific paradigm, but this is not our main intention. Our real goal is to see how sensitive the conclusions of these studies might be to a slight change in the theoretical mechanisms whose location is being sought.

Our overall goal, then, is to use this new framework as a tool with which to try to break the conclusions of brain imaging studies that purport to tell us something about localization of cognitive functions.

A Molecular Framework for Cognition

The alternative framework we wish to put forward is a "molecular" model of cognition. It has connections to many previous lines of thought in cognitive science, but it is most closely inspired by Douglas Hofstadter's *Jumbo* model, which was originally intended to explore the cognitive processes at work in an experienced anagram solver (Hofstadter 1995).

The framework is intended to describe only the higher, more abstract, levels of cognition, above the level at which purely data-driven processing occurs.

The Core Concept: Instances

At the heart of this framework lies one key idea: a distinction between *instance* and *generic* versions of the concepts stored in the system. In much of cognitive science the idea of a concept is used as if there were only one entity encoding the concept; so, for example, theorists will talk about *the* [coin] node becoming strongly activated, or about the priming effect this can have on *the* [bank] node. It is tempting to imagine a large network of nodes (or even neurons), with a [coin] node and a [bank] somewhere in the network, and with vast numbers of connections between all the nodes.

But any complete model of a cognitive system must include *instance* nodes that represent the particular entities involved in our thoughts at a given moment: nodes that represent, not coin in general, but the particular instance of the word *coin* that is being witnessed right now. Any realistic model of cognition must make explicit allowance for these instances, and it turns out that this can have a drastic effect on our theorizing. Instance nodes do not sit quietly in a fixed network; they are created on the fly, they have a relatively short lifetime, and the connections between them are extremely volatile. Furthermore, a complete model should explain how the generic concepts are built up from repeated exposure to specific instances.

The primacy of instances is the core concept behind the proposed molecular framework. There is a deep assumption that, in practical terms, the place where these instances are created, interact, and have their effects on the rest of the system is likely to be far more important than the passive network of generic concepts.

In other respects, the framework is little more than a conjunction and distillation of the most common features of many local theories, though with a bias toward the abstract motivations that drove, among others, McClelland and Rumelhart (McClelland et al. 1986).

Foreground and Background

In our framework there is one main type of object, and two main places.

The objects are called *atoms*, and their main purpose is to encode the smallest packets of knowledge (concept, symbol, node, etc.). Atoms come in two sorts: *generics* and *instances*. For each concept, there is only one generic atom, but there can be many instance atoms. In what follows, the term *atom* on its own will usually be understood to mean an instance atom.

The two main "places" in this framework are the *foreground* and the *background*.

The foreground roughly corresponds to working memory, and is the place where instance atoms are to be found. The foreground is an extremely dynamic place: Atoms are continually being created, and while they are active they can move around and form rapidly changing bonds with one another. The sum total of all the atoms in the foreground, together with the bonds between them, constitute what the system is currently thinking about, or aware of.

The background is approximately equivalent to long-term memory, and is just a store of all the generic atoms from which instance atoms can be made. When an instance atom is in the foreground, it maintains a link back to its generic parent in the background. The background is more or less passive; the foreground is where everything happens.

Note that atoms do not necessarily encode concepts that have names. Some of them capture regularities at a subcognitive level, and for this reason the foreground contains some activity that the system is not routinely aware of, or that it does not find easy to introspect or report on (see Harley 1998, for more detail on this point).

Active Representations and Constraints

So far, this is all sufficiently general that it could be the outline of many different theories of how the cognitive system is structured. But now we will make a commitment that distinguishes this framework from many others: The representations in the foreground are not passive tokens of the sort that are meant to be assembled and used by some external mechanisms, they are *active* representations. In other words, although the atoms encode knowledge about the world in just the way you might expect, they also encapsulate a set of mechanisms that implicitly define how this knowledge is used by the system.

How do the foreground atoms do this? Broadly speaking, each atom contains (and continually updates) a set of constraints that it would like to see satisfied by its neighbors in the foreground. For example, the [chair] atom would prefer to see a group of atoms around it that encode the characteristics and components of a typical chair, and these preferences, encoded inside the atom, are what we refer to as the *constraints* it is seeking to satisfy.

An atom will not just passively seek a place where its constraints are satisfied, it will actively try to force its neighbors to comply with its constraints. Its behavior is a mixture of "Do my neighbors suit me?" and "Can I change my neighbors to better suit me?" An atom can engage in several kinds of activity in pursuit of its goals: It can try to activate new atoms that it would like to see in its neighborhood, or deactivate others that it does not want to see, or change its internal state, change the connections it makes, and so on.

Not all of the atoms in the foreground are successful in their attempts to satisfy their constraints. Many get woken up because something thinks they might be relevant, but after doing their best to fit, they fail to establish strong bonds and become deactivated. A substantial number of atoms, however, do find themselves able to connect to an existing structure and thereafter play a role in how that structure develops.

As a general rule, the constraints inside an atom are supposed to encode a "regularity" about the world—say, the regularity that if something is a chair, it must possess constituent parts that could be construed as legs.

Relaxation

The process in which an atom looks around and tries to take actions to satisfy some local constraints can be characterized as *relaxation*. Everything that happens in the foreground is driven by relaxation. If a change occurs somewhere in the foreground, atoms adjacent to the change will try to accommodate to it, and this accommodation will propagate out from the starting point like a wave, or domino effect.

There does not have to be only one type of relaxation happening at every place; several such processes can occur simultaneously, originating in different parts of the foreground. Almost everything that happens in the foreground can be attributed to changes that occur in a particular place and then send waves of relaxation that propagate across the foreground. Strictly speaking, this is dynamic relaxation, because the foreground never settles into a quiescent state where everything is satisfied; it is always on the boil.

The Foreground Periphery

At the edge of the foreground are a number of areas that connect to structures outside the foreground. One part of the periphery has input lines coming from sensory receptors, while another has output lines that go to motor output effectors. These two patches on the edge of the foreground are responsible for much of the activity among the atoms. When a signal arrives from a low-level sensory detector (or more likely a data-driven system that preprocesses some raw input signals), the result is that one or more atoms are automatically attached to the foreground periphery to represent the signal. These initial atoms then have an effect on nearby atoms.

Another important part of the periphery is a connection to mechanisms that govern the goals, drives, and motivations the system is trying to satisfy. These can be thought of as lying "underneath" the foreground, in the sense that they are more primitive than the cognitive work that goes on in the foreground proper. The work of these motivational/drive systems is not simple, but the effect of their actions is to bias the activity in one direction or another.

Sources of Action

So far, atoms have been characterized as if their role is just to encode knowledge, but in fact, representing the world is only part of what they can do: Some atoms initiate *actions*, and some may encode mixtures of action and representation.

How does the system "do" an action? In the part of the foreground periphery where input arrives from the motivational/drive system, there is a unique spot—the "make-it-so" place—that drives all actions. If an action atom can get itself attached here, this triggers an outward-moving relaxation wave that will (usually) result in signals being sent from the motor output area that cause muscles to do something. The make-it-so place, in the part of the foreground periphery we have called the motivation area, is the place where the buck starts.

Neural Implementation

Nothing has been said, so far, about how this framework is realized in the brain's neural hardware. There are many possibilities here, because this framework is primarily designed to specify high-level mechanisms. The framework itself is neutral with respect to neural implementation.

With that qualification, what follows is a quick sketch of one way it could be realized in the brain. This neural implementation will be assumed in the rest of the chapter.

The cortex could be an overlapping patchwork of "processors," each of which can host one active atom, and the sum total of all these processors is the thing that we have called the *foreground*. Each processor is a large structure with quite complex functionality, and is capable of doing such things as hosting a particular atom for a while, transferring a hosted atom to an adjacent processor if there is pressure for space, and setting up rapidly changing communication links to other atoms located some distance away across the cortex. One possibility is that the central core of each processor corresponds to a cortical column.

The generic, passive atoms that are stored in the background (long-term memory) are colocated with the processors that were just described, but each processor can hold a large number of generics. Each of these passive atoms is encoded in distributed form inside the processor. At the level of the entire cortex, then, a generic atom would seem localized (because it is within one processor), but since each processor is quite extensive, the atom is not at all localized within the processor.

The activation of an instance atom involves a call to the processor that hosts the generic, which causes the processor to find a spare processor that can host the instance atom. The parent processor itself might be able to play host, but if not, then it passes the atom to some other processor (possibly a neighbor) for hosting. One way or another, an activated atom is quickly copied into a processor that can handle it, in much the same way that a computer program might be transferred across a network to a computer that can run it.

In summary, then, the cortex can be viewed in two completely different ways. It can be seen as the foreground, in which case it is effectively a space within which the extremely volatile instance atoms arrive, set up a rapidly changing set of links to other instance atoms, and then depart. Alternatively the cortex can be seen as the place where the contents of long-term memory are stored, since the generic atoms are also located in the processors.

Example 1: Visual Object Recognition

We conclude this summary of the molecular framework with two examples of the kinds of activity that go on in the foreground. The first involves the recognition of an object perceived with the eyes, and the other is the carrying out of an action.

Suppose the system were to start in a thought-free, meditative state, in a darkened room, and then suddenly a light comes on and illuminates a single chair. The foreground would start out relatively empty, and when the light is turned on a sequence of atoms would come into the foreground until, at the end of the process, the [chair] atom would be activated.

This process would begin with the arrival at the foreground periphery of signals along the lines coming from the visual system. When these signals arrive, they trigger the activation of instance atoms representing some low-level features of the visual input. When these atoms appear in the foreground, they attach to the places on the periphery where their features occur, and then they look around at their closest neighbors. If a pair (or perhaps a group) of these atoms recognize that they have occurred together before, they will know about some other atoms that they could call into the foreground, which on those previous occasions represented their co-occurrence. They will activate those second-level atoms, and these in turn will try to attach themselves strongly to the first-level atoms. The ones that succeed in making bonds will then feel confident enough to look around at their neighbors and repeat the process by calling in some even higher-level atoms. An inverted tree of atoms thus develops over the part of the foreground periphery where the chair image came in, and at the top end of this inverted tree, finally, will be the [chair] element.

This picture of the recognition of a chair is extremely simplified, but it gives a rough picture of the kind of activity that occurs: atoms being activated by others, then each atom trying to fit into a growing structure in a way that satisfies its own internal constraints about the roles it can play. As a whole, the system tries to relax into a state in which some atoms have self-consistently interpreted the new information that arrived.

Example 2: Sitting Down

Suppose the person who just recognized the chair next hears the experimenter ask them to sit down. The atoms representing this request will (after an auditory recognition process very similar to the visual recognition event previously described) bump into, and interact with, the large cluster of atoms hovering around the motivation area of the foreground periphery. This cluster represents the mind's complex stack of goals and intentions, all the way from its most nebulous motivations (stay safe, seek warmth, get food, etc.) to its most specific action schemas (accept this experimenter as a trusted friend whose requests should be obeyed). As a result of this interaction between the atoms representing the request and the atoms around the motivation area, a new atom that encodes the sitting action is activated and attached to the make-it-so place on the foreground periphery, and this gives the [perform-a-sitting-action] atom enough strength to cause a cascade of other atoms to be brought in, which then elaborate the sitting plan in the context of where the body currently is, where the chair is, and so on.

In the case of the sitting-down action, a wave of relaxation emerges from the [perform-a-sitting-action] atom and causes a sequence of atoms to spread toward the motor output area. When these atoms arrive at the periphery, muscles move and the sitting action occurs. The only difference between this and visual recognition is that the wave of relaxation does not come from the sensory input area and end with the activation of the [chair] atom, but starts with one atom at the make-it-so place and ends with a broad front of new atoms hitting the motor output area.

Applying the Framework

With this theoretical framework in hand, it is time to examine the claims made in each of our target brain imaging papers, to try to understand those claims in the context of both a regular interpretation of cognition, and the new framework.

Study 1: "'Bottleneck' Slows Brain Activity"

Dux, Ivanoff, Asplund, and Marois (2006) describe a study in which participants were asked to carry out two tasks that were too hard to perform simultaneously. In these circumstances, we would expect (from a wide range of previous cognitive psychological studies) that the tasks would be serially queued, and that this would show up in reaction-time data. Some theories of this effect interpret it as a consequence of a modality-independent "central bottleneck" in task performance.

Dux et al. used time-resolved fMRI to show that activity in a particular brain area—the posterior lateral prefrontal cortex (pLPFC)—was consistent with the queuing behavior that would be expected if this place were the locus of the bottleneck responsible for the brain's failure to execute the tasks simultaneously. They also showed that the strength of the response in the pLPFC seemed to be a function of the difficulty of one of the competing tasks, when, in a separate experiment, participants were required to do that task alone. The conclusion Dux et al. drew is that this brain imaging data tell us the location of the bottleneck: It's in the pLPFC. So this study aspires to be level 2, perhaps even level 3: telling us the absolute location of an important psychological process, perhaps telling us how it relates to other psychological processes.

Rather than immediately address the question of whether the pLPFC really is the bottleneck, we would first like to ask whether such a thing as "the bottleneck" exists at all. Should the psychological theory of a bottleneck be taken so literally that we can start looking for it in the brain? And if we have doubts, could imaging data help us to decide that we are justified in taking the idea of a bottleneck literally?

What Is a "Bottleneck"? Let's start with a simple interpretation of the bottleneck idea. We start with mainstream ideas about cognition, leaving aside our new framework for the moment. There are tasks to be done by the cognitive system, and each task is some kind of package of information that goes to a place in the system and gets itself executed. This leads to a clean theoretical picture: The task is a package moving around the system, and there is a particular place where it can be executed. As a general rule, the "place" has room for more than one package (perhaps), but only if the packages are small, or if the packages have been compiled to make them automatic. In this study, though, the packages (tasks) are so big that there is room for only one at a time.

The difference between this only-room-for-one-package idea and its main rival within conventional cognitive psychology is that the rival theory would allow multiple packages to be executed simultaneously, but with a slowdown in execution speed. Unfortunately for this rival theory, psychology experiments have indicated that no effort is initially expended on a task that arrives later, until the first task is completed. Hence, the bottleneck theory is accepted as the best description of what happens in dual-task studies.

Theory as Metaphor This pattern of theorizing—first a candidate mechanism, then a rival mechanism that is noticeably different, then some experiments to tell us which is better—is the bread and butter of cognitive science. However, it is one thing to decide between two candidate mechanisms that are sketched in the vaguest of terms (with just enough specificity to allow the two candidates to be distinguished), and making a categorical statement about the precise nature of the mechanism. To be blunt, very few cognitive psychologists would intend the idea of packages drifting through a system and encountering places where there is only room for one, to be taken that literally.

On a scale from metaphor at one end to mechanism blueprint at the other, the idea of a bottleneck is surely nearer to the metaphor end. How many cognitive theorists would say that they are trying to pin down the mechanisms of cognition so precisely that every one of the subsidiary assumptions involved in a theory are supposed to be taken exactly as they come? In the case of the bottleneck theory, for instance, the task packages look suspiciously like symbols being processed by a symbol system, in old-fashioned symbolic-cognition style. But does that mean that connectionist implementations are being explicitly ruled out by the theory? Does the theory buy into all of the explicit representation issues involved in symbol processing, where the semantics of a task package is entirely contained within the package itself, rather than distributed in the surrounding machinery? These and many other questions are begged by the idea of task packages moving around a system and encountering a bottleneck, but would theorists who align themselves with the bottleneck theory want to say that all of these other aspects must be taken literally?

We think not. In fact, it seems more reasonable to suppose that the present state of cognitive psychology involves the search for metaphorlike ideas that are described *as if* they were true mechanisms, but which should not be taken literally by anyone, and especially not by anyone with a brain imaging device who wants to locate those mechanisms in the brain.

Molecular Model of the Bottleneck   How would the molecular framework explain the apparent bottleneck in dual task performance?

When the cognitive system decides to carry out an action—like responding to an aural cue with a finger press—what happens in the foreground is that the cluster of atoms that encode the finger-response action get attached to the make-it-so spot on the edge of the foreground. By design, this spot is not allowed to play host to more than one controlled action sequence, where a "controlled" action is one that requires attention.

But now, what is "attention"? One part of the foreground contents (not the foreground itself, notice, but a subset of the atoms that inhabit the foreground) always has a special status: This is the *attentional patch*. The attentional patch can move around, but it is defined by the fact that atoms in the patch are able to spawn large numbers of associated atom clusters, which means that whatever the attentional patch is representing, it is representing it in exceptional detail. Another way to say the same thing is that this is a region of high *elaboration density*.

Now consider an atom that encodes an action that has only recently been learned (say, the pressing of a button in response to an aural cue). Because this atom is relatively young, it needs to attract the attentional patch to it in order to function; in other words, it cannot be executed unless it is explicitly attended to. If an action atom becomes well learned (like the action of sitting down), it does not need the extra boost of being at the center of the attention patch, so the action is allowed to happen while the attentional patch is elsewhere.

When the first task arrives, in this experiment, the atom encoding the response becomes attached to the make-it-so place, then grabs the attentional patch and does not let go of it until the task is completed. Only when the first task relinquishes control is the second task allowed to become attached to the make-it-so place.

What does this mean for the conclusion of the Dux et al. experiment? One possibility is that the pLPFC lights up when a second task atom arrives, asking to be executed as soon as the first is done. Perhaps the pLPFC is just part of the mechanism that manages a competing task, or perhaps it is a buffer where the atoms encoding the second task await their turn to be executed. Under these circumstances, the pLPFC would not be the "location" of the bottleneck at all, but just a region encoding part of the mechanism related to the bottleneck.

Most important of all, the fact that the pLPFC is involved would tell us nothing about the competing theoretical ideas for explaining the bottleneck: the not-enough-room-for-two-packages mechanism, and the molecular mechanism that involves the management of the attentional patch and the make-it-so attachment point. It is certainly not correct to say that discovering the role of the pLPFC tells us where the bottleneck is, or that there is such a thing as a simple bottleneck. Without having an adequate psychological theory first, the imaging data tells us much less than it first seems to.

It might be worth showing the popular-science interpretation of this study, which appeared on the BBC website on January 29, 2007:

US researchers have discovered a likely reason why people find it hard to do two things at once. A "bottleneck" occurs in the brain when people attempt to carry out two simultaneous tasks, the research shows. The study found the brain slows down when attempting a second task less than 300 milliseconds after the first. The findings support the case for a complete ban on the use of mobile phones when driving, the team said.

This same conclusion could have been reported on the strength of cognitive psychological studies alone, and has nothing to do with the specific facts reported in this experiment. Did the researchers discover the "reason" why people find it hard to do two tasks at once? Sadly, no.

Study 2: "Love Activates the Same Brain Areas as Cocaine"

Aron, Fisher, Mashek, Strong, Li, and Brown (2005) used fMRI to try to distinguish between two possible interpretations of what happens when a person is afflicted with the early stages of romantic love. They asked if this kind of love is a strong emotion, or an overwhelming desire to achieve an objective. The researchers showed pictures of the object of affection to a number of individuals who claimed to have been recently smitten, and their main finding was that "romantic love uses subcortical reward and motivation systems to focus on a specific individual." They declared that "romantic love engages a motivation system involving neural systems associated with motivation to acquire a reward rather than romantic love being a particular emotion in its own right."

The interpretation, then, is that the subjects are not just experiencing a strong feeling, they are wanting to acquire something. If correct, the study is telling us something new at the psychological level, so it is apparently a level-4 (functional) study.

Hence, this study is potentially important and useful. But does it, in fact, tell us something important and new about the mechanisms involved in romantic love?

If the molecular framework is accurate, then the thing that drives a cognitive system to do something is activity coming from deep systems (outside the foreground), which impinge on the motivation part of the foreground periphery, and the way that these drives affect the foreground is through relaxation effects on atoms near the motivation area. Exactly how this works is an open question, but does the Aron et al. study help us to settle this question? Well, it tells us that when reward/motivation systems are active, dopamine is involved, and that romantic love involves activity in those dopamine-rich areas. But does this tell us that dopamine release *causes* the motivational mechanism to kick in? or that dopamine release is a side effect of the motivational mechanism doing something? None of these questions are clarified by the experimental result that some particular areas are activated when the subject looks at a picture of his or her beloved.

The molecular framework could explain romantic love by postulating that there is a specialized slot at the edge of the foreground that has room for precisely one atom that encodes a person, and that when an atom manages to get into that slot it stays there for a long time, kicking in a powerful drive mechanism that tends to force the foreground to engage in certain kinds of thoughts about that person. The original function of this mechanism is to make human beings form a sudden, strong bond to an individual for mating and child-nurturing purposes. Given the amount of activity involved in this unusual mechanism, the framework predicts that there is probably a place in the brain that lights up when this happens, but that prediction by itself is trivial. What matters is exactly how this mechanism exerts its effects.

Is it surprising that a person in early-stage romantic love is experiencing a strong motivation to get various rewards associated with the beloved (wanting to touch, wanting to possess, wanting to receive attention and affection, etc.)? Psychological studies, both formal and informal, tell us that this must surely be the case.

Is there any sign, in this study, that we know more about how the motivational mechanisms work, after finding out that motivational areas are involved in romantic love? As far as we can see, there is no hint of such further information.

Study 3: "Why Your Brain Has a 'Jennifer Aniston Cell'"

Quiroga, Reddy, Kreiman, Koch, and Fried (2005) studied signals coming from an array of several hundred electrodes in the brains of subjects who were undergoing exploratory tests to find an epileptic focus, prior to surgery. When pictures of famous people, landmark buildings, animals, and objects were shown, the experimenters were able to find strong responses to several of the images: On average, fourteen out of ninety-four images elicited a significant response.

Having found some images that caused a response, the experimenters then carried out a testing session in which they showed a number of views of the people or things in those images—and in some cases, they showed only the name of what was in the image. What they found was that the same neurons that responded in the first phase of the experiment also responded strongly to different views of the same subject, and even to the name of the subject written in words. These neurons were very specific: By and large, they did not respond to any other images, only to variants of the one that first triggered them.

The conclusion that Quiroga et al. draw from this is that perhaps grandmother cells (Barlow 1972), which encode single concepts in an abstract way, do exist after all. On the face of it, it seems unlikely that the results could be explained if a distributed representation encodes these images. In the classic type of distributed representation, many units would encode a set of features, and any single image such as Jennifer Aniston's face would be represented only by a pattern of activation across many neurons. Quiroga et al. would have us believe that the brain represents these concepts in a sparse, rather than distributed manner, with a small number of neurons being specifically dedicated to each concept. Although this was not an imaging study, this is clearly an important result, if the preceding interpretation is correct, and could be described as a level-2 account, perhaps being capable of extension to level 3. But are there alternative explanations?

Observations   The first thing to note about this study is the strange fact that the experimenters found some neurons that just happened to respond to the chosen pictures. Who would have thought that when you put several hundred electrodes into the brain, and then show the brain roughly a hundred different images, that some 14% of the images would score a direct hit? If the experimenters' conclusion about sparseness of encoding is correct, the chances of finding the particular neurons that respond *just* to, say, Jennifer Aniston must be very small indeed. Multiply that by 14 (since, on average, fourteen out of ninety-four pictures elicited a significant response in the screening part of the experiment), and we seem to have a problem.

Sparseness of encoding is a conjunction of two ideas. First, there has to be some strong specificity in the response of the neurons: A neuron that fires strongly to Jennifer Aniston's face cannot also respond to the faces of the (superficially similar) Julia Roberts or (thematically related and quite similar) Courtney Cox. Second, sparseness means that there cannot be too many neurons doing the same job. That doesn't necessarily mean there should only be one neuron per job (the mythical grandmother cell that is the only neuron encoding your grandmother's face), but there shouldn't be a million of them, either, or the "sparse" label would start to look inappropriate.

If the experimenters in this study were lucky enough to find neurons that encoded for 14% of the small sample of pictures shown to subjects, then one possibility is that large numbers of duplicate neurons encode each image. This leads to the following problem: If there are so many duplicate neurons encoding image-concepts (enough to enable hits on 14% of the ninety-four pictures), then how much room is there in the brain for the many thousands of other images and concepts to which we can give a name, or that we know, or that we might ever have to distinguish, or might come across in the future? If each neuron represents only one image-concept, and if Jennifer Aniston neurons are so common that a random probe easily finds one, then how much room can there be for other stuff? And what happens when we come across a new face, or object? Do we have a bank of idle neurons waiting to be recruited for the face of the next starlet? Or do we kidnap others that have been doing other jobs that have lapsed into obsolescence?

The simple conclusion the researchers drew in this case is not supportable without further argument. It has significant theoretical ramifications that were not addressed by the authors.

A Molecular Account   What happens when we try to account for this experiment using our molecular framework? Recall that when an instance atom is activated it tries to find a processor, somewhere near where its generic parent lives, where it can start work. We now make a reasonable assumption: Suppose that the atoms tend to be instantiated in roughly the same places each time they come up. So if I see an image of Jennifer Aniston now, and then again in ten minutes, the instance atoms for Jennifer Aniston will tend to be in the same place in my foreground (i.e., hosted by the same processor) on each of the two occasions.

The total number of atom-processors in the foreground is relatively small (perhaps in the thousands, as opposed to the hundred billion neurons in the whole brain), so if Quiroga et al. were looking at a part of the brain that was mostly doing high-level processing (as was indeed the case: they kept well away from the low-level vision areas), it would be reasonable to suppose that a random probe would be relatively likely to score a hit on the processor hosting the instance atom that represents Jennifer Aniston.

This idea could explain the results. If the physical structure occupied by an active atom (what we have referred to as the "processor" that hosts the atom) had a moderately large footprint in the foreground, the chance of an electrode landing somewhere in that processor would be quite reasonable. Then, when different views of the same image are shown in the second part of the experiment, the atom for that image would tend to be instantiated in the same spot, and the same neuron would fire strongly each time. Also, since this is the area where high-level concepts are active, the words "Jennifer Aniston" would be just as likely to invoke the same atom.

Now compare this with the conclusion drawn by the experimenters. There are no grandmother cells in this molecular picture; the generic concepts from which the atoms are spawned could be encoded in any way at all, because the electrodes were picking up instances (the active atoms), not the generics. The distinction between generic and instance representations, in fact, is entirely missing from the interpretation of this experiment (a deficit that is shared by many neuroscience studies).

Whichever way we turn, then, there is no evidence for grandmother cells or sparse encoding in this study. If we try to take the sparse encoding idea literally, the results seem strangely improbable, and if we look at our alternative theoretical explanation, the results have no relevance to long-term memory encoding at all.

Study 4: "Subliminal Images Impact on Brain"

Bahrami, Lavie, and Rees (2007) gave participants a visual task to perform, but varied the amount of attention the task demanded. At the same time, participants would see images of tools in peripheral visual areas, but with one eye getting the tool images and the other eye getting a flashing mask in the same place. Because of the masks, the tool images could not be consciously seen, but an analysis of fMRI data from the retinotopic V1 area showed that these tool images were indeed being detected and processed at that stage of the visual pathway. The crucial result was that the amount of activity in V1 associated with the nonconscious tool images was modulated by the amount of attention the main task required: When the attentional load was high, there was less activity in V1.

The immediate conclusion of Bahrami et al. was that unconscious processing of visual stimuli could depend on the degree to which attentional resources were available. This enabled them to say that "These findings challenge previous suggestions that attention and awareness are one and the same (Baars 2005; Mandler 2005) or that attention acts as the gate-keeper to awareness (Block 1996; Lamme 2003)."

If this interpretation is correct, this study should count as level 4 (functional), in that it uses localization data to relate brain function and location and psychological processes, and furthermore enabling us to distinguish between theories at the cognitive level of theorization. Although these conclusions were among the most robust of those we studied in our brief survey, the molecular framework would nevertheless give a slightly different interpretation of the results—and the difference might be enough for those advocating the two rival accounts listed by Bahrami et al. (Baars 2005 and Mandler 2005; Block 1996 and Lamme 2003) to claim that their theories were not necessarily inconsistent with the results after all.

To see why, consider what might be happening if the foreground zone encompasses visual area V1. As described earlier, there is an attentional area, which is a moving patch of high "elaboration" density in the atoms that inhabit the foreground—a subset of the atoms that are able to call up large numbers of others, so as to build a more detailed representation than would otherwise be the case. But when the attentional patch becomes large (as would happen when a task is attentionally demanding), it causes a corresponding thinness in the density of atoms available elsewhere. This thinning of the atoms could stretch out as far as V1. This, in turn, would mean that the atoms being activated in V1 to represent the peripheral tool images would be struggling to form a strong, coherent representation, because strength is partly governed by weight of numbers.

This is straightforward enough, and it gives an interpretation of why there might be clusters of atoms in V1, representing the tool images, that were stronger and more noticeable to the fMRI scan when the attentional load was not as high.

But what determines whether these tool images make it to conscious awareness? This can happen only if the foreground atoms can switch from their current mode (in which the foreground is dominated by atoms related to the primary task) to a new mode in which the system tries to recall and reassemble the atoms that, a few moments ago, were trying to represent the peripheral tools. If the foreground brings back enough of those atoms (which will include those representing both the tool and the intrusive flashing mask), there is a chance that they can cohere enough to form a representation of the tool, at which point the system would move toward a valid conclusion about where the tool image was located. But if the mask created enough noise (in the form of spurious atoms not related to the tool image), then this reconstruction may fail, and when the participants do this introspective examination of their awareness, they may come up with nothing. The tool images would be invisible, not because they caused nothing to happen in the foreground, but because when the foreground attempts to give attention to the place where the tool images might be, it comes up with nothing but noise.

What is interesting about this molecular account is that attention and awareness are *processes*, not places, and they are extremely closely coupled. Bahrami et al. are correct to reject the claim that "attention and awareness are one and the same," but the fact remains that terms like *attention* and *awareness* are used in the literature in widely differing ways, and so this study's conclusion is not as clear as it might seem. If someone were to interpret the Bahrami et al. result to mean that there are two distinct places that control attention and awareness, that conclusion would be false if the molecular account turns out to be correct, because the latter predicts that the two are almost completely enmeshed in one another and separate only under special circumstances.

These questions beg for further theoretical and experimental clarification, but while this particular study makes an interesting and (within limits) valid point about a separation between attention and awareness, the knowledge of that separation does not do much, if anything, to illuminate the detailed differences between the molecular framework and other possible models of attention. Again, we find that the usefulness of the imaging data is circumscribed by the lack of a sufficiently detailed psychological theory.

Study 5: "Brain Scans Can 'Read Your Mind'"

Haynes, Sakai, Rees, Gilbert, Frith, and Passingham (2007) wanted to know if they could decode their subjects' *intentions* (not their explicit motor activity, or preparation to perform a motor activity, but their intention to carry out an abstract idea) from the spatial layout of brain activity in the prefrontal cortex. The subjects were intending to perform either an addition operation or a subtraction, and Haynes et al. did indeed find that they could recognize distinct patterns corresponding to the two intentions.

Two conclusions emerged. One was that the intention manifested itself in a spatial pattern of activity, rather than in the overall level of activity in a particular area. The second conclusion was that the location of this pattern differed in the two cases of (a) thinking about the intention and (b) carrying out the intention: During task execution, a more posterior region of prefrontal cortex was involved, whereas during the intention phase the medial prefrontal cortex showed a clearer pattern. So, reflecting on an intention and carrying out the intention might happen in two different places. These conclusions appear to place this study at level 3, possibly even level 4.

Does this result help us discriminate between any functional-level accounts of cognition? It does tell us that an intention like "I am going to do an addition" is encoded in such a way that it causes changes across a large area of neural circuitry, rather than just in one small patch below the resolution of the scanner. After all, the intention could have been encoded in just a handful of neurons in the prefrontal cortex, with the rest doing unrelated processing, so that the difference would have been undetectable.

Notice, however, that this study, like many of the others, gives us information that seems to be locked in at the neural level alone, without coming up to the functional level and telling us something about how the mechanism of "intending to do an action" actually works. Both empirical conclusions—about the distributed spatial pattern and the change of location between intention and execution—are just giving us different kinds of location data without telling us what kind of mechanism is operating and how it is doing its work.

This study is straightforwardly consistent with our molecular framework. The spatially distributed pattern of atoms that encode the intention to perform an action would be very similar each time that same intention occurred (for the same reason that, earlier, we argued that the Jennifer Aniston atom would likely appear in the same place each time it was activated). If a particular spatial distribution of atoms gave rise to a particular spatial distribution of brain activity (not a foregone conclusion, but quite plausible nonetheless), then a brain scan could distinguish the patterns resulting from two different intentions.

Study 6: "Scientists Discover Brain Trigger for Selfish Behavior"

This study is somewhat different from the others. Knoch, Pascual-Leone, Meyer, Treyer, and Fehr (2006) used low-frequency repetitive transcranial magnetic stimulation (rTMS) to disrupt the dorsolateral prefrontal cortex (DLPFC) in subjects who were trying to play something called the "Ultimatum Game."

This game is a test of the subject's willingness to make a tradeoff between accepting an unfair offer of money (it is unfair because the person making the offer will get a bigger cut than the subject) and rejecting the offer (in which case neither person will get anything). If the unfair offer is accepted, then this indicates that the selfish motive of just taking the money is the one that dominates. If the offer is rejected, this would show that the person has given greater weight to the need to maintain reciprocity—the social custom of rewarding fairness and showing disapproval of unfairness.

The researchers had reason to believe that the DLPFC was involved in the decision-making process here, but there was a question about whether (a) an impulse to reject the unfair offer was coming from somewhere, and the role of the DLPFC was to control that impulse, or (b) an impulse to be selfish and accept the money was coming from elsewhere, with the DLPFC moderating that impulse. The way to decide, according to Knoch et al., was to disrupt the DLPFC during the decision making, and see what happened. More acceptances of unfair offers would imply that this region had previously been acting as a brake on selfish impulses, but if the acceptance rate dropped, this would indicate that the usual role of the DLPFC was to moderate the unfairness motive.

The experimental results indicated that the right DLPFC (but not the left) was involved in suppressing selfish impulses, because the acceptance rate went up when it was disrupted. Subjects still said that they judged the offers to be unfair, when asked, but they felt less inclined to reject them. We consider this study to be concerned with locating where in the brain functions happen, and is therefore level 2.

Observations   Two observations can be made about this experiment. First, the role of the DLPFC might not be to act as a "gate" on the signals coming from the source of selfish impulses: There may be a separate structure that adds up the motives coming from various sources, with the DLPFC sending a vote for reciprocity and another structure sending a vote for selfishness. This kind of architecture would look very different from one in which the DLPFC was specifically designed to gate the signals coming from a selfishness module.

The second observation is about whether the DLPFC is specialized to do the job of enforcing fairness (as Knoch et al. imply), or whether it might simply be part of a mechanism for considering complex motivational issues.

The easiest way to see how this could be so is to go back to the molecular framework again. In the part of the foreground periphery that we have called the "motivation" area substantial numbers of atoms are building representations of the system's goals, drives, and desires. In times of simplicity (I am hungry, there is a cream puff in front of me, and it's mine), there is not much complexity in the structures hanging around the motivation area. But when difficult decisions have to be made, as in the tradeoffs of the Ultimatum Game, a good deal of activity may occur, during which large complexes of atoms must represent complex, abstract ideas and decide between rival impulses coming from outside the foreground. All this activity takes up space in the foreground, so these complex decisions might require larger amounts of cortical real estate.

Now consider one more feature that might be built into the design of the foreground: As far as possible, it needs to be robust against dithering. It must have default plans ready to go if more complex decision-making fails. So, in trying to make a decision to follow one impulse or another, the foreground probably builds representations for several different options, in parallel.

In the present case, the option to obey a selfish impulse is fairly simple, not involving much thought or emotion, so the atoms representing the "take the money" plan may be quite compact and easily assembled. But the processing of fairness and reciprocity concepts is likely to be more extensive, and it may also trigger some strong emotions that trigger yet more action plans. This combination of abstractness and a strong cluster of emotional responses could mean that a larger amount of the foreground needs to be taken up by the processing of the impulses coming from an "unfairness" signal.

If the role of the DLPFC is to accommodate large clusters of atoms involved in difficult decisions, and if simple, default decisions (like just going with the selfish motive) are handled elsewhere, then a disruption of the DLPFC might cause the foreground to go for the simple, selfish option; not because the DLPFC was specialized for fairness, but because its job was to act as an overspill area for complex motivational decisions.

This idea could be consistent with the observation that subjects still say the offer is unfair even when, with their DLPFC disrupted, they decide not to do anything about it. This would happen because the DLPFC is located near the motivational area of the foreground periphery, and is primarily involved in hosting atoms that deal with the flood of signals coming from the "drives"—the cluster of lower-level brain mechanisms that push the foreground to attend to different priorities such as food, comfort, sex, stimulation, and threat. The abstract representation of the idea [this offer is unfair] will take place in the main part of the foreground, where the recognition of other abstract objects occurs. But having abstract knowledge of unfairness is not the same as using that knowledge as an ingredient in the complicated process of weighing the relative merits of different drives, and it is the latter process that the DLPFC might be specifically responsible for. So the DLPFC would get the information that "this offer is unfair" from the main part of the foreground, but if it were disrupted it might not host the complex set of motivation-related atoms triggered by the "unfairness" signal coming from below, and so the default "selfishness" signal wins the day.

Summary This study is a good illustration of how the conclusion of a brain imaging experiment can depend on subtle aspects of the theoretical mechanisms that the experiment is supposed to be localizing. A simple interpretation of the result, in this case, might lead us to believe that the DLPFC is responsible for implementing fairness or reciprocity behaviors. Our alternative molecular framework, however, might give the same structure the role of considering all kinds of complex problems related to the resolution of drives and motivations, not just fairness.

Discussion

In this analysis of the theoretical integrity of six randomly chosen, influential brain imaging experiments, we have found that in no case did the experimental conclusions give us new information about the structure or function of any mechanisms in the human cognitive system. Where we learned anything, we learned only that some known mechanisms are located in a particular place. In no case did a location-fact non-contentiously give us a new functional-fact. So, although at first sight three of these studies aspired to at least level 2, and three even to level 4, in fact we are forced to conclude that when we put them under the microscope they all end up at level 2—localization studies. Even then, we have argued that, because there are alternative accounts of what is happening during the cognitive processing involved in these tasks, we are not sure what exactly is being localized in these brain regions. The strongest conclusion that can be justified in each of the studies appears to be that brain region X "has something to do with" cognitive function Y. There is no reason to assume that these particularly famous studies are other than representative of the entire field.

In the Quiroga et al. experiment (study 3) we also found that the conclusion about sparse encoding in neurons was simply not theoretically coherent. Our alternative "molecular" framework could explain the results of that experiment, but the explanation was orthogonal to the one the authors gave.

In two cases where the authors made strong claims about the location of a functionally defined mechanism—study 1 (claiming that the pLPFC is the location of the dual-task performance bottleneck) and study 6 (claiming that the right DLPFC is specialized for enforcing the fairness motive)—we were able to nullify the reported conclusion by shifting to our molecular framework. In another case, study 4, we were able to at least reduce the clarity of the conclusion by giving a molecular-framework interpretation of what was happening.

Overall, we believe these six studies showed an alarming sensitivity to the theories in cognitive psychology that generated the mechanisms these authors tried to locate. By changing the theoretical framework to one that was slightly out of the mainstream, we were able to show that the conclusions changed. Indeed, in those cases where the conclusions were not perturbed (studies 2 and 5), this may only have been because the claims were too dilute to be susceptible to attack.

If it was this easy for us to propose a framework that made some of the localization results seem less secure, then how vulnerable might these localization studies be to other, as yet unheard-of theoretical frameworks?

Looking Back

Let us return to the questions we raised in the introduction and try to fill in some answers:

- Is where-it-happens information of any use to present-day psychology? Not at the moment, because our cognitive models are insufficiently specified.
- Are the claims about neural localization internally and theoretically coherent? Not always: In one of the six cases we examined, the claim was theoretically incoherent.
- Do the localization claims refer to components of the mind that are clearly defined? No. Many of our current models we consider too constrained by the language of description, so such lay labels as "attention" are sometimes treated as if they correspond in a simple way to cognitive mechanisms. For this reason, we advocate computational modeling, where cognitive processes may have no simple correspondence with our intuitions and labels, as the way forward. Note, we are not saying that where-it-happens is never going to be interesting or useful!
- Are the inferences made by researchers theory-laden? A definite yes to this one.
- Are today's studies, which give us only crude localization data (both spatially and temporally), just a prelude to later research that will pin down location and function precisely, or is crude localization all we can ever expect from brain imaging technology? This question is an important one to which we return in the following sections.

By pointing out that our new framework often conflicts with these localization results, we are implying that more work needs to be done, somewhere. But in any of the cases where our framework raises new questions, should those questions be addressed by more studies of the localization of function? Is the solution really just more brain imaging?

The Stages of Cognitive Science

Cognitive science is destined to go through three phases in its history. In phase 1 we do our best to produce metaphorlike descriptions of functional-level mechanisms. The language we use to articulate theories at this level will contain descriptions of things that sometimes look as if they could be mechanisms at the implementational level, but this is often an illusion.

In the future (and perhaps starting already) we would hope to move toward a complete outline theory of the human cognitive system. At this stage, we would expect the basic processes and structures to be clear enough that no drastic changes would be arriving to disrupt the outline theory in the future. This then would be phase 2; but this stage would still be only a functional-level description of the mind.

In phase 3, we would commit to how the complete functional-level theory was implemented in the particular neural hardware we find in our brains. Instead of just completely describing how the "atoms" of our framework interacted with one another to give rise to all known psychological data, for example, we would go on to say how those atoms were implemented in specific neural circuits. These three stages are not expected to be completely separate, of course, but we nevertheless believe that extensive phase 3 work is not very useful or appropriate when we are still struggling to move from phase 1 to phase 2.

Are all studies of the brain a waste of time? Certainly not, but a great deal hinges on the granularity of the information being gathered. If today's brain imaging studies were just a warm-up for new types of investigation that promise to yield detailed circuit diagrams and real-time behavior of large networks of human neurons, with such things as precise tracking of synapse strengths and dendritic tree layouts, then we could perhaps see how today's crude localization studies might be laying the groundwork for future scientific cornucopias.

But nothing remotely like such a level of neural detail is on the horizon, and so we are in a bind. On the one hand, the resolution of these brain imaging studies is not enough to tell us useful things about the functional level, and future improvements in the technology do not appear to offer the granularity of information that we need. On the other hand, the level of specificity of the cognitive theories is currently not good enough to make coarse-grained localization theories useful.

The Way Forward
Would it be reasonable for someone working in imaging to say "so we're in this pickle because of psychology—how are they going to get us out of it?" We don't think that psychology, in the sense of being just an experimental science, can solve the problem by itself. In all the preceding cases, where our molecular framework gives an idiosyncratic view of what might be happening at the functional level, there are many questions we could ask about what might be going on, but the best way to answer those questions would be to increase the sophistication of our computer simulations of the functional-level mechanisms (Loosemore 2007), and to perform human behavioral experiments to test the predictions those simulations made. We can see how answers to these kinds of questions would advance our understanding of psychology immeasurably. But right now, we are being flooded with accurate answers to questions about the brain location of mechanisms that we do not believe in and inaccurate answers to questions about the brain location of mechanisms that are currently not terribly interesting. This state of affairs seems to us to be a great leap backwards.

18 Neuroimaging as a Tool for Functionally Decomposing Cognitive Processes

William Bechtel and Richard C. Richardson

Both those who extol and those who castigate neuroimaging studies and their invocation in cognitive science often misconstrue the contribution neuroimaging is seeking to make, and is capable of making, to cognitive science. We do believe that advances in neuroimaging, including functional magnetic resonance imaging (fMRI), as well as such techniques as single cell recording, are important contributions to the experimental repertoire of cognitive science. We also anticipate that neuroimaging's importance will increase with improvements in imaging technologies and techniques.

Our objective here, however, is neither to extol nor to castigate neuroimaging, but to make clear what sort of contribution neuroimaging, when done well, can make to understanding and explaining mental phenomena. Many of those who adopt extreme views of neuroimaging are not themselves practitioners of the technique and fail to appreciate principles that are commonplace or platitudes among the expert practitioners. Of course, some who adopt extreme views are practitioners. Accordingly, though we are by no means expert practitioners, we start with some commonplaces that are not always transparent in reports of neuroimaging, but are generally understood by the researchers conducting the research (see, for example, Logothetis 2008) and need to be taken into account by those evaluating it:

1. The brain contains some regions that are specialized for processing specific types of information. This is most clearly established in sensory and motor regions, though we expect the conclusion is more general; yet even these regions integrate information from a large number of other regions with which they engage in complex dynamical interaction. Some of those regions are colloquially thought of as "downstream" in the visual system.

2. Functional MRI, by identifying particular areas of increased blood flow, may seem to support the idea that there are highly specialized regions, some kind of modules, but much of this is illusory. Measures of BOLD activity show differences in regional activation, and the impression of modules is enhanced by the often vivid illustrations. Finding differences in activation, coupled with BOLD signals, is not tantamount to

identifying modules; and the typical and very vivid coloring is but an illustrative artifact.

3. Even though there are specialized processing regions (commonplaces 1 and 2), these regions are not encapsulated or insulated from one another. A given region may process a particular type of information and thereby be differentiated from other regions, but it processes information generated in other areas with which it is connected and outputs information to yet other regions. This is often accompanied by elaborate feedback (even in the sensory areas). The network of connections is crucial to the operation of the brain (commonplace 7). Though there is often talk of centers, the real interest is in seeing how various areas interact in a given task. What is wanted is an understanding of populations of neurons, their connections, and ultimately their dynamics.

4. The fact that a given brain region displays increased activation to a stimulus or in performing a specified task does not at all imply that the same region does not respond to many other stimuli or cannot engage in other tasks (commonplace 3). In fact, aside from more peripheral areas, regions commonly respond to many different stimuli; there is also a great deal of spontaneous activity. This is one implication of emphasizing that BOLD signals tell us about *changes* in activation.

5. Lack of a BOLD signal in a region doesn't mean the region lacks activation. This is true for a number of reasons: (a) Though it is true that enhanced activation increases blood flow, it is possible for functionally significant regions to go undetected (a voxel includes thousands of neurons, and it takes increased activity in many to "light up" a region); (b) some neurons may be more efficient than others, and thus have a less visible BOLD signal; (c) some regions have very high blood flow in general, and their BOLD signal may increase only marginally even when active.

6. The activity in any given region of the brain is a function of both excitation and inhibition; any changes in the balance—whether the result is an increase or a decrease in activity—will affect the BOLD signal. (Increased inhibition can lead to increased metabolism, and not to a negative signal.)

7. Imaging studies are invoked not primarily to answer the question of where in the brain an operation is performed, but to determine what operations are performed and how they matter to the overall outcome. Moreover, they are not intended to address global issues (e.g., what sort of information processing system the brain is) but local issues (e.g., whether two activities invoke the same neural processes, or whether some area is implicated in some cognitive activity).

We take these to be uncontroversial ideas among those whose research deploys fMRI systematically. We also do not take these to be unconnected observations. Indeed, they form a more or less integrated set of practices. Unfortunately, some interpretations of fMRI work defy one or more of the commonplace assumptions within the field.

We emphasize these commonplaces at the outset because we think it is important to keep the overall framework in mind when discussing the use and abuse of fMRI. We will return to specific commonplaces in our discussion, which focuses on Loosemore and Harley's challenges to invoking neuroimaging results that engage cognitive phenomena. Loosemore and Harley's challenges are representative of those who castigate neuroimaging as useless for understanding the mind/brain (for other recent critics, see Coltheart 2004; Uttal 2001; van Orden and Paap 1997). Their critique has two major parts: (1) an argument that neuroimaging is premature, since its results can only be properly construed once cognitive psychology has reached a more mature state; and (2) an analysis of six studies (four involving neuroimaging, one single-cell recording, one transcranial magnetic stimulation) that are meant to demonstrate the inability of neuroimaging to contribute to the maturation of cognitive theories. In the following sections we address these points. In the second section, we contrast Loosemore and Harley's conception of how sciences progress with a different conception grounded on analysis of progress in sciences devoted to discovering the mechanisms responsible for phenomena of interest. In the third section, we examine the neuroimaging studies Loosemore and Harley criticize and argue that the objections the researchers raise against them are not warranted.

The Contribution of Neuroimaging to Discovering Cognitive Mechanisms

Loosemore and Harley offer what we take to be an extremely problematic account of how scientific inquiry progresses as it attempts to identify the mechanisms responsible for a given phenomenon. They present three stages cognitive science is "destined" to go through in its history. Stage 1 involves advancing "metaphor-like descriptions of functional-level mechanisms." At stage 2, researchers agree on a "complete outline theory of the human cognitive system." At this stage, Loosemore and Harley further claim, "we would expect the basic processes and structures to be clear enough that no drastic changes would be arriving to disrupt the outline theory in the future." Finally, at stage 3 researchers can identify how this complete account is realized in the human brain.

The talk of the stages of cognitive science as a matter of destiny is theirs rather than ours, though it is not developed in their paper to any significant extent. Apparently, the stages are inflexible in ordering, and determine the usefulness of information from the neurosciences. We regard their stage theory with skepticism. Loosemore and Harley maintain that cognitive science is currently only at stage 1 and until it progresses through stage 2, neither neuroimaging nor any other investigation of the brain is capable of providing any significant contributions. In this view, the role for neuroimaging would essentially be limited to identifying the structures that realize a given cognitive process; neuroimaging would not contribute substantially toward elaborating the structure of cognitive models, and would be useful only at stage 3. (Presumably, other sources of information about neurophysiological mechanisms would also not contribute, in the absence of at least a stage 2 psychology.) In our view, this both underestimates the contributions neuroimaging can make to the development of cognitive models and overestimates the prospects of progress for cognitive science in the absence of information about neural processing. Integration of behavioral, psychological and neuroscientific perspectives is, on our view, much more promising as a research program (Bechtel and McCauley 1999; Craver 2007; McCauley 2007; McCauley and Bechtel 2001; Richardson 2009). It would be a mistake to postpone inquiries into cognitive neuroscience while we wait on the emergence of a completed psychology; moreover, it is possible for the use of imaging data to discriminate between cognitive models (Henson 2006).

Figuring out the basic processes or operations through which a complex mechanism is able to generate some phenomenon of interest—in this case, some aspect of human behavior or some cognitive capacity—is, in fact, a critical part of developing a mechanistic explanation. Guidance in discovering these operations often comes from identifying the component parts of the system and using their identity as a tool in identifying the operations they perform. Cognitive psychology, through much of its history (from the 1950s through the late 1980s), was constrained to attempting to identify the operations involved in producing cognitive phenomena without benefit of information about the brain regions that perform these operations.[1] This was a result of the lack of research tools and techniques that enable identification of human brain areas involved in performing cognitive activities.

During the same period, researchers in neuroscience developed not only detailed accounts of the brain areas involved in processes such as visual perception, but also elaborated serious proposals as to the specialized operations (commonplace 1) these areas perform (van Essen and Gallant 1994). They did this working with other species in which invasive techniques such as single-cell recording, direct electrical stimulation, and localized lesions could be employed (Logothetis and Pfeuffer 2004). It is important to realize that these neuroscientific inquiries were concerned with determining the identity of brain areas (using tools such as neural connections and the patterns of topographical projection of the visual field onto different maps), systematically mapping out the projections to and from a given area (using, for example, retrograde stains to detect regions projecting to an area of interest), and figuring out what operations the delineated areas performed. The last objective was accomplished primarily by determining the nature of the visual stimuli that would specifically produce action potentials in neurons in a particular brain region (edges in V1, illusory contours in V2, motion in V4, color and shape in V5, etc.). The research produced some quite surprising discoveries about the functional processes involved in vision, including the differentiation of two relatively independent processing streams (dorsal and ventral) that process different information about visual stimuli—the identity of the objects perceived and the location and potential for acting on the objects (see Bechtel 2008, for a historical review).

The results of these investigations, mostly done on monkeys (also mice, rats, and rabbits), have been generalized to humans, although often only via the use of neuro-imaging since research comparable to that done on other mammals cannot be performed on humans (for ethical and political reasons). Arguably, these accounts of visual processing generated in approximately fifty years of research are the most detailed characterizations of the operations involved in a cognitive activity (commonplace 1). Moreover, these results are among those least likely to be disrupted (radically at least) by further research. This was due in no small measure to the fact that research identifying brain regions went hand-in-hand with research identifying the operations these regions performed: As researchers differentiated brain areas, for example, on the basis of their containing a topological map of the visual field, they also investigated what stimuli would enhance the spiking rate of neurons in the area. The elaboration of this research depended on coordinating research from a variety of scientific research specialties. It was, emphatically, not true that psychologists first developed a detailed and defensible cognitive model, which was only afterward shown to be realized in the brain.

Stepping back a bit, we can place research seeking mechanisms for cognitive phenomena in the broader context of the discovery of mechanisms in the life sciences (Bechtel 2008; Bechtel and Richardson 1993). Developing a mechanistic explanation requires, in part, decomposing the mechanism into its parts and operations. Another extremely important challenge in developing a mechanistic explanation is to determine how the parts and operations are organized, both spatially and temporally, so as to produce the phenomenon. This is crucial to understanding the discovery of mechanisms, but perhaps not so crucial in the current context, except in the emphasis on uncovering system dynamics.

Typically, different research techniques are required to decompose a system functionally into its operations or structurally into its parts, and one set of tools may be available when another is not. Brodmann (1909; 1994), for example, made major progress in differentiating brain regions using neuroanatomical tools. Despite hoping the areas he delineated would be functionally significant, he had no tools for identifying the operations they performed. Likewise, gene sequencing has provided detailed maps of the genomes of many species, but cannot itself inform us about the functionality of various strands of DNA. On the other hand, decomposing the mechanism functionally into its operations can also be pursued without information about the structures involved. Like cognitive psychologists, biochemists initially had no tools for discovering the structures they took to be responsible for catalyzing reactions and had to proceed to identify the reactions employing purely functional techniques. Whereas cognitive psychologists have had limited tools for developing functional decompositions (e.g., dissociations in reactions times, error patterns, or cognitive deficits), biochemists were able to be more invasive by, for example, inhibiting reactions with poisons and identifying the product that built up. Nonetheless, the fundamental logic of the cases is similar.

The fact that researchers have made progress in developing a functional decomposition independently of a structural decomposition, or vice versa, however, does not make it a virtue to proceed with one before the other. Though psychology did manage to make progress in the middle decades of the last century in identifying cognitive processes, the virtue was born of necessity. Without access to an independent source of evidence, psychologists made the best of what was possible. Proposing that operations are performed by identifiable parts often serves to significantly advance inquiry into both parts and operations. Typically, neither the functional analysis nor the structural analysis reaches a mature form before operations are identified with parts; neither can it reach a mature form the organization of the system is understood. It is not uncommon for researchers to realize, after they have linked an operation with a part, that the part in question cannot perform the whole operation and, in fact, multiple operations are involved in what seemed to be a simple operation. In some cases, knowledge of the structure and capacities of a part suggest that the characterization of the operation itself needed to be revised. For example, biochemists spent 20 years seeking a high-energy chemical intermediate that transferred energy released in the electron transport chain to adenosine triphosphate (ATP). The recognition that this reaction occurs in the cristae membranes in mitochondria suggested a very different operation for energy transfer, one involving the creation of a proton gradient across a membrane. Likewise, recognition of the importance of long-term potentiation (LTP) in the 1960s involved both anatomical work and electrophysiological research integrating both structural and functional information (Craver 2003).

Linking operations to parts is thus often an important aspect of developing both the functional and structural decompositions (commonplace 1). Since the structural decomposition often involves specifying spatially where the parts are, and the connections among those parts, integrating the two often takes the form of localizing operations within the overall mechanism (accordingly, we employ the term *localization* for hypotheses identifying structures with functions). The point of localization, however, is not simply to figure out *where* operations take place, but to draw on what is known about the structures involved and their relation to other structures to provide evidence and often heuristic guidance in characterizing operations and unearthing the systemic organization. As we emphasize in our commonplaces (3 and 7), the point is to understand how the system functions, how it works dynamically, and that is not just a matter of finding what, if anything, realizes a particular function. Thus, one should not construe fMRI, or other means of localizing cognitive processes in the brain, as simply revealing how an independently developed psychological theory is implemented, or where some cognitive capacity is realized.[2]

The process of developing a mature mechanistic account may involve numerous iterations of localization combined with further articulations of functional and structural decompositions, along with independent assessments of the functional capacities of components. For example, initial attempts to identify where in the brain a supposed operation involved in a particular task occurs may reveal multiple structures; it may also fail to reveal some structures that are involved (commonplace 5). This is a powerful spur to discovery. It is possible that several of the brain areas perform the same operation. There is sometimes substantial redundancy. It is also possible that each of the brain areas performs a different function, which complement one another.[3] Typically, researchers tend to suspect that each distinct part is performing a somewhat different operation and that the initial functional account needs to be amended. Since invasive research on brain areas in humans is restricted, researchers need to pursue other strategies for revealing the operations involved. An important clue is often the discovery that one of the brain areas is involved in a variety of different tasks (commonplace 4). Researchers can then explore what operation might be employed in these different tasks, what different tasks have in common, and how differences can be managed. Having connected one of the areas to a specific operation, they can then return to the first task and ask what operations are required besides that associated with the given area. The process now iterates as researchers explore these other areas. The important point to emphasize is that localization need not come at the end of inquiry (stage 3 in Loosemore and Harley's picture), but may come early in inquiry, where it can function as a discovery heuristic (Wimsatt 2007). Another way to press the point is to emphasize that functional decompositions both respond to and shape structural decompositions.

Although Loosemore and Harley emphasize the stage account for developing cognitive psychology in their abstract, it is not totally clear to us how committed they really are to it. As we have said, we are skeptical. Nothing much here hinges on the skepticism over stages. The paper included here does not do much to elaborate the account. Instead, they articulate four levels at which "imaging the localization of function of components of anything—parts of cars, computers, or brains—can be described": tokenism, absolute location, relative location, and functional. Tokenism is the use of brain images just because they are available and impressive, not because they contribute to the scientific investigation. Of course, we recognize that sometimes the imaging doesn't substantially contribute to research, aside from providing a vivid presentation. We suppose that is tokenism. Absolute location provides the locus of an operation, whereas relative localization appeals to how operations are situated with respect to each other to support claims about how they act on each other. Loosemore and Harley note that, in the case of the brain, relative location can be further articulated in terms of neural connectivity, since it is connected brain areas that are likely to interact with each other in generating the phenomenon. The functional location uses the location where an operation is performed to develop the decomposition into operations—the contribution of a component to systemic function. As soon as they introduce this level, Loosemore and Harley return to their central criticism: "you already need to know mostly what each component does before you can begin to make sense of it." This rests on the assumption that the only real use of neuroimaging would be to provide information about the implementation or realization of already well-understood cognitive processing. We regard this as their central mistake.

If this charge were true, it would not be necessary to examine actual imaging studies to show that, although they might seem to be at level 4, they really are only at level 2 because they do not contribute to the further articulation of a functional decomposition. All that would be necessary would be to show that a detailed functional decomposition (that was unlikely to be further changed) was not already available in cognitive psychology to demonstrate that imaging studies were limited to stage 2 or 3. The most Loosemore and Harley would need to show is that the psychology is so impoverished that it cannot sustain any attempt at neural realization. The critical focus would be on the psychology rather than the neuroscience. As an analogy, absent a developed phenomenological theory of inheritance (such as the patterns supposedly unearthed by Mendel), it might make little sense to inquire into the mechanisms of inheritance (though that was actually attempted). The actual history is more interesting, and surely does not sustain the top-down picture that dominates in Loosemore and Harley.

In analyzing the cases, they argue that the imaging studies have not contributed toward a better functional decomposition. Thus, implicitly at least, Loosemore and Harley seem to be granting that imaging studies could contribute to functional decomposition, as we have suggested, but in fact they fail to fulfill this promise. To address this, we need to go beyond a general characterization of a mechanistic research program and the role localization plays in it to a detailed examination of the contribution of localization arising from neuroimaging.

Reexamination of the Neuroimaging Studies

A major portion of Loosemore and Harley's discussion is devoted to six target neuroimaging studies (two, in fact, do not employ imaging but either single-cell recording or transcranial magnetic stimulation to suppress operations). They choose the studies, they explain, on the basis that they were discussed in the popular press—a selection strategy they defend on the grounds that they "wanted to generate a sample of what the popular press finds interesting about psychology and the brain." This strikes us as a peculiar way of identifying neuroimaging studies that have the best chance of contributing to a functional decomposition of cognitive processes. Even if, as Loosemore and Harley claim, the press is interested in research that purports to explain behavior, it might not be the best evaluator of what research is contributing positively to current research objectives any more than the popularity of a topic is indicative of its importance (think of flying saucers or Bigfoot). It is also clear that reports in the public press tend to distort the studies at issue, either emphasizing what the studies do not, or actively distorting their impact. The best research is more complex, and more focused, than the press is comfortable reporting. For those who have any doubt, the interest of the press in claims of finding genes for particular functions and underlying specific diseases, rather than in the complex regulatory mechanisms involved in gene expression that are increasingly being identified, should be a cautionary note. We regard the popular reports of brain regions "for" this or that cognitive activity with comparable skepticism. Irrespective of how these studies were chosen, however, we will argue that each aims at contributing to functional decomposition of mental processes and so escapes the charges Loosemore and Harley make.

Before turning to the studies themselves, we need to comment briefly on a peculiar feature of Loosemore and Harley's critique of these studies. Part of their critiques is directed to the details of the studies themselves, and for the most part, we'll be occupied with this part. However, a second part of their critiques is devoted to arguing that an alternative framework they put forward, employing a very different functional decomposition, is compatible with the results of each of the studies. As a result, they claim that the functional decompositions of cognitive phenomena are underdetermined by the evidence and any imputed functional contributions of the imaging studies are unsupported. We would be remiss to ignore this second part.

Loosemore and Harley present their framework, which they call a *molecular model of cognition*, as "a new, unified framework that describes the overall architecture of the human cognitive system." They evidently do not think of this as a serious model of cognition, but as a kind of toy structure they can use critically. The architecture consists of a dynamic working memory in which active "concept units" representing instances interact with each other based on constraints incorporated in each concept, and a background long-term memory in which concept units representing generic categories reside. The model is presented very sketchily, with no empirical backing and no substantive constraints. Loosemore and Harley describe qualitatively how their model might be applied to recognizing visual objects and the activity of sitting down, but offer no detailed results to demonstrate that the model could accommodate even the most accepted empirical results about recognition or control. From Loosemore and Harley's perspective, this is not a serious problem, since their goal is simply to show that the neuroimaging results underdetermine the functional decomposition of cognitive mechanisms. As they explain, "our real goal is to see how sensitive the conclusions of these studies might be to a slight change in the theoretical mechanisms whose location is being sought." One might think that if research results can be equally accommodated by newly constructed and untested qualitative models, this is a reason not to trust the imaging researchers' interpretation of their results. This, however, is a cartoon of serious science. Scientists do not need to defend the interpretation of their research against any underspecified model, but only those that are taken to be serious alternative models. (If Loosemore and Harley were right, then evolutionary biologists would need consistently to defend themselves against Creationist contentions. That would hardly improve the state of the biological sciences.) The alternative models that are taken seriously are those for which evidence already points to their plausibility. In the absence of any articulated models, perhaps speculation is sufficient. Normally, though, there is a more or less well-articulated set of alternatives, and the point of experimentation is to discriminate among them (commonplace 7). We'll see that this is a pattern Loosemore and Harley miss in some of the studies they condemn.

Loosemore and Harley indicate that their alternative cognitive model is in the tradition of computational models in cognitive science. Serious computational modelers, however, provide detailed accounts of operations and demonstrate that the resulting models, minimally, can accommodate behavioral data about the phenomena being modeled. There is increasing interest in computational models linking their results to knowledge of the brain, often based on neuroimaging results (see, for example, Anderson 2007). These efforts, however, are highly demanding, and importantly, when they attempt to draw on neuroimaging studies to evaluate their models, the project is essentially comparable to that in the imaging studies Loosemore and Harley review. Our point is not to defend this sort of modeling. Computational models are sometimes dramatically underdetermined by the evidence, so that many computational models are compatible with both behavioral profiles and capabilities. This renders the endeavor extremely challenging. For those engaged in such research, the goal is to reduce the degree of underdetermination over time as new evidence eliminates previously plausible models. This underdetermination is different from that resulting from an underspecified and untested model such as Loosemore and Harley invoke.

Before leaving Loosemore and Harley's molecular model, it is worth noting that one of its more novel features is the proposal that the representations of instances are "created on the fly." There are interesting similarities here with Larry Barsalou's account of concepts, but the differences in how Barsalou has developed and defended his account are also noteworthy. In his early research on concepts Barsalou (1987) demonstrated, using behavioral data, that prototypicality judgments for both goal-directed and ordinary taxonomic concepts vary substantially over time, and proposed that they were constructed anew and differently on each occasion of use. Barsalou (1999) advanced an account according to which concepts are grounded in perceptual-motor processing. Accordingly, unlike many traditional psychological accounts of concepts that treat them as amodal representations, Barsalou argues that concepts are essentially modal. More recently, he has defended a view that reasoning with concepts involves simulation, where simulation is understood as

... the reenactment of perceptual, motor, and introspective states acquired during experience with the world, body, and mind. As an experience occurs (e.g., easing into a chair), the brain captures states across the modalities and integrates them with a multimodal representation stored in memory (e.g., how a chair looks and feels, the action of sitting, introspections of comfort and relaxation). Later, when knowledge is needed to represent a category (e.g., chair), multimodal representations captured during experiences with its instances are reactivated to simulate how the brain represented perception, action, and introspection associated with it. (Barsalou 2008, 618–619)

Unlike Loosemore and Harley, who contend that the full functional account of these processes needs to be developed *in advance* of finding neural realizers, Barsalou has embraced neural studies, including imaging, as a tool for developing his account. In his hands, fMRI results are employed in much the same manner as purely behavioral evidence in determining the linkages between the operations involved in conceptual tasks and those figuring in sensory motor tasks. For example, in a purely behavioral study that supported the claim that simulation figures in perceptual processing, Solomon and Barsalou (2004) took advantage of the fact that larger properties are more difficult to verify perceptually to predict that it should be more difficult to evaluate whether larger properties apply to a given concept (a property verification task) than smaller properties. This is a prediction an amodal account of concepts would not make, but turned out to be true. Similarly, Pecher, Zeelenberg, and Barsalou (2004) found that switching modalities in successful property identification trials impaired performance. Simmons et al. (2007) turned to fMRI to show that areas in left fusiform gyrus that are active in color perception are more active in tasks requiring subjects to verify that properties are related to a concept when subjects are queried with color properties than with motor properties. These are results that would be expected if concepts are modally grounded, but not otherwise. Note that Barsalou had little interest in the specific brain areas involved but rather was interested in whether the same brain areas are involved in sensory processing and categorization tasks, as this could contribute to characterizing the operations involved in the categorization task. Again, this is a commonplace (3).

We turn now to the specific studies Loosemore and Harley review and criticize. Of course, criticism of such studies is welcome and often informative. Studies are sometimes well constructed and sometimes not. We had no prior conviction about whether or not the studies Loosemore and Harley criticized are well constructed. In fact, we find some more interesting than others and have ordered the four neuroimaging studies in ascending order of interest (taking up the two nonimaging studies last). Our concern, though, is with whether the sort of criticism Loosemore and Harley offer is probative—whether it sheds light on the use or abuse of neuroimaging. Let us look at the cases Loosemore and Harley selected.

Dux, Ivanoff, Asplund, and Marois

The first study discussed by Loosemore and Harley is one by Dux, Ivanoff, Asplund and Marois (2006). It has long been known that tasks may compete for cognitive resources, and when interference occurs, tasks appear to be queued rather than performed in parallel. Behaviorally, this was explored with studies of reaction time. What was generally seen is that competing tasks tended to be delayed if they were presented within a suitably short timeframe. The delay was both a measure of the interference and suggestive of a mechanism. The question Dux et al. ask concerns the neural basis of this interference. Until their study, attempts to localize the "bottleneck" had relied on the amplitude of BOLD responses to identify the source of the interference. The result is that different studies have emphasized a wide array of "putative neural substrates," including lateral, frontal, prefrontal and dorsal regions. The novel contribution of Dux et al. was to turn to time-resolved fMRI, allowing them to discern the relative timing across regions. They argue that the posterior lateral prefrontal cortex (pLPFC) is crucially implicated in the limitations on processing. They do not claim that it is solely implicated in the limitations on processing.

Loosemore and Harley say this is a level-2 or level-3 study, telling us the absolute location of some process, and perhaps something about its relation to other psychological processes. Loosemore and Harley express some skepticism about whether bottlenecks are real or not. Of course, if they are not, then the Dux et al. study can hardly reach even level 2, since there would be no process to localize. We are not certain what weight to give this skepticism.[4] The existence of interference is a robustly resilient psychological effect, quite apart from the use of imaging studies. We are inclined to take the allusion to a "bottleneck" as simply shorthand for the interference effects evident in competing tasks. At other places, Loosemore and Harley seem to relax their skepticism, at least acknowledging that there are interference effects. They notice that "cognitive psychological studies alone" are sufficient to underscore the fact that there is interference. They also note that the Dux et al. study does not allow the researchers to "discover the 'reason' people find it hard to do two tasks at once." With that conclusion we have no quarrel. Dux et al. also do not claim to have found such a "reason."

As we've said, we take the point of the Dux et al. study to adjudicate between the several proposals for the locus of the "bottleneck," using time-resolved fMRI. The pLPFC exhibited behavior consistent with it being a "bottleneck." A bottleneck needs to satisfy several criteria: (1) it must be shared by tasks that do not share either input or output modalities; (2) it must be "involved" in response selection; and (3) it must exhibit serial queuing. The third is, of course, what makes a bottleneck a bottleneck. It is important that being a bottleneck at all depends on the structure being connected in appropriate ways to both input and output modalities. If there were not multiple inputs, there would likewise be no possibility for being a bottleneck (criteria 1 and 2). This is not a matter so much of finding a location for some process as of finding an appropriately linked brain structure (commonplace 7). Dux et al. cautiously observe that this does not mean no other regions play a role in dual task interference (commonplace 4); it is simply *not* true that the failure to detect activation in their experiment indicates there is no activation in the alternative regions, or that other regions are not functionally involved (commonplace 2). As they notice, in addition, this region is recruited by quite diverse cognitive tasks. Finally, the Dux et al. study doesn't actually pretend, as far as we can see, to tell us anything about the specific cognitive function(s) in the pLPFC (commonplace 7) aside from the fact that it is, in one way or another, involved in response selection (criterion 2). It is nonetheless a functional study, geared to identifying the network of connections involved in performance.

Aron, Fisher, Mashek, Strong, and Brown

For Aron, Fisher, Mashek, Strong, and Brown (2005), the goal is to understand the type of mental operations involved in early stages of romantic love, which would seem to situate their study at level 4. The main alternatives they consider are that romantic love is a distinct emotion (as has been defended by Gonzaga et al., 2001) or that it involves operations that figure more generally in the pursuit of rewards. Loosemore and Harley mischaracterize these alternatives as "a strong emotion" or "an overwhelming desire to achieve an objective," missing the point of relating romantic love to the broader set of processes involved in pursuing rewards. To evaluate these alternatives Aron et al. consider two predictions that would follow from the second alternative but not from the first: (1) "romantic love would specifically involve subcortical regions that mediate reward, such as the ventral tegmental area (VTA) and ventral striatum/nucleus accumbens," and (2) "the neural systems involved in early-stage romantic love ... would be associated with other goal and reward systems, such as the anterior caudate nucleus." The imaging results they present support these predictions. Note how Aron et al. state their conclusion:

[T]he results lead us to suggest that early-stage, intense romantic love is associated with reward and goal representation regions, and that rather than being a specific emotion, romantic love is better characterized as a motivation or goal-oriented state that *leads to* various specific emotions such as euphoria or anxiety. (p. 335)

Thus, Aron et al. present their study as identifying parts of a network of processes involved in romantic love, not, as Loosemore and Harley suggest, as equating romantic love with a particular process (commonplace 7). Notice, the thought is not that there are not specialized regions (commonplace 1), but that romantic love involves the VTA, which "mediates" reward. The thought is also not that the VTA is a center that "realizes" reward mechanisms. In fact the study is focused on *denying* there is a distinct emotion, and situating the response in a more general network of responses.

One of the reasons Aron et al. find it significant that the VTA and related areas are involved is that these areas are dopamine rich. Loosemore and Harley criticize this part of the study for not specifying the relation between dopamine release and motivation. However, that was not Aron et al.'s objective. Rather, the point of identifying these areas as dopamine rich is to be able to link the imaging results with a broad array of results from other techniques for investigating dopamine function and to relate romantic love to other activities that involve these dopamine-rich brain areas. Loosemore and Harley question whether the study shows anything more than that early stages of romantic love involve desire for the object of love. What the study actually purports to show is that the desire involved in romantic love involves the same mechanisms of desire as figure in such phenomena as desire for cocaine and so is not unique to romantic love. If these results are correct, they advance the functional study of romantic love by relating it to a broader class of mental activities and the network involved in those activities. Of course, much more research is required to identify the component parts and operations within this network, and here we are skeptical; but determining what network to examine is an important step in developing a functional account. Our point is that the focus of the study is on networks rather than loci (commonplace 7).

Bahrami, Lavie, and Rees

Bahrami, Lavie, and Rees (2007) addressed the question of whether modulating attentional load in one task could affect the processing in early visual areas of stimuli of which the subjects lacked conscious awareness. The study is clearly about the relation of one process (attention) to another (visual processing). This is made apparent by the motivation for the study. Bahrami et al. turned to imaging to address a possible confound in earlier attempts to address this issue behaviorally by measuring priming effects through reaction times (Chun and Jiang 1998; Dehaene et al. 1998). The effects of priming on reaction time could result from the effects of attention on early processing or from modulating the strength of motor response associations. The latter option was not an idle worry, as there is independent psychological evidence for the effects of priming on motor responses (Sumner et al. 2006). Also, the previous evidence that high perceptual load modulates V1 activity did not distinguish between conscious and unconscious perception: "Indeed, some have even claimed that V1 activity related to feedback from extrastriate cortices serves as the arbiter of conscious awareness" (Bahrami et al. cite Silvanto et al. 2005). Given the effects they were able to show on processing in V1 under conditions where they prevented subjects from becoming aware of the visual stimuli while otherwise modulating their attentional load, Bahrami et al. concluded the following:

The present findings are the first to show that neural processes involved in the retinotopic registration of stimulus presence in V1 depend on availability of attentional capacity, even when they do not invoke any conscious experience.... Importantly, our new findings that the level of attentional load in a central task determines retinotopic V1 responses to invisible stimuli clarify both that unconscious processing depends on attentional capacity (which is reduced in conditions of high load) and that availability of attentional capacity for stimulus processing (in the low load conditions) cannot be a sufficient condition for awareness. (p. 510)

It is hard not to see this study as directed at level 4, the functional level in Loosemore and Harley's hierarchy. The objective was to find out whether one process (attentional demands in one task) affected another (early visual possessing). The only reason Loosemore and Harley offer for it not being at this level is that their molecular framework could offer a different interpretation. At best, this would show that the Bahrami et al. study was not conclusive, not that it was not a level-4 study. Since they later claim that none of the studies they review rise above level 2, there must be another reason for downgrading the study. Our best guess is that Loosemore and Harley infer from the fact that Bahrami et al. invoke processing in a place in the brain that it is only a localization study, rather than a contribution to a functional analysis (commonplace 7). But it is clear that location of processing was used here only to situate the activity of interest in an already developed functional model of visual processes so as to gain evidence about the impact of attention on that processing.

Haynes, Sakai, Rees, Gilbert, Frith, and Passingham

The goal of Haynes et al. (2007) is likewise to resolve a functional question, one that had been posed by earlier imaging studies revealing prefrontal activities in human goal-related activities. These studies failed to resolve whether the activity in prefrontal cortex reflected an intention to perform a certain type of activity or planning for task execution. The alternatives are straightforward. Is forming an intention a separate mental operation? Or are forming an intention and planning for execution part of a singular process? To determine whether this activity could be differentiated, Haynes et al. first had subjects choose which task to perform (add or subtract two numbers) before they were given the numbers themselves and required to select the answer. They then searched in multiple prefrontal areas for a distinctive pattern during the delay corresponding to the subjects' choice to add versus subtract. They identified an area in the medial prefrontal cortex within which distributed patterns for intending to add or subtract could be differentiated. From these, they could predict the subjects' later response with 71% accuracy. Moreover, these distinctive patterns were no longer present during task execution, although an area more posterior was active in execution.

From this evidence, Haynes et al. concluded that intention was encoded separately from preparation of action: "Our new findings resolve this crucial question by showing for the first time that prefrontal cortex encodes information that is specific to a task currently being prepared by a subject, as would be required for regions encoding a subject's intentions" (p. 324). They also found activity in lateral prefrontal cortex from which they could make an above-chance prediction of subsequent action, and so their ultimate claim is that a network of areas is involved in task-specific representations. They suggested further that the contributions of medial and lateral areas might be differentiated, with the medial region representing the subject's choosing the action, since other studies had indicated a role for medial prefrontal cortex in making choices.

So clearly there are some specialized regions, but they are nothing like modules (otherwise a 71% prediction would be too low).

Loosemore and Harley complain that

> ... this study, like many of the others, gives us information that seems to be locked in at the neural level alone, without coming up to the functional level and telling us something about how the mechanism of "intending to do an action" actually works. Both empirical conclusions—about the distributed spatial patterns, and the change of location between intention and execution—are just giving us different kinds of location data without saying what kind of mechanism is operating, and how it is doing its work.

Loosemore and Harley seem to be looking for a mechanism at a lower level than Haynes et al. were addressing—asking how intending is accomplished, whereas the goal was simply to demonstrate that intending could be distinguished from specific motor planning. This is the apparent conflict between the idea that fMRI reveals modules and the idea that there is substantial interaction (commonplaces 1 and 3). Given this simple goal, there would be no reason to think that the study could have revealed the "mechanism" of intending. It could have turned out, though, that there was no difference in the areas that encoded a specific intention during the delay interval and during execution. Although a researcher might have still argued, in that situation, that the two operations were different but performed in the same brain area, that seems less plausible given the ability to read the intention off the pattern of activation. The more plausible conclusion would have been to reject the distinction between intention and planning the actual response. Further evidence of their interest in functional organization at this level is Haynes et al.'s attempts to link the medial and lateral activity with other results suggesting choosing to specifically involve medial prefrontal activity.

Knoch, Pascual-Leone, Meye, Treyer, and Fehr

Although Loosemore and Harley claim their paper focuses on brain imaging studies, two of the studies they describe involve other techniques. We do not object to the inclusion of other studies, since we believe multiple means of accessing complex functions is desirable. Knoch, Pascual-Leone, Meyer, Treyer, and Fehr (2006) employ transcranial magnetic stimulation (TMS), which temporarily suppresses the operation of a brain area. The main reason they use a technique to suppress the operation of an area that had been shown in neuroimaging studies to be active when subjects are performing a task is to analyze functionality (commonplace 6). Inhibiting a region can be revelatory (cf. Bechtel and Richardson 1993; Craver 2007). Whereas fMRI imaging can reveal whether blood flow is altered when subjects perform a task, it leaves open the possibility that the neural processing was directly involved in the task (as opposed to being a downstream effect of a region more functionally involved). If task performance is altered in a manner indicative of a missing operation when the area is suppressed, one has more compelling evidence about the operation the area performed.

The cognitive activity Knoch et al. explored shows up in what is called the "ultimatum game." Humans often reject deals they find to be unfair even if they thereby end up worse off. (Economists and decision theorists claim this to be an irrational pattern in human reasoning.) This tendency of humans (not chimpanzees) to reject unfair deals even at personal cost is well established in the behavioral literature, and imaging studies relatively consistently show activity in the dorsolateral prefrontal cortex (DLPFC) as well as the anterior insula when subjects are deciding whether to accept the deal (Sanfey et al. 2003). To determine whether the DLPFC was critically involved in evaluating fairness, Knoch et al. suppressed it with repetitive TMS (rTMS). They also introduced a further manipulation—in some trials the unfair deal was chosen by the computer, in some by another human being who stood to profit. Presumably, subjects do not regard an "offer" by a computer as fair versus unfair, though they do assess offers by human subjects in these terms.

Knoch et al. found that impairment of the right DLPFC resulted in higher rates of acceptance of unfair deals proposed by other humans than when it was not suppressed (even though subjects still judged the deals to be unfair). It also eliminated the increased reaction time subjects showed when confronting unfair deals. But it had no effect on the rate of acceptance of unfair deals selected by the computer, where judgments of fairness do not come into play. These results not only demonstrated that the right DLPFC was contributing to the rejection of unfair offers, it also enabled the researchers to reject the alternative hypothesis Sanfey et al. had offered as to the operation it performed—controlling the emotional impulse (originating elsewhere) to reject the unfair offer. If that were correct, under rTMS, subjects should have been even more inclined to reject, rather than to accept, unfair deals. They interpreted the results they did obtain as indicating that the right DLPFC served to override selfish impulses in the service of culturally based conceptions of fairness (for which Henrich et al. [2001] had argued on anthropological grounds).

Loosemore and Harley view this study as at level 2, concerned only with the absolute location of a function. This misrepresents the goal of the study—to establish the inhibitory operation performed by right DLPFC and to decide between two processing models in which inhibition is viewed as operating on two different processes. In applying their own model to these results, Loosemore and Harley seem to simply accept Knoch et al.'s conclusion that DLPFC plays a role in inhibiting selfish responses (that we do not doubt), though not recognizing that this was the main question the study addressed. Loosemore and Harley also mischaracterize Knoch et al., construing them as treating the DLPFC as a "gate" (a term that never appears in the Knoch et al. paper) "specialized to do the job of enforcing fairness." Knoch et al., however, explicitly construe the DLPFC as "part of a network that modulates the relative impact of fairness motives and self-interest goals on decision-making." Fairly clearly, they are thinking in terms of a network of brain areas and seeking only to determine what operation one known brain area performs (commonplaces 3 and 7).

In fact, the alternative accounting Loosemore and Harley offer does not seem all that different from the one Knoch et al. put forward—they suggest that the DLPFC houses "atoms involved in difficult decisions," and when these are inhibited, the default simple, selfish action is pursued. They say little about what it would be to be involved in difficult decisions—it simply mediates between the "abstract knowledge of unfairness" and the pursuit of the default action. That is, it is involved in applying the abstract knowledge to inhibit the default selfish action, exactly what Knoch et al. set out to demonstrate in countering the interpretation of Sanfrey et al.

Quiroga, Reddy, Kreiman, Koch and Fried

The study by Quiroga, Reddy, Kreiman, Koch, and Fried (2005) is also not an imaging study. It has as a backdrop other work that shows selective responses in the human medial temporal lobe to faces and objects (e.g., Kreiman et al. 2000). In the current study, electrodes were implanted in eight subjects within the amygdala, the hippocampus, the entorhinal cortex, and the parahippocampal gyrus. (The purpose was diagnostic, intended to identify foci for epileptic seizures.) They previously had seen that some of these implants recorded a consistent pattern of response, so that, for example, one showed a response to Bill Clinton's face from several different perspectives. The researchers suggested that these "neurons might encode an abstract representation of an individual" (Quiroga et al. 2005, 1102). One alternative hypothesis they considered was that the representations might be distributed, depending on patterns of simple features. Thus, they seem to have two hypotheses in mind: (1) that neuronal responses are to fairly specific "low-level" features and the responses to faces are distributed responses; and (2) that neuronal responses are "abstract." The fact that responses were relatively independent of the perspective does not fit well with the former view.[5]

Loosemore and Harley suggest this is a level 2 or level 3 study, presumably because of the specificity of response Quiroga et al. observe. Loosemore and Harley tell us that the "sparse encoding" endorsed by Quiroga et al. requires a very specific response, so that "a neuron that fires strongly in response to Jennifer Aniston's face cannot also respond to the faces of the (superficially similar) Julia Roberts or (thematically related and quite similar) Courtney Cox" (pp. 14–15). However, Quiroga et al. are careful to observe: "We do not mean to imply the existence of single neurons coding uniquely for discrete percepts" (p. 1106) (commonplace 4). Some units actually responded to pictures of different individuals; and even if a probe records a response to only one face in the test set, that does not show it would not also respond to other faces.

The actual point is that neuronal encoding/response has the interesting feature that, though the response is to a person, it is "abstract" insofar as it is a response to the face from many perspectives, including drawings, and even the person's name itself.[6] Of course, as we've pointed out, it's one thing to show that there's a response to, say, Jennifer Aniston from various perspectives; it's another to show that no other stimuli could elicit a response (commonplace 4). In any case, the former is what is important to make the researcher's fundamental point, which concerns the "invariant" response of some units to some visual stimuli independent of significant variation in the visual features. Again, the purpose is to distinguish the functional response of the neurons. The point is surely not simply to identify the location of some unit, but to discriminate the possible functional analyses.

The key methodological complaint from Loosemore and Harley about this study is how unlikely the result is. It would, Loosemore and Harley suggest, be unlikely to find so many hits. Quiroga et al. say that some images were chosen after an interview with the subjects. Presumably, these images were chosen because of some interest the subject had. If you found that the subject was a Johnny Cash fan, you wouldn't pick pictures of Jennifer Aniston. Loosemore and Harley spend a good deal of time pointing out how unlikely it is to find the right pictures, but that would make sense only if, for example, the images were a random draw from the Internet. That's not at all what the paper suggests.

In their alternative molecular account, the active atoms will tend to be instantiated in the same areas; and if this is so, then the same atom would tend to be activated in the same place in response to the various pictures of Jennifer Aniston. Whatever the merits of their molecular account, this seems simply to embrace the conclusion of Quiroga et al., that the representations are relatively abstract.

General Observation Regarding Imaging Studies

Our defense of construing these studies as contributing to the functional decomposition of mental processes is not meant to deny that it is possible to challenge the functional interpretation of any of them. We do not know, or pretend to know, whether any of these studies will stand the test of time. Neither do we intend to offer a blanket defense for the use of fMRI, or any other imaging techniques. We actually think that convergence of multiple independent lines of evidence is likely to produce results in cognitive science (Henson 2006; Poldrack 2006). Functional MRI is no magic bullet. It is a tool in an arsenal. The methodological moral is perhaps crucial to our takes on the specific studies. We see them as focused on resolving specific issues, and not on determining where cognitive functions are "realized." The pertinent challenges for researchers are those that advance well-defined and conceptually motivated competing accounts of the operations involved in generating the cognitive phenomena. Indeed, most of these studies were conducted to evaluate just such competing accounts. Progress in developing mechanistic explanations often stems from discovering that existing proposals for mechanisms are overly simplified and require incorporation of additional parts, operations, and more complex organization. (In Bechtel and Richardson [1993], we endeavored to show through examples how such progress is often obtained.) The studies Loosemore and Harley criticize, as well as much work using neuroimaging, is engaged in just this quest.

Conclusion: The Use and Abuse of fMRI

We offer no grand conclusions. We intend no general endorsement of fMRI studies, though we do embrace the technology as one among many. We also recognize that as the power of fMRI increases, and the techniques for using fMRI improve, it will become increasingly useful. We do offer a cautionary moral, based on the sort of common-places we began with: fMRI studies are often overinterpreted, by both critics and en-thusiasts. We've focused here on one pair of critics, Loosemore and Harley, but we see similar threats from enthusiasts. Although we think Loosemore and Harley offer chal-lenges that are important in locating overinterpretations of fMRI research, we do not think they manage to address the specific concerns those studies aim to resolve. This should not be taken as an endorsement of the specific outcomes of the focal studies, but an acknowledgment of their focus and limitations. From a philosophical perspec-tive, the problem is that the specific studies are targeted at resolving very specific ques-tions, whereas Loosemore and Harley treat them as much more general. These studies are pieces of what Kuhn called "normal science," working within a paradigm.

Within that paradigm, there are commonplaces that Loosemore and Harley ignore. Fundamentally, we think the tendency to ignore the commonplaces follows from a mistaken picture of the character of interlevel research programs and the history of science. Within philosophy, this picture treats the history of science as a tendency toward greater articulation, and progress as a matter of reduction. In this picture, we look to the more fundamental sciences to capture the results of higher-level inquiries. In Loosemore and Harley's criticisms of fMRI studies, this is reflected in the thought that one must have a well-articulated and well-confirmed psychological theory before it is worthwhile to conduct research into the neuroscientific details. The point of the neuroscience would then be to reduce, or capture, the psychological results. It should be clear that we think waiting for a completed psychology, or even the outlines of a completed psychology, is likely to be like waiting for Kafka's gatekeeper. In other cases, we think that the idea that fMRI, or other work driven by techniques from the neuro-sciences alone, is sufficient to reveal cognitive mechanisms suffers from the same sort of errors. We do think there is a better picture of interlevel research programs that captures both the history of science and the conduct of research involving fMRI. We've certainly not enforced that alternative picture here, though we've suggested how it might generate a different take on the character of fMRI research.

Notes

1. The exception is, of course, information derived from traumatic insults (or surgical ablations) that result in sometimes quite dramatic deficits associated with massive damage to the brain. The fact that these did contribute to our understanding of cognitive function should be enough to give us pause concerning the usefulness of neuroscientific information to cognitive science. We devote some space on this in Bechtel and Richardson (1993).

2. In what is called *reverse inference*, the activation of a brain region is used to infer that some cognitive operation is happening. Such inferences are problematic, and depend crucially on how selective the region is (Poldrack 2006); even when they are legitimate, however, this should not be understood to imply that the region "realizes" the cognitive function. See the discussion of Haynes et al. (2007) in the text.

3. Vision once again offers a useful exemplar. Distance is discerned not only by binocular disparity, but by such things as shift in hue. This reveals itself in a variety of interesting illusions, as Richard Gregory has illustrated.

4. Loosemore and Harley offer a metaphorical rendering of the idea of a bottleneck that would make anyone skeptical; but that doesn't play any role in the Dux et al. study. It is invented by Loosemore and Harley.

5. On the surface, this result appears to be in tension with Barsalou's approach to concepts discussed earlier—abstract representations are not, on the face of it, modal. Resolving this and related issues is a topic for further research; we would note, though, that posing such tensions to be resolved is an important benefit of adopting multiple research strategies, neural and behavioral.

6. The most striking case, we think, is actually the responses to Halle Berry, which included responses to displays of her name, her face in various poses, a pencil sketch, and her in the Catwoman costume. In terms of features, there is very little common ground.

19   What Is Functional Neuroimaging For?

Max Coltheart

Functional neuroimaging consists of imaging brain activity using positron emission tomography (PET), functional magnetic resonance imaging (fMRI), or MEG while the person whose brain is being imaged is performing some cognitive task. Scrutiny of the functional neuroimaging literature suggests that such work has so far pursued three (not mutually exclusive) goals:

1. Neuroanatomical localization of cognitive processes   Here, the goal is to discover something about the role of particular brain regions in cognitive processing, by seeking "to determine which particular brain regions or systems exhibit altered activity in response to the engagement of particular cognitive, emotional, or sensory processes" (Poldrack, this volume, p. 147). Loosemore and Harley (chapter 17, this volume) use the term "level 2 studies" to refer to this kind of functional neuroimaging work.

2. Testing theories of cognition   Cognitive-theory testing using neuroimaging data can take either of two forms. Some functional neuroimaging studies are concerned with one particular theory expressed in cognitive terms, and seek to test that theory. In contrast, other neuroimaging studies are concerned with competing theories expressed in cognitive terms, and seek to adjudicate between such theories. Loosemore and Harley (chapter 17, this volume) use the term "level 4 studies" to refer to this kind of functional neuroimaging work.

3. Testing neural models   A neural model (Horwitz et al. 1999) is a proposal as to which regions of the brain are activated when some task is being performed, what pathways of communication are used between these regions, and what the functional strengths of these pathways are (see Horwitz et al. 1999, figure 1 for an example). If the model is purely neural, it says nothing about what processing function is performed by each of the brain regions, just as, if a model is purely cognitive, it says nothing about what brain region is used to perform each of the processing functions it proposes.

Poldrack (chapter 13, this volume) refers to localization (goal 1 above) as *the* goal of functional neuroimaging, which might be taken to express the view that studies using this technique have not pursued the other goals listed here. However, this isn't so: for example, Loosemore and Harley (chapter 17, this volume) refer to "rival accounts" of the relationship between attention and consciousness, and these rival accounts are competing theories that can be expressed solely in cognitive terms: One theory proposes that attention affects processing only when the relevant stimuli are conscious, and the other theory claims that varying attentional load can affect the processing of stimuli of which the subject is unaware. Bahrami and colleagues explicitly presented their study as an attempt to adjudicate between these two cognitive theories of the relationship between attention and consciousness—that is, their study is an example of one that pursued goal 2. The neuroimaging literature contains many other examples of studies that pursued this goal (the cognitive theory testing goal, as distinct from the localization goal), some of which are discussed in this chapter.

I will put aside for the moment the neural-modeling goal, and focus specifically on the two goals that seek to tell us something about cognition itself rather than just about brain processes.

Neuranatomical Localization of Cognitive Processes (Goal 1)

In many of the chapters in this volume (e.g., the chapters by Poldrack, Roskies, Loosemore and Harley, and Mole and Klein), the view is emphatically expressed that a specific cognitive-level theory or model of how processing is accomplished in the relevant cognitive domain is *always* required as a guide for any attempts to localize cognition with neuroimaging. For example "Whether one uses standard subtractive techniques or more recent event-related designs, having a functional decomposition of a task is essential to good experimental design as well as interpretation" (Roskies, this volume, p. 204); "in any fMRI design, an understanding of how neural activity relates to cognitive processes requires that the task be decomposed into particular processes, in essence requiring a theory of how the task is performed" (Poldrack, this volume, p. 157). Similarly, "in order to localize the modules of a cognitive system, one must first know what the system's modules actually are. So we must begin with a model and then seek to do localization research" (Coltheart 2004, 23).

If reference to some existing cognitive theory of processing in the relevant cognitive domain is always an essential foundation for localization studies using neuroimaging, how often is this requirement actually honored in such studies? Very rarely, according to Poldrack: "Unfortunately, such task analyses are very rarely presented in neuroimaging papers. Whereas formal theories from cognitive psychology could often provide substantial guidance as to the design of such tasks, it is uncommon for neuroimaging studies to take meaningful guidance from such theories" (this volume, p. 149). A look at all of the localization studies published in any annual volume of any journal specializing in functional neuroimaging work shows that Poldrack's analysis is correct.

Why is this so? One possibility, raised by Loosemore and Harley in their chapter, is that cognitive psychology is not (yet?) able to provide such formal theories to help localization endeavors in functional neuroimaging: "Is where-it-happens information of any use to present-day psychology? Not at the moment, because our cognitive models are insufficiently specified" (p. 239), and they go on to advocate the practice of computational modeling of cognition as a way of guaranteeing that models are sufficiently specific and explicit, a practice also recommended by Poldrack in his chapter.

But surely this is not correct. Many domains of cognition have been explored by functional neuroimaging for which cognitive psychology can already supply specific, explicit, and often even computational models. including the following examples:

1. Speech production (e.g., Harley 1993; Roelofs 1997)
2. Speech recognition (e.g., the Shortlist model of Norris and McQueen 2008, and the TRACE model, Strauss et al. 2007)
3. Face recognition (Burton et al. 1990)
4. Spelling (Glasspool et al. 1995)
5. Music processing (Peretz and Coltheart 2003)
6. Reading (Coltheart et al. 2001, Plaut et al. 1996)
7. Working memory (Lewandowsky and Farrell 2002)

There are many other such examples. Indeed, I doubt that a single domain of cognition remains in which functional neuroimaging has been done but no explicit modular information-processing cognitive models are available. All of these models provide highly detailed proposals about what the specific information-processing modules of a particular cognitive system are, and could therefore be used to guide functional localization research. So, though Poldrack is quite correct that little use is made of such models in functional neuroimaging work, this is not because such models don't exist. Why is it so, then? I don't know. But I do suggest that the reason we have not yet learned much about cognition from functional neuroimaging studies intended to localize cognitive processes in the brain (i.e., to achieve goal 1) is their almost universal failure to use contemporary modular information-processing models of cognition.

Testing Current Theories of Cognition (Goal 2)

The theory that face recognition is performed by the fusiform face area is not a cognitive theory, that is, not a theory about the mind: It is a theory about the brain. A theory of cognition can be expressed in purely cognitive terms—that is, without mentioning the brain. The theory that face recognition depends on holistic rather than feature-based processing is an example of a cognitive theory. So the question here (Coltheart 2006a) is how functional neuroimaging data can be used to test theories that are expressed in purely cognitive terms.

As mentioned earlier, such testing of cognitive theories can either focus on a single cognitive theory, seeking to obtain neuroimaging evidence that supports or weighs against that theory, or consider two or more theories, seeking neuroimaging evidence that favors one of these theories and weighs against the other or others.

I'll first consider the former scenario. I have argued elsewhere that to show neuro-imaging evidence is compatible with some cognitive theory does not in itself provide any evidence for that theory. Referring to a particular neuroimaging study of working memory, I pointed out that "All possible results of this study are compatible with [the theory] and so no result could have contradicted the theory" (Coltheart 2006b, 423). A demonstration that some data, D, are consistent with some theory, T, cannot be offered as support for that theory. Suppose the theory T is "Most Australian men are particularly fond of beer," and data D show that the proportion of Muslim people who drink beer is very low. Here, D is consistent with T, but no one would offer it as evidence in support of T's being true. Something more is needed than the data merely being consistent with the theory: No data can be offered as evidence for any theory unless one can show that the method of data collection might have yielded data in-consistent with the theory. That condition is obviously not satisfied in the beer exam-ple, because no pattern of data from a study of Muslim people can affect our opinion of any theory about the drinking predilections of Australian men. The condition is also often not satisfied in functional neuroimaging studies aimed at testing some cognitive theory, as in the working memory example mentioned earlier.

This point is elegantly elaborated in the chapter by Mole and Klein in this volume:

[T]he fact that a body of data is *consistent with* a hypothesis is not enough to show that the data provide a reason to believe that the hypothesis is true ... an informative body of data is a body of data that enables us to rule out certain possibilities.... To provide evidence for a hypothesis, the data must not only be consistent with the hypothesis, they must also count against the contradic-tory of the hypothesis. (pp. 100–102; cf. "What's needed is to show that Theory A predicts X while Theory B predicts ~X, where X is some pattern of neuroimaging data," in Coltheart 2006a, 325)

What this means is that in any functional neuroimaging study aimed at testing some cognitive theory, it must be demonstrated that the study *could plausibly have yielded* a pattern of data that would have counted against the theory. Studies in which this is not demonstrated, and which claim to support some theory solely because the data are consistent with the theory, commit what Mole and Klein call *the consistency fallacy*: This is the argument from a demonstration that a set of data are consistent with a theory to the claim that these data provide evidence in support of the theory. Such studies are rife in the functional neuroimaging literature; Mole and Klein discuss sev-eral examples.

This point also applies to the second scenario I consider here, where two or more competing cognitive theories are available and a functional neuroimaging study is carried out to adjudicate between them. Here, it needs to be the case for every one of the theories concerned that there was a plausible possible outcome of the study which is inconsistent with—would weigh against—that theory. For any theory where this is not so, no data, no matter how consistent with the theory, could count as supporting that theory.

Note here that I am not proposing that crucial experiments that conclusively refute one theory and prove another to be true can be done. I take the same view as Mole and Klein: "data rarely refute a ... hypothesis absolutely or unconditionally. They merely weigh against it." A study that successfully adjudicates in favor of theory A over theory B is a study whose data weigh against theory B but are as predicted by theory A. For me, as for Mole and Klein, the question "What can neuroimaging tell us about cognition?" is to be construed as "What hypotheses about cognition can neuroimaging data provide us with reasons to believe?" *and* its corollary, "What hypotheses about cognition can neuroimaging data provide us with reasons to doubt?"

Additional challenges arise when multiple-theory adjudication rather than single-theory testing is the aim of a functional neuroimaging study. One cannot seek to adjudicate between theories unless these theories are contradictory, that is, could not both be true. When this relationship of contradiction holds, evidence in favor of one theory can be evidence against the other. One instructive example of a functional neuroimaging study that aimed to adjudicate between competing cognitive theories is that by Vuilleumier, Henson, Driver, and Dolan (2002) concerning object recognition. Their paper begins by describing two theories of object recognition, both expressed purely in cognitive terms:

Theory A: "[T]he visual system builds abstract three-dimensional (3D) models of objects from two-dimensional retinal images, and stores visual information independent of momentary viewing parameters such as orientation or scale" (p. 491; the reference given for this theory is Biederman 1987).

Theory B: "recognition relies primarily on view-specific processes, and is based on past encounters with an object" (p.491; the references given for this theory are Wallis and Bulthoff 1999, and Tarr et al. 1998).

Vuilleumier and colleagues used the phenomenon of neural repetition priming in their attempt to adjudicate between these two theories. Many neuroimaging studies have shown that when a visually presented object is re-presented, the neural response to it is diminished. Would this happen if the second presentation differed in viewpoint from the first? The answer was, yes and no. Priming-induced decreases in neural activity in the right fusiform cortex depended on whether the repetitions had a common viewpoint, whereas priming-induced decreases in neural activity in the left fusiform cortex were uninfluenced by whether the repetitions had a common viewpoint or different viewpoints.

What conclusions should we draw about theory A and theory B from these findings? According to Vuilleumier, "Our findings suggest that view-independent and view-invariant accounts of object recognition should be reconciled, as both may exist in distinct and differentially lateralized brain systems" (Vuilleumier et al. 2002, 498). Did they mean to assert that both theory A and theory B were wrong?

Their data can be taken as weighing against theory A only if that theory denies there is a viewpoint-specific level of representation in the object recognition system, and similarly their data can be taken as weighing against theory B only if that theory denies a viewpoint-independent level of representation in the object recognition system. But Biederman (1987), while asserting that there is a viewpoint-independent level of representation in the system, nowhere denies that there is also a viewpoint-specific level; and Wallis and Bulthoff (1999) and Tarr et al. (1998), while asserting that a viewpoint-specific level of representation exists in the system, nowhere deny that there is also a viewpoint-independent level.

This is not a straightforward example of Mole and Klein's consistency fallacy, because there are possible outcomes of the study that could have been obtained and would have counted against one or the other of the theories. I will consider two of these.

Outcome 1: Suppose repetition priming had been observed in some brain areas, but it was *never* affected by a change of viewpoint. This outcome has nothing to say about theory A since it is merely consistent with theory A, but it does weigh against theory B, since theory B does lead one to expect to find regions of the brain where repetition effects are affected by change in viewpoint.

Outcome 2: Suppose repetition priming had been observed in some brain areas, but it was *always* affected by a change of viewpoint. This outcome has nothing to say about theory B since it is merely consistent with theory B, but it does weigh against theory A, since theory A leads one to expect to find regions of the brain where repetition effects are unaffected by change in viewpoint.

But the actual outcome of the study (repetition was observed in some brain regions, and it was affected by viewpoint change in some of these areas, but not in the others) is inconclusive with respect to adjudication between the two theories. This is an example of a general problem: In these kinds of adjudication studies, it is necessary to make explicit what the theories state is *not* the case, not just what they say *is* the case. Imagine if the theories had been formulated thus:

Theory A: The visual system builds abstract three-dimensional (3D) models of objects from two-dimensional retinal images, and stores visual information independent of momentary viewing parameters such as orientation or scale; it does not represent objects in a viewpoint-specific way.

Theory B: Recognition relies primarily on viewpoint-specific processes, and is based on past encounters with an object; it does not represent objects in a viewpoint-independent way.

Now the actual outcome *would* have been conclusive: It provides evidence against both theories. But if the theories had been formulated in this way, a different problem would have emerged—the question of whether either theory had ever been proposed. Who has proposed that the visual system does not represent objects in a viewpoint-specific way? Who has proposed that the visual system does not represent objects in a viewpoint-independent way? I think the answer to both questions is, no one. Requiring that the theory formulations specify what the theories say is *not* the case has thus revealed a hitherto hidden gulf between the theories and their ostensible predictions.

So I am suggesting that two reasons we have as yet not learned much about cognition from functional neuroimaging studies intended to test cognitive theories (i.e., to achieve goal 2) are (1) the widespread commission of Mole and Klein's consistency fallacy, and (2) the widespread failure to design studies that could have yielded results that would count against the theories being considered.

Where Has the Field of Functional Neuroimaging Got So Far?

The contributors to this volume have widely different views about this. According to Loosemore and Harley, "But right now, we are being flooded with accurate answers to questions about the brain location of mechanisms that we do not believe in and inaccurate answers to questions about the brain location of mechanisms that are currently not terribly interesting. This state of affairs [in psychology] seems to us to be a great leap backwards" (p. 240), and they give examples supporting this argument. In contrast, Roskies asserts that "Neuroimaging is in its early days, and though there is remarkable promise . . ." (p. 213), but she does not give any examples of what she regards as remarkable promise in this field. Poldrack's chapter surveys many of the methodological difficulties that confront the field and, while not offering a view as to how well the field has progressed, provides no examples of such progress (though he does suggest that some recent meta-analyses offer "glimmers of hope"; p. 158).

Poldrack's verdict after his review is similar to that offered by Downing, Liu, and Kanwisher (2001) in their review of functional neuroimaging work on attention. This review begins in a very upbeat way: "Neuroimaging can be used . . . to test cognitive theories of attention. . . . We consider four classic questions in the psychology of visual attention. . . . We describe studies from our laboratory that illustrate the ways in which fMRI and MEG can provide key evidence in answering these questions" (Downing et al. 2001, 1329). Then, as the paper progresses there is a diminuendo, leaving us with just a series of promissory notes at the end of the paper:

Substantial challenges remain. Can neuroimaging studies provide converging evidence on some of the key theoretical debates in the field? For example, feature integration theory and the biased-competition model represent alternative frameworks that interpret the same data in terms of substantially different mechanisms. Perhaps neuroimaging will some day be able to distinguish between such theories, an achievement that would represent a major contribution.

. . .

The promise of cognitive neuroscience is that findings from different methodologies will cross-fertilise.

. . .

If successful, these techniques could provide the most powerful tool yet for investigating the mechanisms underlying visual attention. (Downing et al. 2001, 1340)

I have been suggesting (Coltheart 2004, 2005, 2006a, b, 2008a, b) that a sensible way to assess just how much progress this field has made *so far* is to ask for specific examples where there is reasonably general agreement that a functional neuroimaging study has successfully localized some specific cognitive function in the brain, or has provided good reason to believe that some particular theory of cognition is correct when the study was capable of providing evidence that would weigh against that theory, or has provided good reason to prefer one cognitive theory over a competing theory. None of the examples offered to me so far has seemed at all compelling (Coltheart 2006b). Does this volume contain any examples that its readers find compelling?

Four Questions to Ask of Any Existing or Proposed Functional Neuroimaging Study, and Why They Should Be Asked

I sum up by suggesting this set of four questions that, I have found, generate considerable enlightenment when asked about any particular cognitive neuroimaging study:

1. If a goal of the study is functional localization of cognition, ask yourself: What well-accepted model of cognitive processing in that cognitive domain does the study presume? This question should be asked because, as so many contributors to this volume have emphasized, such localization studies can be interpreted only if what particular components of cognition the study is seeking to localize is stated, and such a statement amounts to a model of cognitive processing.
2. If a goal of the study is to test some model of cognitive processing, ask yourself: What plausible outcome of the neuroimaging study might have been obtained that would have counted as evidence *against* that model? This question needs a satisfactory answer if one is to demonstrate that the consistency fallacy has been avoided.
3. If a goal of the study is to adjudicate between competing models of cognitive processing, ask yourself: What is it about each model that is contradicted by the other(s)—are the models genuinely incompatible? Unless this question is answered, we cannot

be sure that the theories actually are competing, and if they aren't, then adjudication between them isn't a possible goal.

4. And, of course, for each of these competing models, ask yourself: What plausible outcome of the neuroimaging study might have been obtained that would have counted as evidence against that model? Again, this is to show that the consistency fallacy has been avoided.

What About Neural Modeling?

The study by Williams, Baker, Op de Beeck, Shim, Dang, Triantafyllou, and Kanwisher (2008) provides an excellent example of what neural modeling is and how it is distinct from cognitive modeling. The stimuli in this study were exemplars of three visually distinct categories of nonsense objects: "spikies," "smoothies," and "cubies." On each trial, the subject saw a pair of such objects, always drawn from the same object category, and was asked to judge whether the two objects were identical or not. The objects were presented peripherally, on either side of the fixation point and 7 degrees away from it.

Although stimuli were never presented to the fovea, fMRI showed that the region of primary visual cortex corresponding to the fovea was activated, and what is more, the pattern of foveal activation varied according to object category. Moreover, this presence of object category–specific information in foveal retinotopic cortex was task specific, because

1. when the task was changed to a same/different comparison of color rather than shape, using the same objects, this object category–specific information was no longer detectable in foveal retinotopic cortex; and

2. in the shape-comparison task, the degree to which activation of foveal retinotopic cortex contained object category–specific information increased monotonically over trial blocks.

Percent correct same/different judgment performance also increased monotonically over trial blocks, suggesting that the presence of the object category–specific information in foveal retinotopic cortex assisted in the performance of the shape task.

These results seem to require that feedback was operating from higher cortical areas (perhaps from the lateral occipital complex, or LOC) to foveal retinotopic cortex, and that this feedback occurs only when the task is shape judgment. This conclusion implies a model, but not a cognitive model, since the terms used to express this model are not cognitive terms. They are neural terms, and so the model being proposed is a neural model rather than a cognitive model.

The data of Williams and colleagues suggest a neural model that includes two distinct brain regions (LOC and foveal retinotopic cortex) and a feedback pathway from the former to the latter, a pathway that operates when the task is shape comparison but not when it is color comparison. Clearly, it would be nice to know what the functional significances of these two regions and this pathway are for the shape comparison task. Any attempt to answer that question would consist of superimposing a processing —even a cognitive-processing—interpretation over the neural model, to create what one might appropriately term a neurocognitive model of how the shape comparison task is performed. Williams and colleagues make some interesting suggestions as to how this might be done. The key question, of course, is in what way feedback of information to foveal retinotopic cortex helps performance of the task. What is the information-processing function of this brain region for the shape comparison task? "One possibility is that foveal retinotopic cortex may serve as a kind of scratch pad to store or compute task-relevant information" (Williams et al. 2008, 1444). One component of the Baddeley-Hitch model of working memory (Baddeley and Hitch 1974) is a visuospatial scratch pad, and many tasks have been developed that are intended to tap the operation of that subsystem of working memory. Might one observe activation of foveal retinotopic cortex whenever one of these tasks is being performed? An especially interesting point here is that some tasks that tap this component of the working memory model don't require presentation of visual stimuli, for example, the task of counting how many uppercase letters of the alphabet contain a curve (Coltheart et al. 1975). If foveal retinotopic cortex is the neural site of the visuospatial scratch pad, then that brain region would be more active in the curve-counting task than in a comparable control task, counting how many letters of the alphabet contain the sound "ee" in their names, even though no visual stimulation had occurred.

Suppose, though, that Williams and colleagues had not been interested in suggesting any functional interpretation of their neural model. In that case, their work would not have addressed the first two of the three goals of functional neuroimaging stated at the beginning of this chapter; and in general any neuroimaging work aimed solely at creating a neural model—and there is much such work—does not address either of these two goals. Naturally, it would be absurd to criticize such work for this reason.

This functional neuroimaging study by Williams and his colleagues has told us something new (and exciting) about the brain. In contrast, I have argued, in common with several other contributors to this volume, that functional neuroimaging has not yet told us anything new and exciting about cognition; and I have suggested several reasons for this lack.

Acknowledgment

I thank Mark Williams for much valuable discussion of issues with which this chapter is concerned.

References

Adler, J., and Carmichael, M. 2004. Mind reading. *Newsweek* 144.1: 42–47.

Aguirre, G. K., and D'Esposito, M. 1999. Experimental design for brain fMRI. In: C. T. W. Moonen and P. A. Bandettini (Eds.) *Functional MRI* (pp. 369–380). New York: Springer.

Amunts, K., Schleicher, A., Burgel, U., Mohlberg, H., Uylings, H. B., and Zilles, K. 1999. Broca's region revisited: Cytoarchitecture and intersubject variability. *Journal of Comparative Neurology* 412.2: 319–341.

Amunts, K., Weiss, P. H., Mohlberg, H., Pieperhoff, P., Eickhoff, S., Gurd, J. M., et al. 2004. Analysis of neural mechanisms underlying verbal fluency in cytoarchitectonically defined stereotaxic space—The roles of Brodmann areas 44 and 45. *NeuroImage* 22.1: 42–56.

Amunts, K., and Zilles, K. 2001. Advances in cytoarchitectonic mapping of the human cerebral cortex. *NeuroImaging Clinics of North America* 11.2: 151–169.

Anderson, J. R. 2007. *How Can the Human Mind Occur in the Physical Universe?* Oxford: Oxford University Press.

Andresen, D. R, Vinberg , J. and Grill-Spector, K. 2009. The representation of object viewpoint in human visual cortex. Neuroimage. 45.2: 522–536

Aron, A., Fisher, H., Mashek, D. J., Strong, G., Li, H., and Brown, L. L. 2005. Reward, motivation, and emotion systems associated with early-stage intense romantic love. *Journal of Neurophysiology* 94.1: 327–337.

Arthurs, O. J., and Boniface, S. J. 2003. What aspect of the fMRI BOLD signal best reflects the underlying electrophysiology in human somatosensory cortex? *Journal of Clinical Neurophysiology* 114.7: 1203–1209.

Ashburner, J., and Friston, K. J. 1999. Nonlinear spatial normalisation using basis functions. *Human Brain Mapping* 7: 254–266.

Ashburner, J., Friston, K. J., and Penny, W. (Eds.) 2004. *Human Brain Functions* (2nd Ed.). Burlington, MA: Academic Press.

Baars, B. J. 2005. Global workspace theory of consciousness: Toward a cognitive neuroscience of human experience. *Progress in Brain Research* 150: 45–53.

Baddeley, A. D., and Hitch, G. J. L. 1974. Working memory. In G. A. Bower (Ed.), *The Psychology of Learning and Motivation: Advances in Research and Theory, Volume 8* (pp. 47–89). New York: Academic Press.

Bahrami, B., Lavie, N., and Rees, G. 2007. Attentional load modulates responses of human primary visual cortex to invisible stimuli. *Current Biology* 17.6: 509–513.

Baker, C. I., Hutchison, T. L., and Kanwisher, N. 2007. Does the fusiform face area contain sub-regions highly selective for nonfaces? *Nature Neuroscience* 10.1: 3–4.

Baker, C. I., Simmons, W. K., Bellgowan, P. S., and Kriegeskorte, N. 2007. Circular inference in neuroscience: The dangers of double dipping. Paper presented at the Society for Neuroscience, San Diego.

Bandettini, P. A., Wong, E. C., Hinks, R. S., Tikofsky, R. S., and Hyde, J. S. 1992. Time course EPI of human brain function during task activation. *Magnetic Resonance in Medicine* 25: 390–397.

Barlow, H. 1972. Single units and sensation: A neuron doctrine for perception. *Perception* 1: 371–394.

Barsalou, L. W. 1987. The instability of graded structure: Implications for the nature of concepts. In U. Neisser (Ed.), *Concepts Reconsidered: The Ecological Intellectual Bases of Categories*. Cambridge: Cambridge University Press.

Barsalou, L. W. 1999. Perceptual symbol systems. *Behavioral and Brain Sciences* 22: 577–660.

Barsalou, L. W. 2008. Grounded cognition. *Annual Review of Psychology* 59.1: 617–645.

Bartels, A., and Zeki, S. 2000. The neural basis of romantic love. *NeuroReport* 11.17: 3829–3834.

Bartels, A., and Zeki, S. 2004. The neural correlates of maternal and romantic love. *NeuroImage* 21: 1155–1166.

Bartholomew, D. 1999. *Latent Variables and Factor Analysis*. New York: Oxford University Press.

Beauchamp, M. S., Argall, B. D., Bodurka, J., Duyn, J. H., and Martin, A. 2004. Unraveling multisensory integration: Patchy organization within human STS multisensory cortex. *Nature Neuroscience* 7: 1190–1192.

Bechtel, W. 2002a. Aligning multiple research techniques in cognitive neuroscience: Why is it important? *Philosophy of Science* 69: S48–S58.

Bechtel, W. 2002b. Decomposing the mind-brain: A long-term pursuit. *Brain and Mind* 3: 229–242.

Bechtel, W. 2008. *Mental Mechanisms: Philosophical Perspectives on Cognitive Neuroscience*. London: Routledge.

Bechtel, W., and McCauley, R. N. 1999. Heuristic identity theory (or back to the future): The mind-body problem against the background of research strategies in cognitive neuroscience. In

M. Hahn and S. C. Stoness (Eds.), *Proceedings of the 21st Annual Meeting of the Cognitive Science Society* (pp. 67–72). Mahwah, NJ: Lawrence Erlbaum Associates.

Bechtel, W., and Richardson, R. C. 1993. *Discovering Complexity: Decomposition and Localization as Strategies in Scientific Research.* Princeton, NJ: Princeton University Press.

Belliveau, J. W., Kennedy, D. N., McKinstry, R. C., Buchbinder, B. R., Weisskoff, R. M., Delcanton, J. J., et al. 1991. Functional mapping of the human visual cortex by magnetic resonance imaging. *Science* 254: 716–719.

Berns, G. S., Chappelow, J., Fink, C. F., Pagnoni, G., Martin-Skurski, M. E., and Richards, J. 2005. Neurobiological correlates of social conformity and independence during mental rotation. *Biological Psychiatry* 58: 245–253.

Berridge, M. J., and Rapp, P. E. 1979. A comparative survey of the function, mechanism and control of cellular oscillations. *Journal of Experimental Biology* 81: 217–279.

Bichot, N. P., Rao, C. S., and Schall, J. D. 2001. Continuous processing in macaque frontal cortex during visual search. *Neuropsychologia* 39: 972–982.

Biederman, I. 1987. Recognition-by-components: A theory of human image understanding. *Psychological Review* 94. 115–147.

Biederman, I., and Gerhardstein, P. C. 1993. Recognizing depth-rotated objects: Evidence and conditions for three-dimensional viewpoint invariance. *Journal of Experimental Psychology: Human Perception and Performance* 19: 1162–1182.

Binder, J. R., Frost, J. A., Hammeke, T. A., Bellgowan, P. S., Rao, S., and Cox, R. W. 1999. Conceptual processing during the conscious resting state. A functional MRI study. *Journal of Cognitive Neuroscience* 11: 80–95.

Biswal, B., Bandettini, P. A., Jesmanowicz, A., and Hyde, J. S. 1993. Time-frequency analysis of functional EPI time-course series. *Proceedings of SMRM, 12th Annual Meeting* (p. 722) New York.

Biswal, B., DeYoe, E. A., and Hyde, J. S. 1996. Reduction of physiological fluctuations in FMRI using digital filters. *Magnetic Resonance in Medicine* 35: 107.

Biswal, B. B., and Hudetz, A. G. 1996. Synchronous oscillations in cerebrocortical capillary red blood cell velocity after nitric oxide synthase inhibition. *Microvascular Research* 52: 1–12.

Biswal, B. Hudetz, A. G., Yetkin, F. Z. Haughton, V. M., and Hyde, J. S. 1997a. Hypercapnia reversibly suppresses low-frequency fluctuations in the human motor cortex during rest using echo-planar MRI. *Journal of Cerebral Blood Flow & Metabolism* 17: 301.

Biswal, B. B., and Hyde, J. S. 1997. Contour-based registration technique to differentiate between task-activated and head motion-induced signal variations in fMRI. *Magnetic Resonance in Medicine* 38.3: 470–476.

Biswal, B. B., and Hyde, J. S. 1998. Functional connectivity during continuous task activation. *Proceedings of 6th ISMRM* (p. 2132) Sydney.

Biswal, B. B., and Ulmer, J. L. 1999. Blind source separation of multiple signal sources of FMRI data sets using independent component analysis. *Journal of Computer Assisted Tomography* 23: 265–271.

Biswal, B. B., Van Kylen, J., and Hyde, J. S. 1997b. Simultaneous assessment of flow and BOLD signals in resting-state functional connectivity maps. *NMR in Biomedicine* 10: 165–170.

Biswal, B., Yetkin, F. Z., Haughton, V. M., and Hyde, J. S. 1995. Functional connectivity in the motor cortex of resting human brain using echo-planar MRI. *Magnetic Resonance in Medicine* 34: 537.

Biswal, B. B., Yetkin, F. Z., Ulmer, J. L., Haughton, V. M., and Hyde, J. S. 1997c. Detection of abnormal task-activation signal changes in Tourette Syndrome using FMRI. *NeuroImage* 5: 308.

Biswal, B. B., Yetkin, F. Z., Ulmer, J. L., Haughton, V. M., and Hyde, J. S. 1997d. Detection of abnormal functional-connectivity in Tourette Syndrome using FMRI. *Proceedings of the 5th ISMRM* (p. 733)Vancouver.

Blessed, G., Tomlinson, B. E., and Roth, M. 1968. The association between quantitative measures of dementia and senile change in the cerebral grey matter of elderly subjects. *British Journal of Psychiatry* 114: 797–811.

Block, N. 1996. How can we find the neural correlate of consciousness? *Trends in Neurosciences* 19: 456–459.

Booth, R., Charlton, R., Hughes, C., and Happe, F. 2003. Disentangling weak coherence and executive dysfunction: planning drawing in autism and attention-deficit/hyperactivity disorder. *Philosphical Transactions of the Royal Society of London B: Biological Sciences* 358.1430: 387–392.

Braak, H., and Braak, E. 1996. Development of Alzheimer-related neurofibrillary changes in the neocortex inversely recapitulates cortical myelogenesis. *Acta Neuropathologica* 92: 197–201.

Braver, T. S., Cohen, J. D., Nystrom, L. E., Jonides, J., Smith, E. E., and Noll, D. C. 1997. A parametric study of prefrontal cortex involvement in human working memory. *NeuroImage* 5: 49–62.

Bressler, S. 1996. Large-scale cortical networks and cognition. *Brain Research Reviews* 20: 288–304.

Brett, M., Johnsrude, I. S., and Owen, A. M. 2002. The problem of functional localization in the human brain. *Nature Reviews Neuroscience* 3.3: 243–249.

Brewer, J. B., Zhao, Z., Desmond, J. E., Glover, G. H., and Gabrieli, J. D. 1998. Making memories: Brain activity that predicts how well visual experience will be remembered [see comments]. *Science* 281: 1185–1187.

Brodmann, K. 1909; Reprinted 1994. Vergleichende Lokalisationslehre der Grosshirnrinde (L. J. Garvey, Translator). Leipzig: J. A. Barth.

Brown, J. W., and Braver, T. S. 2005. Learned predictions of error likelihood in the anterior cingulate cortex. *Science* 307: 1118–1121.

Buchel, C. 2004. Perspectives on the estimation of effective connectivity from neuroimaging data. *Neuroinformatics* 2: 169–174.

Buchel, C., Coull, J. T., and Friston, K. J. 1999. The predictive value of changes in effective connectivity for human learning. *Science* 283.5407: 1538–1541.

Buchel, C., and Friston, K. J. 1998. Dynamic changes in effective connectivity characterized by variable parameter regression and Kalmanfiltering. *Human Brain Mapping* 6.5–6: 403–408.

Buchel, C., and Friston, K. J. 2000. Assessing interactions among neuronal systems using functional neuroimaging. *Neural Networks* 13: 871–882.

Buckner, R. L., Bandettini, P. A., O'Craven, K. M., Savoy, R. L., Petersen, S. E., Raichle, M. E., and Rosen, B. R. 1996. Detection of cortical activation during averaged single trials of a cognitive task using functional magnetic resonance imaging. *Proceedings Of The National Academy Of Sciences U.S.A.* 93: 14878–14883.

Bullmore, E. T., Horwitz, B., Honey, G. D., Brammer, M. J., Williams, S. C. R. and Sharma, T. 2000. How good is good enough in path analysis of fMRI data? *NeuroImage* 11: 289–301.

Bulthoff, H. H., and Edelman, S. 1992. Psychophysical support for a two-dimensional view interpolation theory of object recognition. *Proceedings of the National Academy of Sciences U. S. A* 89: 60–64.

Bulthoff, H. H., Edelman, S. Y., and Tarr, M. J. 1995. How are three-dimensional objects represented in the brain? *Cerebral Cortex* 5: 247–260.

Bunge, S. A., Dudukovic, N. M., Thomason, M. E., Vaidya, C. J., and Gabrieli, J. D. E. 2002. Immature frontal lobe contributions to cognitive control in children: Evidence from fMRI. *Neuron* 33: 301–311.

Burton, A. M., Bruce, V., and Johnston, R. A. 1990. Understanding face recognition with an interactive activation model. *British Journal of Psychology* 8: 361–380.

Buxton, R. B. 2002. *Introduction to Functional Magnetic Resonance Imaging: Principles and Techniques.* Cambridge: Cambridge University Press.

Cabeza, R. 2002. Hemispheric asymmetry reduction in older adults: The HAROLD model. *Psychology of Aging* 17: 85–100.

Callicott, J. H., Mattay, V. S., Bertolino, A., Finn, K., Coppola, R., Frank, J. A., et al. 1999. Physiological characteristics of capacity constraints in working memory as revealed by functional MRI. *Cerebral Cortex* 9: 20–26.

Cantlon, J. F., Brannon, E. M., Carter, E. J., and Pelphrey, K. A. 2006. Functional imaging of numerical processing in adults and 4-y-old children. *PLoS Biology* 4.5: e125.

Cape, E. G., and Jones, B. E. 1998. Differential modulation of high-frequency-electroencephalogram activity and sleep-wake state by noradrenaline and serotonin microinjections into the region of cholinergic basalis neurons. *Journal of Neuroscience* 18.7: 2653–2666.

Caplan, D., and Moo, L. 2004. Cognitive conjunction and cognitive functions. *NeuroImage* 21: 751–756.

Carlson, T. A., Schrater, P., and He, S. 2003. Patterns of activity in the categorical representations of objects. *Journal of Cognitive Neuroscience* 15.5: 704–717.

Casey, B. J., Cohen, J. D., Jezzard, P., Turner, R., Noll, D. C., Trainor, R. J., et al. 1995. Activation of prefrontal cortex in children during a nonspatial working memory task with functional MRI. *NeuroImage* 2.3: 221–229.

Chan, A. W., Peelen, M. V., and Downing, P. E. 2004. The effect of viewpoint on body representation in the extrastriate body area. *Neuroreport* 15.15: 2407–2410.

Chu, T., Glymour, C., Scheines, R., and Spirtes, P. 2003. A statistical problem for inference to regulatory structure from associations of gene expression measurements with microarrays. *Bioinformatics* 19: 1147–1152.

Chun, M. M., and Jiang, Y. 1998. Contextual cueing: Implicit learning and memory of visual context guides spatial attention. *Cognitive Psychology* 36.1: 28–71.

Ciuciu, P., Poline, J. B., Marrelec, G., Idier, J., Pallier, C., and Benali, H. 2002. Unsupervised robust non-parametric estimation of the hemodynamic response function for any fMRI experiment. *Technical Report, submitted to IEEE Transactions on Medical Imaging*, SHFJ/CEA, Orsay, France.

Cohen, J., and Meskin, A. 2004. On the epistemic value of photographs. *Journal of Aesthetics and Art Criticism* 62.2: 197–210.

Coltheart, M. 2004. Brain imaging, connectionism, and cognitive neuropsychology. *Cognitive Neuropsychology* 21: 21–25.

Coltheart, M. 2005. What has functional neuroimaging told us about the mind? Paper presented to the European Cognitive Neuropsychology Workshop, Bressanone, Italy.

Coltheart, M. 2006a. What has functional neuroimaging told us about the mind (so far)? *Cortex* 42: 323–331.

Coltheart, M. 2006b. Perhaps cognitive neuroimaging has not told us anything about the mind (so far). *Cortex* 42: 422–427.

Coltheart, M. 2008a. What is cognitive neuroimaging for? Human Brain Mapping Conference, Melbourne, Australia.

Coltheart, M. 2008a. What is cognitive neuroimaging for? International Congress of Psychology, Berlin, Germany.

Coltheart, M., Hull, E., and Slater, D. 1975. Sex differences in imagery and reading. *Nature* 253: 438–440.

Coltheart, M., Rastle, K., Perry, C., Langdon, R., and Ziegler, J. 2001. DRC: A Dual Route Cascaded model of visual word recognition and reading aloud. *Psychological Review* 108: 204–256.

Cooper, R., Crow, H. J., Walter, W. G., and Winter, A. L. 1966. Regional control of cerebral vascular reactivity and oxygen supply in man. *Brain Research* 3: 174.

Corbetta, M., and Shulman, G. L. 1998. Human cortical mechanisms of visual attention during orienting and search. *Philosophical Transactions of the Royal Society of London B: Biological Sciences* 353: 1353–1362.

Coulon, O., Mangin, J. F., Poline, J. B., Zilbovicius, M., Roumenov, D., Samson, Y., et al. 2000. Structural group analysis of functional activation maps. *NeuroImage* 11: 767–782.

Cox, D. D., and Savoy, R. L. 2003. Functional magnetic resonance imaging (fMRI) "brain reading": Detecting and classifying distributed patterns of fMRI activity in human visual cortex. *NeuroImage* 19: 261–270.

Cox, D. D., and Savoy, R. L. 2003. Functional magnetic resonance imaging (fMRI) "brain reading": Detecting and classifying distributed patterns of fMRI activity in human visual cortex. *NeuroImage* 19.2: 261–270.

Craver, C. 2003. The making of a memory mechanism. *Journal of the History of Biology* 36: 153–195.

Craver, C. 2007. *Explaining the Brain: What a Science of the Mind-Brain Could Be.* New York: Oxford University Press.

Crivello, F., Schormann, T., Tzourio-Mazoyer, N., Roland, P. F., Zilles, K., and Mazoyer, B. M. 2002. Comparison of spatial normalization procedures and their impact on functional maps. *Human Brain Mapping* 16.4: 228–250.

Crivello, F., Tzourio, N., Poline, J. B., Woods, R. P., Mazziotta, J. C., and Mazoyer, B. 1995. Intersubject variability in functional neuroanatomy of silent verb generation: Assessment by a new activation detection algorithm based on amplitude and size information. *NeuroImage* 2.4: 253–263.

Culham, J. C. 2006. Functional neuroimaging: Experimental design and analysis. In R. Cabeza and A. Kingstone (Eds.), *Handbook of Functional Neuroimaging of Cognition* (2nd ed.). Cambridge, MA: MIT Press.

Culham, J. C., Brandt, S. A., Cavanagh, P., Kanwisher, N. G., Dale, A. M., and Tootell, R. B. 1998. Cortical fMRI activation produced by attentive tracking of moving targets. *Journal of Neurophysiology* 80.5: 2657–2670.

Culham, J. C., Danckert, S. L., DeSouza, J. F., Gati, J. S., Menon, R. S., and Goodale, M. A. 2003. Visually guided grasping produces fMRI activation in dorsal but not ventral stream brain areas. *Experimental Brain Research* 153.2: 180–189.

Dang-Vu, T. T., Desseilles, M., Albouy, G., Darsaud, A., Gais, S., Rauchs, G., Schabus, M., et al. 2005. Dreaming: A neuroimaging view. *Schweizer Archiv für Neurologie und Psychiatrie* 156.8: 415–425.

Danks, D. 2005. Scientific coherence and the fusion of experimental results. *British Journal for the Philosophy of Science* 23: 141–156.

Dapretto, M., Davies, M. S., Pfeifer, J. H., Scott, A. A., Sigman, M., Bookheimer, S. Y., et al. 2006. Understanding emotions in others: Mirror neuron dysfunction in children with autism spectrum disorders. *Nature Neuroscience* 9.1: 28–30.

Daubechies, I. 1992. *Ten Lectures on Wavelets.* Philadephia: SIAM Press.

Davies, P. W., and Bronk, D. W. 1957. Oxygen tension in mammalian brain. *Federal Proceedings* 16: 689.

Dehaene, S., Naccache, L., Le Clec'H, G., Koechlin, E., Mueller, M., Dehaene-Lambertz, G., et al. 1998. Imaging unconscious semantic priming. *Nature* 395.6702: 597–600.

Delis, D. C., Freeland, J., Kramer, J. H., and Kaplan, E. 1988. Integrating clinical assessment with cognitive neuroscience: Construct validation of the California Verbal Learning Test. *Journal of Consulting and Clinical Psychology* 56: 123–130.

De Martino, B., Kumaran, D., Seymour, B., and Dolan, R. J. 2006. Frames, biases, and rational decision-making in the human brain. *Science* 313.5787: 684–687.

Demb, J. B., Desmond, J. E., Wagner, A. D., Vaidya, C. J., Glover, G. H., and Gabrieli, J. D. 1995. Semantic encoding and retrieval in the left inferior prefrontal cortex: A functional MRI study of task difficulty and process specificity. *Journal of Neuroscience* 15: 5870–5878.

den Ouden, H. E., Frith, U., Frith, C., and Blakemore, S. J. 2005. Thinking about intentions. *NeuroImage* 28.4: 787–796.

Dimiralp, S., and Hoover, K. 2003. Searching for the causal structure of a vector autoregression. *Oxford Bulletin of Economics and Statistics* 65: 745.

Dodel, S., Golestani, N., Pallier, C., Elkouby, V., Le Bihan, D., and Poline, J. B. 2005. Condition-dependent functional connectivity: Syntax networks in bilinguals. *Philosophical Transactions of the Royal Society of London B: Biological Sciences* 360.1457: 921–935.

Dolan, R. J., Fink, G. R., Rolls, E., Booth, M., Holmes, A., Frackowiak, R. S. J., and Friston, K. J. 1997. How the brain learns to see objects and faces in an impoverished context. *Nature* 389: 596–598.

Donders, F. C. 1868/1969. On the speed of mental processes. (Trans. W. G. Koster). *Acta Psychologica* 30: 412–431.

Dora, E., and Kovach, A. G. B. 1982. Effect of acute arterial hypo- and hypertension on cerebro-cortical NAD/NADH redox state and vascular volume. *Journal of Cerebral Blood Flow & Metabolism* 2: 209–218.

Downing, P., Liu, J., and Kanwisher, N. 2001. Testing cognitive models of visual attention with fMRI and MEG. *Neuropsychologia* 12: 1329–1342.

Dretske, F. 1981. *Knowledge and the Flow of Information.* Cambridge, MA: MIT Press.

Drzezga, A., Grimmer, T., Peller, M., Wermke, M., Siebner, M., Rauschecker, J. P., et al. 2005. Impaired cross-modal inhibition in Alzheimer's Disease. *PLoS Medicine* 2: 288.

Duncan, J., and Owen, A. M. 2000. Common regions of the human frontal lobe recruited by diverse cognitive demands. *Trends in Neuroscience* 23.10: 475–483.

Dux, P. E., Ivanoff, J., Asplund, C. L., and Marois, R. 2006. Isolation of a central bottleneck of information processing with time-resolved fMRI. *Neuron* 52.6: 1109–1120.

Edelman, S., and Bulthoff, H. H. 1992. Orientation dependence in the recognition of familiar and novel views of three-dimensional objects. *Vision Research* 32: 2385–2400.

Eickhoff, S. B., Stephan, K. E., Mohlberg, H., Grefkes, C., Fink, G. R., Amunts, K., and Zilles, K. 2005. A new SPM toolbox for combining probabilistic cytoarchitectonic maps and functional imaging data. *NeuroImage* 25.4: 1325–1335.

Eisenberger, N. I., Lieberman, M. D., and Williams, K. D. 2003. Does rejection hurt? An FMRI study of social exclusion. *Science* 302.5643: 290–292.

Eldridge, L. L., Knowlton, B. J., Furmanski, C. S., Bookheimer, S. Y., and Engel, S. A. 2000. Remembering episodes: A selective role for the hippocampus during retrieval. *Nature Neuroscience* 3: 1149–1152.

Ellis, H. D. 2006. Delusions: A suitable case for imaging. *International Journal of Psychophysiology* 63: 146–151.

Elsner, J. B., and Tsonis, A. A. 1996. *Singular Spectrum Analysis: A New Tool in Time Series Analysis*. New York: Plenum Press.

Eme, P. E., and Marquer, J. 1999. Individual strategies in a spatial task and how they relate to aptitudes. *European Journal of Psychology of Education* 14: 89–108.

Epstein, R., and Kanwisher, N. 1998. A cortical representation of the local visual environment. *Nature* 392.6676: 598–601.

Farid, H. 2006. Digital doctoring: how to tell the real from the fake. *Significance* 3: 162–166.

Farid, H. 2009. Digital Doctoring: Can we trust photographs? In B. Harrington (Ed.) *Deception: From Ancient Empires to Internet Dating*. Palo Alto, CA: Stanford University Press.

Fischl, B., Rajendran, N., Busa, E., Augustinack, J., Hinds, O., et al. 2008. Cortical folding patterns and predicting cytoarchitecture. *Cerebral Cortex* 18.8: 1973–1980.

Fischl, B., Sereno, M. I., and Dale, A. M. 1999a. Cortical surface-based analysis: Inflation, flattening and a surface-based coordinate system. *NeuroImage* 9: 195–207.

Fischl, B., Sereno, M. I., Tootell, R. B., and Dale, A. M. 1999b. High-resolution intersubject averaging and a coordinate system for the cortical surface. *Human Brain Mapping* 8.4: 272–284.

Fisher, R. A., Williams, M., Lobo do Vale, R., Lola da Costa , A., & Meir, P. 2006. Evidence from Amazonian forests is consistent with isohydric control of leaf water potential. *Plant, Cell & Environment* 29.2: 151–165.

Flandin, G., Kherif, F., Pennec, X., Malandain, G., Ayache, N., and Poline, J. B. 2002a. Improved detection sensitivity of functional MRI data using a brain parcellation technique. In *Proceedings 5th*

International Conference on Medical Image Computing and Computer Assisted Intervention, LNCS 2488 (Part I, pp. 467–474. Tokyo: Springer Verlag.

Flandin, G., Kherif, F., Pennec, X., Rivière, D., Ayache, N., and Poline, J. B. 2002b. Parcellation of brain images with anatomical and functional constraints for fMRI data analysis. In: *Proceedings 1st International Symposium on Biomedical Imaging*: 907–910. Washington, DC.

Flandin, G., Penny, W., Pennec, X., Ayache, N., and Poline, J. B. 2003. A multisubject anatomo-functional parcellation of the brain. *NeuroImage* 19: 1600.

Fodor, J. A. 1983. *The Modularity of Mind: An Essay on Faculty Psychology*. Boston, MA: MIT Press.

Folstein, M., Folstein, S., and McHugh, P. R. 1975. Mini-mental state: A practical method of grading the cognitive state of patients for the clinician. *Journal of Psychiatric Research* 12: 189–198.

Forman, S. D., Cohen, J D., Fitzgerald, M., Eddy, W. F., Mintun, M. A., and Noll, D. C. 1995. Improved assessment of significant activation in functional magnetic resonance imaging (fMRI): Use of a cluster-size threshold. *Magnetic Resonance in Medicine* 33: 636–647.

Frackowiak, R., Friston, K., Frith, C., Dolan, R., and Maziotta, J. 1997. *Human Brain Function*. Burlington MA: Academic Press.

Friston, K. J. 2003. Learning and inference in the brain. *Neural Networks* 16: 1325–1352.

Friston, K. J., and Buchel, C. 2000. Attentional modulation of effective connectivity from V2 to V5/MT in humans. *Proceedings of the National Academy of Sciences U.S.A.* 97.13: 7591–7596.

Friston, K. J. Frith, C. D., Liddle, P. F. and Frickowiak, R. S. 1993. Functional connectivity: The principal component analysis of large (PET) data sets. *Journal of Cerebral Blood Flow & Metabolism* 13: 5.

Friston, K. J., Frith, C. D., Turner, R., and Frackowiak, R. S. J. 1995. Characterizing evoked hemo-dynamics with fMRI. *NeuroImage* 2: 157–165.

Friston, K. J., Harrison, L., and Penny, W. 2002. Dynamic causal modeling. *Neuroimage* 19: 1273–1302.

Friston, K. J., Holmes, A. P., Price, C. J., Buchel, C., and Worsley, K. J. 1999. Multisubject fMRI studies and conjunction analyses. *NeuroImage* 10: 385–396.

Friston K. J., Jezzard P., and Turner R. 1994. Analysis for functional MRI time-series. *Human Brain Mapping* 1: 153–171.

Friston, K. J., Mechelli, A., Turner, R., and Price, C. J. 2000. Nonlinear responses in fMRI : The Balloon model, Volterra kernels, and other hemodynamics. *NeuroImage* 12.4: 466–477.

Friston, K. J., Price, C. J., Buechel, C., and Frackowiak, R. S. J. 1997. A taxonomy of study design. In R. S. J. Frackowiak, K. J. Friston, C. D. Frith, R. J. Dolanm, and J. C. Mazziotta (Eds.), *Human Brain Function* (pp. 141–162). San Diego, CA: Academic Press.

Friston, K. J., Price, C. J., Fletcher, P., Moore, C., Frackowiak, R. S. J., and Dolan, R. J. 1996. The trouble with cognitive subtraction. *NeuroImage* 4: 97–104.

Friston, K. J., Rotshtein, P., Geng, J. J., Sterzer, P., and Henson, R. N. 2006. A critique of functional localisers. *NeuroImage* 30.4: 1077–1087.

Fujita, I., Tanaka, K., Ito, M., and Cheng, K. 1992. Columns for visual features of objects in monkey inferotemporal cortex. *Nature* 360: 343–346.

Gauthier, I., Skudlarski, P., Gore, J. C., and Anderson, A. W. 2000. Expertise for cars and birds recruits brain areas involved in face recognition. *Nature Neuroscience* 3: 191–197.

Gauthier, I., Tarr, M. J., Anderson, A. W., Skudlarski, P., and Gore, J. C. 1999. Activation of the middle fusiform 'face area' increases with expertise in recognizing novel objects. *Nature Neuroscience* 2: 568–573.

Gazzaniga, M. S., Ivry, R., and Mangun, G. R. 2002. *Cognitive Neuroscience: The Biology of the Mind* (2nd Ed.) New York: W. B. Norton and Co.

Genovese, C. R., Noll, D. C., and Eddy, W. F. 1997. Estimating test-retest reliability in functional MR imaging: Statistical methodology. *Magnetic Resonance in Medicine* 38.3: 497–507.

George, N., Dolan, R. J., Fink, G. R., Baylis, G. C., Russell, C., and Driver, J. 1999. Contrast polarity and face recognition in the human fusiform gyrus. *Nature Neuroscience* 2: 574–580.

Gilaie-Dotan, S., and Malach, R. 2007. Sub-exemplar shape tuning in human face-related areas. *Cerebral Cortex* 17.2: 325–338.

Gillath, O., Bunge, S. A., Shaver, P. R., Wendelken, C., and Mikulincer, M. 2005. Attachment-style differences in the ability to suppress negative thoughts: Exploring the neural correlates. *NeuroImage* 28.4: 835–847.

Gispert, J. D., Pascau, J., Reig, S., Martinez-Lazaro, R., Molina, V., Garcia-Barreno, P., et al. 2003. Influence of the normalization template on the outcome of statistical parametric mapping of PET scans. *NeuroImage* 19.3: 601–612.

Gläscher, J., Tuscher, O., Weiller, C., and Buchel, C. 2004. Elevated responses to constant facial emotions in different faces in the human amygdala: An fMRI study of facial identity and expression. *BMC Neuroscience* 5: 45.

Glasspool, D. W., Houghton, G., and Shallice, T. 1995. Interactions between knowledge sources in a dual-route connectionist model of spelling. In L. S. Smith and P. J. B. Hancock (Eds.), *Neural Computation and Psychology*. London: Springer-Verlag.

Glymour, C. 2003a. Learning, prediction and causal Bayes nets. *Trends in Cognitive Science* 7.1: 43–47.

Glymour, C. 2003b. *The Mind's Arrows: Bayes Nets and Graphical Causal Models*. Cambridge, MA: MIT Press.

Glymour, C., and Cooper, G. 1999. *Computation, Causation and Discovery*. Cambridge, MA: MIT/AAAI Press.

Goebel, R., Roebroeck, A., Kim, D. S., and Formisano, E. 2003. Investigating directed cortical inter-actions in time-resolved fMRI data using vector autoregressive modeling and Granger causality mapping. *Magnetic Resonance Imaging* 21: 1251–1261.

Golanov, E. V., Yamamoto, S., and Reis, D. J. 1994. Spontaneous waves of cerebral blood flow associated with a pattern of electrocortical activity. *American Journal of Physiology* 266: R204–214.

Golarai, G., Ghahremani, D. G., Whitfield-Gabrieli, S., Reiss, A., Eberhardt, J. L., Gabrieli, J. D., and Grill-Spector, K. 2007. Differential development of high-level visual cortex correlates with category-specific recognition memory. *Nature Neurosci*ence 10: 512–522.

Gonzaga, G. C., Keltner, D., Londahl, E. A., and Smith, M. D. 2001. Love and the commitment problem in romantic relations and friendship. *Journal of Personality and Social Psychology* 81.2: 247–262.

Gorno-Tempini, M. L., Price, C. J., Josephs, O., Vandenberghe, R., Cappa, S. F., Kapur, N., and Frackowiak, R. S. J. 1998. The neural systems sustaining face and proper-name processing. *Brain* 121: 2103–2118.

Grady, C. L., McIntosh, A. R., Horwitz, B., Maisog, J. M., Ungerleider, L. G., Mentis, M. J., et al. 1995. Age-related reductions in human recognition memory due to impaired encoding. *Science* 269.5221: 218–221.

Greene, J. D., Sommerville, R. B., Nystrom, L. E., Darley, J. M., and Cohen, J. D. 2001. An fMRI investigation of emotional engagement in moral judgement. *Science* 293: 2105–2107.

Greicius, M. D., Srivastava, G., Reiss, A. L., and Menon, V. 2004. Default-mode network activity distinguishes Alzheimer's disease from healthy aging: Evidence from functional MRI. *Proceedings of the National Academy of Sciences U. S. A* 101.13: 4637–4642.

Grill-Spector, K. 2006. Selectivity of adaptation in single units: Implications for FMRI experiments. *Neuron* 49: 170–171.

Grill-Spector, K., Henson, R., and Martin, A. 2006a. Repetition and the brain: Neural models of stimulus-specific effects. *Trends in Cognitive Science* 10: 14–23.

Grill-Spector, K., Knouf, N., and Kanwisher, N. 2004. The fusiform face area subserves face percep-tion not generic within category identification. *Nature Neuroscience* 7: 555–562.

Grill-Spector, K., Kushnir, T., Edelman, S., Avidan, G., Itzchak, Y., and Malach, R. 1999. Differen-tial processing of objects under various viewing conditions in the human lateral occipital com-plex. *Neuron* 24: 187–203.

Grill-Spector, K., Kushnir, T., Hendler, T., and Malach, R. 2000. The dynamics of object-selective activation correlate with recognition performance in humans. *Nature Neuroscience* 3: 837–843.

Grill-Spector, and K., Malach, R. 2001. fMR-adaptation: A tool for studying the functional proper-ties of human cortical neurons. *Acta Psychologica (Amsterdam)* 107.1–3: 293–321.

Grill-Spector, K., Sayres, R., and Ress, D. 2006b. High-resolution imaging reveals highly selective nonface clusters in the fusiform face area. *Nature Neuroscience* 9: 1177–1185.

Grova, C., Makni, S., Flandin, G., Ciuciu, P., Gotman, J., and Poline, J. B. 2007. Anatomically informed interpolation of fMRI data on the cortical surface. *NeuroImage* 31.4: 1475–1486.

Gurley, J. R., and Marcus, D. K. 2008. The effects of neuroimaging and brain injury on insanity defenses. *Behavioral Sciences and the Law* 26: 85–97.

Gusnard, D. A., and Raichle, M. E. 2001. Searching for a baseline: Functional imaging and the resting human brain. *Nature Reviews Neuroscience* 2: 685–694.

Halchenko, Y. O., Hanson, S. J., and Pearlmutter, B. A. 2004. Fusion of functional brain imaging modalities using L-norms signal reconstruction. *Annual Meeting of the Cognitive Neuroscience Society*, San Francisco, CA.

Hamilton, M. 1960. A rating scale for depression. *Journal of Neurology, Neurosurgery, & Psychiatry* 23: 56–62.

Hampson, M., Olson, I. R., Leung, H. C., Skuldarski, P., and Gore, J. C. 2004. Changes in functional connectivity of human MT/V5 with visual motion input. *Neuroreport* 7: 1315.

Hampson, M., Peterson, B. S., Skuldarski, P., and Gore, J. C. 2002. Changes in functional connectivity using temporal correlations in MR images. *Human Brain Mapping* 15: 247.

Hampton, A. N. Bossaerts, P., and O'Doherty, J. P. 2006. The role of the ventromedial prefrontal cortex in abstract state-based inference during decision making in humans. *Journal of Neuroscience* 26: 8360–8367.

Hanson, S. J., and Bly, B. M. 2001. The distribution of BOLD is non-Gaussian. *NeuroReport*: 1971–1977.

Hanson, S. J., and Halchenko, Y. 2008. Brain reading using full brain support vector machines for object recognition: There is no "face" identification area. *Neural Computation* 20.2: 486–503.

Hanson, S. J., Matsuka, T., Hanson, C., Rebbechi, D., Halchenko, Y., Zaimi, A., and Pearlmutter, B. 2007. Structural equation modeling of neuroimaging data: Exhaustive search and Markov Chain Monte Carlo. *Brain Structure & Function*.

Hanson, S. J, Matsuka, T., and Haxby, J. V. 2004a. Combinatorial codes in ventral medial temporal lobes for objects: Haxby (2001) revisited: Is there a face area?. *NeuroImage* 23.1: 156–166.

Hanson, S. J., and Timberlake, W. 1983. Regulation during challenge. *Psychological Review* 90.3: 261–282.

Hanson, S. J., Matsuka, T., and Haxby, J. V. 2004b. Combinatorial codes in ventral temporal lobe for object recognition: Haxby (2001) revisited: Is there a 'face' area? *NeuroImage* 23: 156–166.

Hanson, S. J., Rebbechi, D., Hanson, C., and Halchenko, Y. 2007. Dense mode clustering in brain maps. *Magnetic Resonance Imaging* 25.9: 1249–1262.

Hariri, A. R., Mattay, V. S., Tessitore, A., Kolachana, B., Fera, F., Goldman, D., et al. 2002. Serotonin transporter genetic variation and the response of the human amygdala. *Science* 297.5580: 400–403.

Harley, T. A. 1993. Phonological activation of semantic competitors during lexical access in speech production. *Language and Cognitive Processes* 8: 291–309.

Harley, T. A. 1995. *The Psychology of Language* (1st Ed.). London: Psychology Press.

Harley, T. A. 1998. The semantic deficit in dementia: Connectionist approaches to what goes wrong in picture naming. *Aphasiology* 12: 299–308.

Harley, T. A. 2004a. Does cognitive neuropsychology have a future? *Cognitive Neuropsychology* 21: 3–16.

Harley, T. A. 2004b. Promises, promises. Reply to commentators. *Cognitive Neuropsychology* 21: 51–56.

Harley, T. A. 2008. *The Psychology of Language* (3rd Ed.). London: Psychology Press.

Harr, J. 1995. *A Civil Action*. New York: Random House.

Harris, L. T., Todorov, A., and Fiske, S. T. 2005. Attributions on the brain: Neuro-imaging dispositional inferences, beyond theory of mind. *NeuroImage* 28.4: 763–769.

Hasher, L., Stoltzfus, E. R., Zacks, R. T., and Rypma, B. 1991. Age and inhibition. *Journal of Experimental Psychology* LMC. 17: 163–169.

Hasson, U., Hendler, T., Ben Bashat, D., and Malach, R. 2001. Vase or face? A neural correlate of shape-selective grouping processes in the human brain. *Journal of Cognitive Neuroscience* 13: 744–753.

Haxby, J. V., Gobbini, M. I., Furey, M. L., Ishai, A., Schouten, J. L., and Pietrini, P. 2001. Distributed and overlapping representations of faces and objects in ventral temporal cortex. *Science* 293.5539: 2425–2430.

Haxby, J. V., Ungerleider, L. G., Clark, V. P., Schouten, J. L., Hoffman, E. A., and Martin, A. 1999. The effect of face inversion on activity in human neural systems for face and object perception. *Neuron* 22: 189–199.

Hayasaka, S., and Nichols, T. E. 2003. Validating cluster size inference: Random field and permutation methods. *NeuroImage* 20.4: 2343–2356.

Haynes, J. -D. 2008. Detecting deception from neuroimaging signals—a data-driven perspective. *Trends in Cognitive Sciences* 12.4: 126–127.

Haynes, J. -D., Driver, J., and Rees, G. 2005. Visibility reflects dynamic changes of effective connectivity between V1 and fusiform cortex. *Neuron* 46: 811–821.

Haynes, J. -D., and Rees, G. 2005. Predicting the orientation of invisible stimuli for activity in human primary visual cortex. *Nature Neuroscience* 8.5: 686–691.

Haynes, J. -D., and Rees, G. 2006. Decoding mental states from brain activity in humans. *Nature Reviews Neuroscience* 7: 523–534.

Haynes, J. -D., Sakai, K., Rees, G., Gilbert, S., Frith, C., and Passingham, R. E. 2007. Reading hidden intentions in the human brain. *Current Biology* 17.4: 323–328.

Hayward, W. G., and Tarr, M. J. 2000. Differing views on views: Comments on Biederman and Bar (1999). *Vision Research* 40: 3895–3899.

Heberlein, A. S., and Saxe, R. R. 2005. Dissociation between emotion and personality judgments: Convergent evidence from functional neuroimaging. *NeuroImage* 28.4: 770–777.

Hempel, C. G. 1945. Studies in the logic of confirmation. Reprinted in *Aspects of Scientific Explanation*. London: Collier-Macmillan, 1965.

Henrich, J., Boyd, R., Bowles, S., Camerer, C., Fehr, E., Gintis, H., et al. 2001. In search of Homo economicus: Behavioral experiments in 15 small-scale societies. *American Economic Review* 91.2: 73–78.

Henson, R. N. A. 2005. What can functional imaging tell the experimental psychologist? *Quarterly Journal of Experimental Psychology* A. 58: 193–233.

Henson, R. N. A. 2006. Forward inference using functional neuroimaging: Dissociations versus associations. *Trends in Cognitive Sciences* 10.2: 64–69.

Henson, R. N. A., Shallice, T., and Dolan, R. 2000. Neuroimaging evidence for dissociable forms of repetition priming. *Science* 287.5456: 1269–1272.

Henson, R. N. A., Shallice, T., Gorno Tempini, M. L., and Dolan, R. J. 2002. Face repetition effects in implicit and explicit memory tests as measured by fMRI. *Cerebral Cortex* 12: 178–186.

Herrmann, C. S., Lenz, D., Junge, S., Busch, N. A., and Maess, B. 2004. Memory-matches evoke human gamma-responses. *BMC Neuroscience* 5: 13.

Hofstadter, D. R. 1995. The architecture of Jumbo. In D. R. Hofstadter, *Fluid Concepts & Creative Analogies: Computer Models of the Fundamental Mechanisms of Thought*. New York: Basic Books.

Holstege, G., Georgiadis, J. R., Paans, A. M. J., Meiners, L. C., van der Graaf, F. H. C. E., and Reinders, A. A. T. S. 2003. Brain activation during human male ejaculation. *Journal of Neuroscience* 23.27: 9185–9193.

Horton, J. C., Dagi, L. R., McCrane, E. P., and de Monasterio, F. M. 1990. Arrangement of ocular dominance columns in human visual cortex. *Archives of Ophthalmology* 108: 1025–1031.

Horwitz, B. 1994. Neural modeling and positron emission tomography. In R. W. Thatcher (Ed.). *Functional Neuroimaging: Technical Foundations*. San Diego, CA: Academic Press.

Horwitz, B., Tagamets, M-A., and McIntosh, A. R. 1999. Neural modeling, functional brain imaging, and cognition. *Trends in Cognitive Sciences* 3: 91–98.

Houdé, O., and Tzourio-Mazoyer, N. 2003. Neural foundations of logical and mathematical cognition. *Nature Reviews Neuroscience* 4: 507–514.

Hudetz, A. G., Roman, R. J., and Harder, D. R. 1992. Spontaneous flow oscillations in the cerebral cortex during acute changes in mean arterial pressure. *Journal of Cerebral Blood Flow & Metabolism* 12: 491.

Hudetz, A. G., Smith, J. J., Lee, J. G., Bosnjak, Z. J., and Kampine, J. P. 1995. Modification of cerebral laser-Doppler flow oscillations by halothane, PCO2, and nitric oxide synthase blockade. *American Journal of Physiology 269, Heart and Circulatory Physiology* 38: H114.

Hyde, J. S., and Biswal, B. 2000. *Functionally Related Correlation in the Noise.* Berlin: Springer Verlag.

James, T. W., Culham, J. C., Humphrey, G. K., Milner, A. D., and Goodale, M. A. 2003. Ventral occipital lesions impair object recognition but not object-directed grasping: An fMRI study. *Brain* 126.11: 2475–2763.

James, W. 1890. *Principles of Psychology, Vol. 1.* New York: Henry-Holt and Co.

Jennings, J. M., McIntosh, A. R., Kapur, S., Tulving, E., and Houle, S. 1997. Cognitive subtractions may not add up: The interaction between semantic processing and response mode. *NeuroImage* 5: 229–239.

Jernigan, T. L., Gamst, A. C., Fennema-Notestine, C., and Ostergaard, A. L. 2003. More "mapping" in brain mapping: Statistical comparison of effects. *Human Brain Mapping* 19.2: 90–95.

Jesmanowicz, A., Bandettini, P. A, and Hyde, J. S. 1998. Single-shot half k-space high resolution gradient recalled EPI for FMRI at 3 Tesla. *Magnetic Resonance in Medicine* 40: 754–762.

Jezzard, P., LeBihan, D., Cuenod, D., Pannier, L., Prinster, A. and Turner, R. 1993. An investigation of the contribution of physiological noise in human functional MRI studies at 1.5 tesla and 4 tesla. *Proceedings of SMRM, 12th Annual Meeting* (1392). New York.

Jiang, X., Rosen, E., Zeffiro, T., Vanmeter, J., Blanz, V., and Riesenhuber, M. 2006. Evaluation of a shape-based model of human face discrimination using FMRI and behavioral techniques. *Neuron* 50: 159–172.

Jiang, Y., and Kanwisher, N. 2003. Common neural mechanisms for response selection and perceptual processing. *Journal of Cognitive Neuroscience* 15.8: 1095–1110.

Jiang, Y., Saxe, R., and Kanwisher, N. 2004. Functional magnetic resonance imaging provides new constraints on theories of the psychological refractory period. *Psychological Science* 15.6: 390–396.

Jobsis, F. F., Keizer, J. H., LaManna, J. C., and Rosenthal, M. 1977. Reflectance spectrophotometry of cytochrome aa$_3$ in vivo. *Journal of Applied Physiology* 43: 858–872.

Johansen-Berg, H., Behrens, T. E., Robson, M. D., Drobnjak, I., Rushworth, M. F., Brady, J. M., et al. 2004. Changes in connectivity profiles define functionally distinct regions in human medial frontal cortex. *Proceedings of the National Academy of Science U.S.A.* 101.36: 13335–13340.

Johnson-Laird, P. N. 2001. Mental models and human reasoning. In E. Dupoux, *Language, Brain, and Cognitive Development: Essays in Honor of Jacques Mehler.* Cambridge, MA: MIT Press.

Joreskog, K. G., and Sorbom, D. 1989. *LISREL 7: A Guide to the Program Applications* (2nd Ed.). Chicago: SPSS.

Kamitani, Y., and Tong, F. 2005. Decoding the visual and subjective contents of the human brain. *Nature Neuroscience* 8.5: 679–685.

Kanwisher, N. G., McDermott, J., and Chun, M. M. 1997. The fusiform face area: A module in human extrastriate cortex specialized for face perception. *Journal of Neuroscience* 17.11: 4302–4311.

Kanwisher, N., Woods, R. P., Iacoboni, M., and Mazziotta, J. C. 1997. A locus in human extrastriate cortex for visual shape analysis. *Journal of Cognitive Neuroscience* 9.1: 133–142.

Kanwisher, N., and Yovel, G. 2006. The fusiform face area: A cortical region specialized for the perception of faces. *Philosophical Transactions of the Royal Society of London B: Biological Sciences* 361: 2109–2128.

Kariman, K., and Burkhart, D. C. 1985. Non-invasive in vivo spectrophotometric monitoring of brain cytochrome aa$_3$ revisited. *Brain Research* 360: 203–213.

Kay, K. N., Naselaris, T., Prenger, R. J., and Gallant, J. L. 2008. Identifying natural images from human brain activity. *Nature* 452: 352–355.

Kennedy, D. P., Redcay, E., and Courchesne, E. 2006. Failing to deactivate: Resting functional abnormalities in autism. *Proceedings of the National Academy of Science U.S.A.* 103.21: 8275–8280.

Kherif, F., Poline, J. B., Meriaux, S., Benali, H., Flandin, G., and Brett, M. 2004. Group analysis in functional neuroimaging: Selecting subjects using similarity measures. *NeuroImage* 20.4: 2197–2208.

Kiani, R., Esteky, H., Mirpour, K., and Tanaka, K. 2007. Object category structure in response patterns of neuronal population in monkey inferior temporal cortex. *Journal of Neurophysiology* 97: 4296–4309.

Knoch, D., Pascual-Leone, A., Meyer, K., Treyer, V., and Fehr, E. 2006. Diminishing reciprocal fairness by disrupting the right prefrontal cortex. *Science* 314.5800: 829–832.

Koechlin, E., Ody, C., and Kouneiher, F. 2003. The architecture of cognitive control in the human prefrontal cortex. *Science* 302: 1181–1185.

Kötter, R., and Wanke, E. 2005. Mapping brain without coordinates. *Philosophical Transactions of the Royal Society of London B: Biological Sciences* 360: 751–766.

Kourtzi, Z., and Kanwisher, N. 2001. Representation of perceived object shape by the human lateral occipital complex. *Science* 293.5534: 1506–1509.

Kreiman, G., Koch, C., and Fried, I. 2000. Category-specific visual responses of single neurons in the human medial temporal lobe. *Nature Neuroscience* 3: 946–953.

Kriegeskorte, N., Mur, M., Ruff, D. A., Kiani R., Bodurka, J., Esteky, H., et al. 2008. Matching categorical object representations in inferior temporal cortex of man and monkey. *Neuron* 60: 1126–1141.

Kruggel, F., and Yves von Cramon, D. 1999. Alignment of magnetic-resonance brain datasets with the stereotactical coordinate system. *Medical Image Analysis* 3.2: 175–185.

Kuhn, T. 1962. *The Structure of Scientific Revolutions*. Chicago: University of Chicago Press.

Kulvicki, J. 2006. *On Images: Their Structure and Content*. New York: Oxford University Press.

Kwong, K. K., Belliveau, J. W., Chesler, D. A., Goldberg, I. A., Weisskoff, R. M., Poncelet, B. P., et al. 1992. Dynamic magnetic resonance imaging of human brain activity during primary sensory stimulation. *Proceedings of the National Academy of Sciences U.S.A.* 89: 5675–5679.

LaConte, S., Anderson, J., Muley, S., Ashe, J., Frutiger, S., Rehm, K., et al. 2003. The evaluation of preprocessing choices in single-subject BOLD fMRI using NPAIRS performance metrics. *NeuroImage* 18.1: 10–27.

Lamme, V. A. 2003. Why visual attention and awareness are different. *Trends in Cognitive Science* 7: 12–18.

Lauritzen, S. 2002. *Graphical Models*. New York: Oxford University Press.

Lautrey, J. 2002. A pluralistic approach to cognitive differentiation and development. In R. J. Steinberg, J. Lautrey, and T. Lubart (Eds), *Models of Intelligence: International Perspectives*. Washington DC: American Psychological Association.

LeBars, P., Katz, M., Berman, N., et al. 1997. A placebo-controlled, double-blind, randomized trial of an extract of gingko biloba for dementia. *JAMA* 278: 1327–1332.

Leonard, M., Eckert, M. A., and Kuldau, J. M. 2006. Exploiting human anatomical variability as a link between genome and cognome. *Genes, Brain and Behavior* 5. S1: 64–77.

Leopold, D. A., and Wilke, M. 2005. Neuroimaging: Seeing the trees for the forest. *Current Biology* 15.8: R766–R768.

Levasseur, J. E., Wei, E. P., Raper, A. J., Kontos, H. A., and Patterson, J. L. 1975. Detailed description of a cranial window technique for acute and chronic experiments. *Stroke 6:* 308–317.

Lewandowsky, S., and Farrell, S. 2002. Computational models of working memory. In L. Nadel, D. Chalmers, P. Culicover, R. Goldstone, and B. French (Eds.), *Encyclopedia of Cognitive Science* (pp. 578–583). London: Macmillan.

Li, S. J., Biswal, B., Li, Z., Risinger, R., Rainey, C., Cho, J. K., et al. 2000. Cocaine administration decreases functional connectivity in human primary visual and motor cortex as detected by functional MRI. *Magnetic Resonance in Medicine* 43: 43–45.

Liou, M., Su, H. -R., Lee, J. -D., Aston, J. A. D., Tsai, A., and Cheng, P. E. 2006. A method for generating reproducible evidence in fMRI studies. *NeuroImage* 29.2: 383–395.

Liou, M., Su, H. R., Lee, J. D., Cheng, P. E., Huang, C. C., and Tsai, C. H. 2003. Bridging functional MR images and scientific inference: Reproducibility maps. *Journal of Cognitive Neuroscience* 15.7: 935–945.

Liu, W. C., Schulder, M., Narra, V., Kalnin, A. J., Cathcart, C., Jacobs, A., et al. 2000. Functional magnetic resonance imaging aided radiation treatment planning. *Medical Physics* 27: 1563–1572.

Logan, G. D. 1990. Repetition priming and automaticity: Common underlying mechanisms? *Cognitive Psychology* 22: 1–35.

Logie, R. H., Della Salla, S., Laiacona, M., Chalmers, P., and Wynn, V. 1996. Group aggregates and individual reliability: The case of short term memory. *Memory and Cognition* 24: 305–331.

Logothetis, N. K. 2003. The underpinnings of the BOLD functional magnetic resonance imaging signal. *Journal of Neuroscience* 23.10: 3963–3971.

Logothetis, N. K. 2008. What we can do and what we cannot do with fMRI. *Nature* 453.7197: 869–878.

Logothetis, N. K., and Pfeuffer, J. 2004. On the nature of the BOLD fMRI contrast mechanism. *Magnetic Resonance Imaging* 22.10: 1517–1531.

Logothetis, N. K., and Sheinberg, D. L. 1996. Visual object recognition. *Annual Review of Neuroscience* 19: 577–621.

Logothetis, N. K., and Wandell, B. A. 2004. Interpreting the BOLD signal. *Annual Review of Physiology* 66: 735–769.

Lohmann, G., and Bohn, S. 2002. Using replicator dynamics for analyzing fMRI data of the human brain. *IEEE Transactions on Medical Imaging* 21.5: 485–492.

Loosemore, R. P. W. 2007. Complex systems, artificial intelligence and theoretical psychology. In B. Goertzel and P. Wang, *Proceedings of the 2006 AGI Workshop*. Amsterdam: IOS Press.

Lowe, M. J., Davidson, R. J., and Orendi, J. 1997a. Intra-hemispheric functional connectivity of FMRI physiological noise correlations: Dependence on attention. *Proceedings of the 5th ISMRM* (p. 1688). Vancouver.

Lowe, M. J., Rutecki, P., Turski, P., Woodard, A., and Sorenson, J. 1997b. Auditory cortex FMRI noise correlations in callosal agenesis. *NeuroImage* 5: S194.

Luo, W. L., and Nichols, T. E. 2003. Diagnosis and exploration of massively univariate neuroimaging models. *NeuroImage* 19.3: 1014–1032.

Madden, D. J., Whiting, W. L., Huettel, S. A., White, L. E., MacFall, J. R., and Provenzale, J. M. 2004. Diffusion tensor imaging of adult age differences in cerebral white matter: Relation to response time. *NeuroImage* 21: 1174–1181.

Malach, R., Reppas, J. B., Benson, R. R., Kwong, K. K., Jiang, H., Kennedy, W. A., et al. 1995. Object-related activity revealed by functional magnetic resonance imaging in human occipital cortex. *Proceedings of the National Academy of Sciences U.S.A.* 92: 8135–8139.

Mandler, G. 2005. The consciousness continuum: From "qualia" to "free will. " *Psychological Research* 69: 330–337.

Mariano, A. J., Chin, T. M., and Özgökmen, T. M. 2003. Stochastic boundary conditions for coastal flow modeling. *Geophysical Research Letters* 30.9: 1457.

Mangin JF, Rivière D, Cachia A, Duchesnay E, Cointepas Y, Papadopoulos-Orfanos D, Scifo P, Ochiai T, Brunelle F, Régis J. 2004. A framework to study the cortical folding patterns. *Neuroimage* 23 Suppl 1: S129–38.

Martinez, J. M., Frouin, V., and Régis, J. 2002. Automatic recognition of cortical sulci of the human brain using a congregation of neural networks. *Medical Image Analysis* 6.2: 77–92.

Mayevsky, A., and Ziv, I. 1991. Oscillations of cortical oxidative metabolism and microcirculation in the ischemic brain. *Neurological Research* 13: 39–47.

McCabe, D. P., and Castel, A. D. 2008. Seeing is believing: The effect of brain images on judgments of scientific reasoning. *Cognition* 107.1: 343–352.

McCauley, R. N. 2007. Reduction: Models of cross-scientific relations and their implications for the psychology-neuroscience interface. In P. Thagard (Ed.*), Handbook of the Philosophy of Science: Philosophy of Psychology and Cognitive Science* (pp. 105–158). New York: Elsevier.

McCauley, R. N., and Bechtel, W. 2001. Explanatory pluralism and heuristic identity theory. *Theory and Psychology* 11.6: 736–760.

McClelland, J. L. 1979. On the time relations of mental processes: An examination of systems in cascade. *Psychological Review* 86: 287–330.

McClelland, J. L., Rumelhart, D. E., and Hinton, G. E. 1986. The appeal of parallel distributed processing. In D. E. Rumelhart, J. L. McClelland, G. E. Hinton, and the PDP Research Group, *Parallel Distributed Processing: Explorations in the Microstructure of Cognition, Vol. 1*. Cambridge, MA: MIT Press.

McGeer, P. L., McGeer, E. G., Akiyama. H, et al. 1990. Neuronal degeneration and memory loss in Alzheimer's disease and aging. In: *The Principles of Design and Operation of the Brain* (pp. 411–426). Berlin: Springer.

Mcgonigle, D. J., Howseman, A. M., Athwal, B. S., Friston, K. J., Frackowiak, R. S. J., and Holmes, A. P. 2000. Variability in fMRI: An examination of intersession differences. *NeuroImage* 11.6: 708–734.

McIntosh, A. R. 1999. Mapping cognition to the brain through neural interactions. *Memory* 7.5/6: 523–548.

McIntosh, A. R. 2000. Towards a network theory of cognition. *Neural Networks* 13: 861–876.

McIntosh, A. R., Bookstein, F. L., Haxby, J. V., and Grady, C. L. 1996. Spatial pattern analysis of functional brain images using partial least squares. *NeuroImage* 3: 143–157.

McIntosh, A. R., and Gonzalez-Lima, F. 1995. Functional network interactions between parallel auditory pathways during Pavlovian conditioned inhibition. *Brain Research* 683.2: 228–241.

McIntosh, A. R., Grady, C. L., Ungerleider, L. G., Haxby, J. V., Rapoport, S. I., and Horwitz, B. 1994. Network analysis of cortical visual pathways mapped with PET. *Journal of Neuroscience* 14.2: 655–666.

McIntosh, A. R., Rajah, M. N., and Lobaugh, N. J. 1999. Interactions of prefrontal cortex in relation to awareness in sensory learning. *Science* 284: 1531–1533.

McKhann, G., Drachman, O., Folstein, M., et al. 1984. Clinical diagnosis of Alzheimer's disease: Report of the NINCDS-ADRDA work group. *Neurology* 34: 939–944.

Mechelli, A., Penny, W. D., Price, C. J., Gitelman, D. R., and Friston, K. J. 2002. Effective connectivity and intersubject variability: Using a multisubject network to test differences and commonalities. *NeuroImage* 17.3: 1459–1469.

Mechelli, A., Price, C. J., Noppeney, U., and Friston, K. J. 2003. A dynamic causal modelling study on category effects: Bottom-up or top-down mediation? *Journal of Cognitive Neuroscience* 15: 925–934.

Mériaux, S., Roche, A., Thirion, B., and Dehaene-Lambertz, G. 2006. Robust statistics for nonparametric group analysis in fMRI. *Proceedings of the 3rd IEEE ISBI*, Arlington, VA.

Meskin, A., and Cohen, J. 2006. Spatially agnostic informants and the epistemic status of photography. In S. Walden (Ed.), *Blackwell Guide to Photographs*. New York: Blackwell.

Miller, J., and Hackley, S. A. 1992. Electrophysiological evidence for temporal overlap among contingent mental processes. *Journal of Experimental Psychology: General* 121: 195–209.

Miller, M. B., Van Horn, J. D., Wolford, G. L., Handy, T. C., Valsangkar-Smyth, M., Inati, S., et al. 2002. Extensive individual differences in brain activations associated with episodic retrieval are reliable over time. *Journal of Cognitive Neuroscience* 14.8: 1200–1214.

Mitchell, J. P., Banaji, M. R., and Macrae, C. N. 2005. General and specific contributions of the medial prefrontal cortex to knowledge about mental states. *NeuroImage* 28.4: 757–762.

Mitchell T. M., Shinkareva S. V., Carlson A., Chang K. M., Malave V. L., Mason R. A., and Just M. A. 2008 Predicting human brain activity associated with the meanings of nouns. *Science* 320: 1191–1195.

Mobbs, D., Hagan, C. C., Azim, E., Menon, V., and Reiss, A. L. 2005. Personality predicts activity in reward and emotional regions associated with humor. *Proceedings of the National Academy of Science U.S.A.* 102.45: 16502–16506.

Mole, C., Kubatzky, C., Plate, J., Waller, R., Dobbs, M., and Nardone, M. 2007. Faces and brains: The limitations of brain scanning in cognitive science. *Philosophical Psychology* 20.2: 197–207.

Moutoussis, K., and Zeki, S. 2002. The relationship between cortical activation and perception investigated with invisible stimuli. *Proceedings of the National Academy of Sciences U.S.A.* 99: 9527–9532.

Mukamel, R., Gelbard, H., Arieli, A., Hasson, U., Fried, I., and Malach, R. 2005. Coupling between neuronal firing, field potentials, and fMRI in human auditory cortex. *Science* 309.5736: 951–954.

Mumford, J. A., and Nichols, T. E. 2008. Power calculation for group fMRI studies accounting for arbitrary design and temporal autocorrelation. *NeuroImage* 39: 261–268.

Munk, M., and Neuenschwander, S. 2000. High-frequency oscillations (20 to 120 Hz) and their role in visual processing. *Journal of Clinical Neurophysiology* 17.4: 341–360.

Murphy, K., and Garavan, H. 2004. An empirical investigation into the number of subjects required for an event-related fMRI study. *NeuroImage* 22.2: 879–885.

Murray, S. O., Kersten, D., Olshausen, B. A., Schrater, P., and Woods, D. L. 2002. Shape perception reduces activity in human primary visual cortex. *Proceedings of the National Academy of Sciences U.S.A.* 99: 15164–15169.

Nee, D. E., Wager, T. D., and Jonides, J. 2007. Interference resolution: Insights from a meta-analysis of neuroimaging tasks. *Cognitive, Affective, & Behavioral Neuroscience* 7: 1–17.

Ng, M., Ciaramitaro, V. M., Anstis, S., Boynton, G. M., and Fine, I. 2006. Selectivity for the configural cues that identify the gender, ethnicity, and identity of faces in human cortex. *Proceedings National Academy of Science U.S.A.* 103: 19552–19557.

Nichols, T., and Hayasaka, S. 2003. Controlling the familywise error rate in functional neuroimaging: A comparative review. *Statistical Methods in Medical Research* 12.5: 419–446.

Nielsen, F. A. 2003. The Brede database: A small database for functional neuroimaging. Presented at the *9th International Conference on Functional Mapping of the Human Brain*, New York, NY.

Norman, K. A., Polyn, S. M., Detre, G. J., and Haxby, J. V. 2006. Beyond mind-reading: Multi-voxel pattern analysis of fMRI data. *Trends in Cognitive Sciences* 10.9: 424–430.

Norris, D., and McQueen, J. M. 2008. Shortlist B: A Bayesian model of continuous speech recognition. *Psychological Review* 115: 357–395.

Nyberg, L., Marklund, P., Persson, J., Cabeza, R., Forkstam, C., Petersson, K. M., and Ingvar, M. 2003. Common prefrontal activations during working memory, episodic memory, and semantic memory. *Neuropsychologia* 41: 371–377.

Oakes, T. R., Johnstone, T., Ores Walsh, K. S., Greischar, L. L., Alexander, A. L., Fox, A. S., and Davidson, R. J. 2005. Comparison of fMRI motion correction software tools. *NeuroImage* 28.3: 529–543.

Ogawa, S., Lee, T., Kay, A., and Tank, D. 1990. Brain magnetic resonance imaging with contrast dependent on blood oxygenation. *Proceedings of the National Academy of Sciences U.S.A.* 87.24: 9868–9872.

Ogawa, S., Tank, D. W., Menon, R., Ellermann, J. M., Kim, S. G., Merkle, H., and Ugurbil, K. 1992. Intrinsic signal changes accompanying sensory stimulation: Functional brain mapping with magnetic resonance imaging. *Proceedings of the National Academy of Sciences U.S.A.* 89: 5951–5955.

Olsson, R. K., and Hansen, L. K. 2006. Linear state-space models for blind source separation. *Journal of Machine Learning Research* 6: 2585–2602.

O'Toole, A. J., Jiang, F., Abdi, H., and Haxby, J. V. 2005. Partially distributed representations of objects and faces in ventral temporal cortex. *Journal of Cognitive Neuroscience* 17.4: 580–590.

O'Toole, A. J., Jiang, F., Abdi, H., Pernard, N., Dunlop, J. P., and Parent, M. A. 2007. Theoretical, statistical, and practical perspectives on pattern-based classification approaches to the analysis of functional neuroimaging data. *Journal of Cognitive Neuroscience* 18: 1735–1752.

Owen, A. M., Coleman, M. R., Boly, M., Davis, M. H., Laureys, S., and Pickard, J. D. 2006a. Detecting awareness in the vegetative state. *Science* 313: 1402.

Owen, A. M., Epstein, R., and Johnsrude, I. S. 2006b. fMRI: Applications to cognitive neuroscience. In P. Jezzard, P. M. Matthews, and S. M. Smith (Eds.), *Functional MRI: An Introduction to Methods* (pp. 311–328). New York: Oxford University Press.

Owen, A. M., McMillan, K. M., Laird, A. R., and Bullmore, E. 2005. N-back working memory paradigm: A meta-analysis of normative functional neuroimaging studies. *Human Brain Mapping* 25: 46–59.

Ozcan, M., Baumgartner, U., Vucurevic, G., Stoeter, P., and Treede, R. D. 2005. Spatial resolution of fMRI in the human parasylvian cortex: Comparison of somatosensory and auditory activation. *NeuroImage* 25.3: 877–887.

Paus, T. 1996. Location and function of the human frontal eye-field: A selective review. *Neuropsychologia* 34.6: 475–483.

Pearl, J. 2000. *Causality*. New York: Oxford University Press.

Pearl, J., and Dechter, R. 1995. Identifying independencies in causal graphs with feedback. *Proceedings of the 1995 Conference on Uncertainty in Artificial Intelligence.*

Pecher, D., Zeelenberg, R., and Barsalou, L. W. 2004. Sensorimotor simulations underlie conceptual representations: Modality-specific effects of prior activation. *Psychonomic Bulletin & Review* 11.1: 164–167.

Peelen, M. V., and Downing, P. E. 2005. Within-subject reproducibility of category-specific visual activation with functional MRI. *Human Brain Mapping* 25.4: 402–408.

Penny, W., Stephan, K. E., Mechelli, A., and Friston, K. J. 2004. Modelling functional integration: A comparison of structural equation and dynamic causal models. *NeuroImage* 23.S1: S264–S274.

Peretz, I., and Coltheart, M. 2003. Modularity of music processing. *Nature Neuroscience* 6: 688–691.

Perini, L. 2005. Explanation in two dimensions: Diagrams and biological explanation. *Biology and Philosophy* 20.2: 257–269.

Pessoa, L., McKenna, M., Gutierrez, E., and Ungerleider, L. G. 2002. Neural processing of emotional faces requires attention. *Proceedings of the National Academy of Sciences U.S.A.* 99.17: 11458–11463.

Pessoa, L., and Padmala, S. 2007. Decoding near-threshold perception of fear from distributed single-trial brain activation. *Cerebral Cortex* 17: 691–701.

Peters, A., and Sethares, C. 2004. Oligodendrocytes, their progenitors, and other neuroglial cells in the aging primate cortex. *Cerebral Cortex* 14: 995–1007.

Petersen, S. E., and Fiez, J. A. 1993. The processing of single words studied with positron emission tomography. *Annual Review of Neuroscience* 16: 509–530.

Petersen, S. E., Fox, P. T., Posner, M. I., Mintun, M., and Raichle, M. E. 1988. Positron emission tomographic studies of the cortical anatomy of single-word processing. *Nature* 331: 585–589.

Petersen, S. E., van Mier, H., Fiez, J. A., and Raichle, M. E. 1998. The effects of practice on the functional anatomy of task performance. *Proceedings of the National Academy of Sciences U.S.A.* 95: 853–860.

Piazza, M., Pinel, P., Le Bihan, D., and Dehaene, S. 2007. A magnitude code common to numerosities and number symbols in human intraparietal cortex. *Neuron* 53.2: 293–305.

Pinel, P., Thirion, B., Mériaux, S., Jobert, A., Serres, J., Le Bihan, D., Poline, J. B., Dehaene, S. 2007. Fast reproducible identification and large-scale databasing of individual functional cognitive networks. *BMC Neuroscience* 31.8: 91.

Plaut, D. C., McClelland, J. L., Seidenberg, M. S., and Patterson, K. E. 1996. Understanding normal and impaired word reading: Computational principles in quasi-regular domains. *Psychological Review* 103: 56–115.

Poeppel, D. 1996. A critical review of PET studies of phonological processing. *Brain and Language* 55: 317–351; discussion: 352–385.

Poggio, T., and Edelman, S. 1990. A network that learns to recognize three-dimensional objects. *Nature* 343: 263–266.

Poldrack, R. A. 2006. Can cognitive processes be inferred from neuroimaging data? *Trends in Cognitive Sciences* 10.2: 59–63.

Poldrack, R. A. 2007. Region of interest analysis for fMRI. *Social Cognitive and Affective Neuroscience* 2.1: 67–70.

Poldrack, R. A, Fletcher, P. C, Henson, R. N., Worsley, K. J., Brett, M., and Nichols, T. E. 2008. Guidelines for reporting an fMRI study. *NeuroImage* 40.2: 409–414.

Poldrack, R. A., and Mumford, J. A. (2009). Independence in ROI analysis: Where's the voodoo? *Social,Cognitive, and Affective Neuroscience* 4: 208–213.

Poldrack, R. A., Sabb, F. W., Foerde, K., Tom, S. M., Asarnow, R. F., Bookheimer, S. Y., and Knowlton, B. J. 2005. The neural correlates of motor skill automaticity. *Journal of Neuroscience* 25: 5356–5364.

Poldrack, R. A., Halchenko, Y., and Hanson, S. J. in press. Decoding the large-scale structure of brain function by classifying mental states across individuals. *Psychological Science.*

Poldrack, R. A., Wagner, A. D., Prull, M. W., Desmond, J. E., Glover, G. H., and Gabrieli, J. D. E. 1999. Functional specialization for semantic and phonological processing in the left inferior frontal cortex. *NeuroImage* 10: 15–35.

Poline, J. B., Strother, S., Dehaene-Lambertz, G., and Lancaster, J. 2006. Motivation and synthesis of the FIAC experiment: The reproducibility of fMRI results across expert analyses. *Human Brain Mapping* 27.5: 351–359.

Polyn, S. M., Natu, V. S., Cohen ,J. D., and Norman, K. A. 2005. Category-specific cortical activity precedes retrieval during memory search. *Science* 310: 1963–1966.

Popper, K. R. 1959. *The Logic of Scientific Discovery*. London: Hutchinson.

Posner, M. I., and Petersen, S. E. 1990. The attention system of the human brain. *Annual Review of Neuroscience* 13: 25–42.

Poupon, C., Clark, C., Frouin., V., Regis, J., Bloch, I., Le Bihan, D., and Mangin, J. F. 2000. Regularization of diffusion-based direction maps for the tracking of brain white matter fascicles. *NeuroImage* 12: 184–195.

Price, C. J., and Friston, K. J. 1997. Cognitive conjunction: A new approach to brain activation experiments. *NeuroImage* 5: 261–270.

Price, C. J., Friston, K. J. 2002. Degeneracy and cognitive anatomy. *Trends in Cognitive Sciences* 6: 416–421.

Quiroga, R. Q., Reddy, L., Kreiman, G., Koch, C., and Fried, I. 2005. Invariant visual representation by single-neurons in the human brain. *Nature* 435.7045: 1102–1107.

Racine, E., Bar-Ilan, F., and Illes, J. 2006. Brain imaging: A decade of coverage in the print media. *Science Communication* 28.1: 122–142.

Raichle, M., MacLeod, A., Snyder, A., Powers, W., Gusnard, D., and Shulman, G. 2001. Blood flow and oxygen delivery to human brain during functional activity. Theoretical modeling and experimental data. *Proceedings of the National Academy of Sciences U.S.A.* 98.12: 6859–6864.

Raichle, M. E., and Mintun, M. A. 2006. Brain work and brain imaging. *Annual Review of Neuroscience* 29: 449–476.

Raizada, R. D., and Poldrack, R. A. 2007. Selective amplification of stimulus differences during categorical processing of speech. *Neuron* 56: 726–740.

Ramus, F. 2006. Genes, brain, and cognition: A roadmap for the cognitive scientist. *Cognition* 101: 247–269.

Rao, S. M., Binder, J. R., Bandettini, P. A., Hammeke, T. A., Yetkin, F. Z., Jesmanowicz, A., et al. 1993. Functional magnetic resonance imaging of complex human movements. *Neurology* 43: 2311.

Rapoport, S. I. 1988. Brain evolution and Alzheimer's disease. *Review of Neurology (Paris)* 144: 79–90.

Reddy, L., and Kanwisher, N. 2007. Category selectivity in the ventral visual pathway confers robustness to clutter and diverted attention. *Current Biology* 17: 1–6.

Rees, G., Frith, C. D., and Lavie, N. 1997. Modulating irrelevant motion perception by varying attentional load in an unrelated task. *Science* 278.5343: 1616–1619.

Reisberg, B., Pattschull-Furlan, A., Franssen, E., et al. 1992. Dementia of the Alzheimer type recapitulates ontogeny inversely on specific ordinal and temporal parameters. In: I. Kostovic, S. Knezevic, and H. M. Wiesniewski, H. M. (Eds.), *Neurodevelopment, Aging and Cognition* (pp. 345–369). Boston: Birkhauser.

Reuchlin, M. 1999. *Evolution de la Psychologie Differentielle*. Paris: Press Universitaire de France.

Richardson, R. C. 2009. Multiple realization and methodological pluralism. *Synthese* 167: 473–492.

Richardson, T. 1996. Graphical Models for Time Series, Ph. D Thesis, Carnegie Mellon University, Pittsburgh, PA.

Richardson, T., and Sprites, P. 1999. Automated discover of linear feedback models. In C. Glymour, and G. Cooper (Eds.), *Computation, Causation and Discovery*. Cambridge, MA: MIT/AAAI Press.

Richardson, T., and Spirtes, P. 2002. Ancestral graph Markov models. *Annals of Statistics* 30: 962–1030.

Richardson, T., and Spirtes, P. 2003. Causal inference via ancestral graph models. In P. Green, N. Hjort, and S. Richardson (Eds.), *Highly Structured Stochastic Systems*. New York: Oxford University Press.

Rivière, D., Mangin, J. F., Papadopoulos-Orfanos, D., Martinez, J.-M., Frouin, V. and Régis, J.. 2002. Automatic recognition of cortical sulci of the human brain using a congregation of neural networks, *Medical Image Analysis* 6.2: 77–92.

Robins, J., Scheines, R., Spirtes, P., and Wasserman, L. 2003. Uniform consistency in causal inference. *Biometrika* 90: 491–515.

Roche, A., Mériaux, S., Keller, M., and Thirion, B. 2007. Mixed-effect statistics for group analysis in fMRI: a nonparametric maximum likelihood approach. *Neuroimage* 38: 501–510.

Roelofs, A. 1997. The WEAVER model of word-form encoding in speech production. *Cognition* 64: 249–284.

Roland, P. E., Larsen, B., Lassen, N. A., and Skinhøj, E. 1980. Supplementary motor areas and other cortical areas in organization of voluntary muscle movements in man. *Journal of Neurophysiology* 43: 118.

Rombouts, S., and Schelten, P. 2005. Functional connectivity in elderly controls and AD patients using resting state fMRI: A pilot study. *Current Alzheimer Research* 2: 115–116.

Rosen, W. G., Terry, R. D., Fuld, P. A., Katzman, R., and Peck A. 1979. Pathological verification of ischemic score in differentiation of dementias. *Annals of Neurology* 7: 486–488.

Roskies, A. L. 2007. Are neuroimages like photographs of the brain? *Philosophy of Science* 74: 860–872.

Roskies, A. L. 2008. Neuroimaging and inferential distance. *Neuroethics* 1.1: 19–30.

Roskies, A. L., and Petersen, S. E. 2001. Visualizing human brain function. In E. Bizzi, P. Calissano and V. Volterra (Eds.), *Frontiers of Life: The Intelligent Systems, Vol. 3:* 87–109. Burlington, MA: Academic Press.

Rosler, A., Mapstone, M., Hays-Wicklund, A., Gitelman, D. R., and Weintraub, S. 2005. The "zoom lens" of focal attention in visual search: Changes in aging and Alzheimer's disease. *Cortex 41*: 512–519.

Rotshtein, P., Henson, R. N., Treves, A., Driver, J., and Dolan, R. J. 2005. Morphing Marilyn into Maggie dissociates physical and identity face representations in the brain. *Nature Neuroscience* 8: 107–113.

Ruff, C. C., Blankenburg, F., Bjoertomt, O., Bestmann, S., Freeman, E., Haynes, J. D., et al. 2006. Concurrent TMS-fMRI and psychophysics reveal frontal influences on human retinotopic visual cortex. *Current Biology* 16.15: 1479–1488.

Rypma, B., Berger, J. S., Genova, H., Rebbechi, D., and D'Esposito, M. 2005. Dissociating age-related changes in cognitive strategy and neural efficiency using event-related fMRI. *Cortex* 41: 582–594.

Rypma, B., and D'Esposito, M. 2000. Isolating the neural mechanisms of age-related changes in human working memory. *Nature Neuroscience* 3: 509–515.

Rypma, B., Prabhakaran, V., Desmond, J. E., and Gabrieli, J. D. E. 2001. Age differences in prefrontal cortical activity in working memory. *Psychology and Aging* 16: 371–384.

Sander, D., Grandjean, D., Pourtois, G., Schwartz, S., Seghier, M. L., Scherer, K. R., et al. 2005. Emotion and attention interactions in social cognition: Brain regions involved in processing anger prosody. *NeuroImage* 28.4: 848–858.

Sanfey, A. G., Rilling, J. K., Aronson, J. A., Nystrom, L. E., and Cohen, J. D. 2003. The neural basis of economic decision-making in the ultimatum game. *Science* 300.5626: 1755–1758.

Sartori, G., and Umilta, C. 2000. How to avoid the fallacies of cognitive subtraction in brain imaging. *Brain and Language* 74: 191–212.

Sawamura, H., Orban, G., and Vogels, R. 2006. Selectivity of neuronal adaptation does not match response selectivity: A single cell study of the fMRI adaptation paradigm. *Neuron* 49: 307–318.

Saxe, R., Brett, M., and Kanwisher, N. 2006. Divide and Conquer: A Defence of Functional Localisers. *NeuroImage* 30.4: 1088–1096.

Saxe, R., Jamal, N., and Powell, L., in press. My body or yours? The effect of visual perspective on cortical body representations. *Cerebral Cortex*.

Saxe, R., and Powell, L., in press. It's the thought that counts: Specific brain regions for one component of Theory of Mind. *Psychological Science*.

Sayres, R., and Grill-Spector, K. 2006. Object-selective cortex exhibits performance-independent repetition suppression. *Journal of Neurophysiology* 95: 995–1007.

Scheines, R. 2003. In S. Turner, and V. McKim (Eds.), *Causality in Crisis*. South Bend, IN: University of Notre Dame Press.

Schuchard, R. A., Cummings, R. W., Ross, D., and Watson, G. 2003. Comparison of SLO perimetry, binocular perimetry, and functional visual field perimetry in patients with macular scotomas. *ARVO Annual Meeting* 44: 2778.

Schwarzlose, R. F., Baker, C. I., and Kanwisher, N. K. 2005. Separate face and body selectivity on the fusiform gyrus. *Journal of Neuroscience* 25: 11055–11059.

Sereno, M. I., Dale, A. M., Reppas, J. B., Kwong, K. K., Belliveau, J. W., Rosen, B. R., and Tootell, R. B. H. 1995. Borders of multiple visual areas in humans revealed by functional magnetic resonance imaging. *Science* 268: 889–893.

Sergent, J., Zuck, E., Levesque, M., and MacDonald, B. 1992. Positron emission tomography study of letter and object processing: Empirical findings and methodological considerations. *Cerebral Cortex* 2: 68–80.

Shallice, T. 1998. *From Neuropsychology to Mental Structure*. New York: Cambridge University Press.

Shallice, T., Marzocchi, G. M., Coser, S., Del Savio, M., Meuter, R. F., and Rumiati, R. I. 2002. Executive function profile of children with attention deficit hyperactivity disorder. *Developmental Neuropsychology* 21: 43–71.

Shimizu, S., Hyvärinen, A., Kano, Y., and Hoyer, P. O. 2005. Discovery of non-gaussian linear causal models using ICA. In *Proceedings of the 21st Conference on Uncertainty in Artificial Intelligence* 526–533.

Shmuel, A., Augath, M., Oeltermann, A., and Logothetis, N. K. 2006. Negative functional MRI response correlates with decreases in neuronal activity in monkey visual area V1. *Nature Neuroscience* 9.4: 569–577.

Shmuel, A., Yacoub, E., Chaimow, D., Logothetis, N. K., and Ugurbil, K. 2007. Spatio-temporal point-spread function of fMRI signal in human gray matter at 7 Tesla. *NeuroImage* 35: 539–552.

Shuman, M., and Kanwisher, N. 2004. Numerical magnitude in the human parietal lobe: Tests of representational generality and domain specificity. *Neuron* 44.3: 557–569.

Silva, R., Scheines, R., Glymour, C., and Spirtes, P. 2006 Learning the Structure of Linear Latent Variable Models. *Journal of Machine Learning Research* 7: 191–246.

Silvanto, J., Cowey, A., Lavie, N., and Walsh, V. 2005. Striate cortex (V1) activity gates awareness of motion. *Nature Neuroscience* 8.2: 143–144.

Simmons, W. K., Matlis, S., Bellgowan, P. S., Bodurka, J., Barsalou, L. W., and Martin, A. 2006. Imaging the context-sensitivity of ventral temporal category representations using high-resolution fMRI. *Society for Neuroscience Abstracts*.

Simmons, W. K., Ramjee, V., Beauchamp, M. S., McRae, K., Martin, A., and Barsalou, L. W. 2007. A common neural substrate for perceiving and knowing about color. *Neuropsychologia* 45.12: 2802–2810.

Simon, O., Kherif, F., Flandin, G., Poline, J. B., Riviere, D., Mangin, J. F., et al. 2004. Automatized clustering and functional geometry of human parietofrontal networks for language, space, and number. *NeuroImage* 23.3: 1192–1202.

Skinner, B. F. 1963. Behaviorism at fifty. *Science* 140: 951–958.

Skudlarski, P., and Gore, J. C. 1998. Changes in the correlations in the FMRI physiological fluctuations may reveal functional connectivity within the brain. *NeuroImage* 3: S600.

Slotnick, S. D., Schwarzbach, J., and Yantis, S. 2003. Attentional inhibition of visual processing in human striate and extrastriate cortex. *NeuroImage* 19: 1602–1611.

Smith, S. M., Beckmann, C. F., et al. 2005. Variability in fMRI: A re-examination of inter-session differences. *Human Brain Mapping* 24.3: 248–257.

Solomon, K. O., and Barsalou, L. W. 2004. Perceptual simulation in property verification. *Memory & Cognition* 32.2: 244–259.

Soon, C. S., Brass, M., Heinze, H.-J., and Haynes, J.-D. 2008. Unconscious determinants of free decisions in the human brain. *Nature Neuroscience* 11.5: 543–545.

Spiridon, M., Fischl, B., and Kanwisher, N. 2005. Location and spatial profile of category-specific regions in human extrastriate cortex. *Human Brain Mapping* 27. 77–89.

Spiridon, M., and Kanwisher, N. 2002. How distributed is visual category information in human occipito-temporal cortex? An fMRI study. *Neuron* 35: 1157–1165.

Spirtes, P. 1995. In P. Besnard and S. Hanks (Eds.), *Proceedings of the Eleventh Conference on Uncertainty in Artificial Intelligence*. San Mateo, CA: Morgan Kaufmann Publishers.

Spirtes, P. 1997. Limits on Causal Inference from Statistical Data. Paper presented at American Economics Association Meeting.

Spirtes, P. 2001. *Proceedings of AI and Statistics*.

Spirtes, P., Glymour, C., and Scheines, R. 2000. *Causation, Prediction, and Search* (2nd Ed.). Cambridge, MA: MIT Press.

Spirtes, P., Meek, C., and Richardson, T. 1996a. *Technical Report CMU-77-Phil*.

Spirtes, P., and Richardson, T. 1996. *Proceedings of the 6th International Workshop on Artificial Intelligence and Statistics*.

Spirtes, P., Richardson, T., and Meek, C. 1996b. *Proceedings of the 6th International Workshop on Artificial Intelligence and Statistics*.

Spirtes, P., Richardson, T., Meek, C. 1997a. *Technical Report CMU-83-Phil*.

Spirtes, P., Richardson, T., Meek, C., Scheines, R., and Glymour, C. 1996c. Using D-separation to calculate zero partial correlations in linear models with correlated errors. *Technical Report CMU-72-Phil*.

Spirtes, P., Richardson, T., Meek, C., Scheines, R., and Glymour, C. 1997b. *Technical Report CMU-82-Phil.*

Sporns, O., Chialvo, D. R., Kaiser, M., and Hilgetag, C. C. 2004. Organization, development and function of complex brain networks. *Trends in Cognitive Sciences* 8: 418–425.

Squire, L. R., Ojemann, J. G., Miezin, F. M., Petersen, S. E., Videen, T. O., and Raichle, M. E. 1992. Activation of the hippocampus in normal humans: A functional anatomical study of memory. *Proceedings of the National Academy of Sciences U.S.A.* 89: 1837–1841.

Stark, C. E., and Squire, L. R. 2001. When zero is not zero: The problem of ambiguous baseline conditions in fMRI. *Proceedings of the National Academy of Sciences U.S.A.* 98: 12760–12766.

Sternberg, S. 1969. The discovery of processing stages: Extension of Donders method. *Acta Psychologica* 30: 276–315.

Strauss, T. J., Harris, H. D., and Magnuson, J. S. 2007. jTRACE: A reimplementation and extension of the TRACE model of speech perception and spoken word recognition. *Behavior Research Methods, Instruments, & Computers* 39: 19–30.

Strother, S. C., Anderson, J., Hansen, L. K., Kjems, U., Kustra, R., Sidtis, J., et al. 2002. The quantitative evaluation of functional neuroimaging experiments: The NPAIRS data analysis framework. *NeuroImage* 15.4: 747–71.

Summerfield, C., Egner, T., Greene, M., Koechlin, E., Mangels, J., and Hirsch, J. 2006. Predictive codes for forthcoming perception in the frontal cortex. *Science* 314.5803: 1311–1314.

Sumner, P., Tsai, P. C., Yu, K., and Nachev, P. 2006. Attentional modulation of sensorimotor processes in the absence of perceptual awareness. *Proceedings of the National Academy of Sciences U.S.A.* 103.27: 10520–10525.

Swallow, K. M., Braver, T. S., Snyder, A. Z., Speer, N. K., and Zacks, J. M. 2003. Reliability of functional localization using fMRI. *NeuroImage* 20.3: 1561–1577.

Talairach, J., and Tournoux, P. 1988. *Co-Planar Stereotaxic Atlas of the Human Brain*: 122. New York: Verlag.

Tanaka, K. 2003. Columns for complex visual object features in the inferotemporal cortex: Clustering of cells with similar but slightly different stimulus selectivities. *Cerebral Cortex* 13: 90–99.

Tarr, M. J., and Bulthoff, H. H. 1995. Is human object recognition better described by geon structural descriptions or by multiple views? Comment on Biederman and Gerhardstein (1993). *Journal of Experimental Psychology: Human Perception and Performance* 21: 1494–1505.

Tarr, M. J., Williams, P., Hayward, W., and Gauthier, I. 1998. Three-dimensional object recognition is viewpoint dependent. *Nature Neuroscience* 1: 275–277.

Thatcher, R. W., Hallet, M., Zeffiro, T., John, E. R., Huerta, M., Jennings, J. M., et al. 1998. Mapping neural interactivity onto regional activity: An analysis of semantic processing and response mode interactions. *NeuroImage* 7.3: 244–254.

Thirion, B., Flandin, G., Pinel, P., Roche, A., Ciuciu, P., and Poline, J. B. 2006a. Dealing with the shortcomings of spatial normalization: Multi-subject parcellation of fMRI datasets. *Human Brain Mapping* 27.8: 678–698.

Thirion, B., Roche, A. Ciuciu, P., and Poline, J. B. 2006b. Improving sensitivity and reliability of fMRI group studies through high level combination of individual subjects results. *Proceedings of the 2006 Conference on Computer Vision and Pattern Recognition Workshop* (p. 62). IEEE Computer Society, Washington, DC.

Thirion, B., Pinel, P., Mériaux, S., Roche, A., Dehaene, S., and Poline, J. B. 2007a. Analysis of a large fMRI cohort: Statistical and methodological issues for group analyses. *NeuroImage* 35.1: 105–120.

Thirion, B., Pinel, P., and Poline, J. B. 2005. Finding landmarks in the functional brain: Detection and use for group characterization. *Proceedings of MICCAI*, Palm Springs.

Thirion, B., Pinel, P., Tucholka, A., Roche, A., Ciuciu, P., Mangin, J. F., and Poline, J. B. 2007b. Structural analysis of fMRI data revisited: Improving the sensitivity and reliability of fMRI group studies. *IEEE Transactions on Medical Imaging* 26.9: 1256–1269.

Thompson, D. J. 1982. Spectral Estimation and harmonic analysis. *IEEE Proceedings* 70: 1055.

Thompson, D. J. 1990. Quadratic-inverse spectrum estimates: Applications to paleoclimatology. *Philosophical Transactions of the Royal Society of London* 332A: 539.

Thompson, J. C., Hardee, J. E., Panayiotou, A., Crewther, D., and Puce, A. 2007. Common and distinct brain activation to viewing dynamic sequences of face and hand movements. *NeuroImage* 37.3: 966–973.

Thyreau, B., Thirion, B., Flandin, G., and Poline, J. B. 2006. Anatomo-functional description of the brain: A probabilistic approach. *ICASP*, Toulouse.

Tobler, P., Fletcher, P., Bullmore, E., and Schultz, W. 2007. Learning-related human brain activations reflecting individual finances. *Neuron* 54: 167–175.

Todd, J. J., and Marois, R. 2004. Capacity limit of visual short-term memory in human posterior parietal cortex. *Nature* 428.6984: 751–754.

Toga, A. W. 2002. Neuroimage databases: The good, the bad and the ugly. *Nature Reviews Neuroscience* 3.4: 302–309.

Tom, S. M., Fox, C. R., Trepel, C., and Poldrack, R. A. 2007. The neural basis of loss aversion in decision-making under risk. *Science* 315.5811: 515–518.

Tong, F., Nakayama, K., Vaughan, J. T., and Kanwisher, N. 1998. Binocular rivalry and visual awareness in human extrastriate cortex. *Neuron* 21. 753–759.

Tootell, R. B., Reppas, J. B., Kwong, K. K., Malach, R., Born, R. T., Brady, T. J., et al. 1995. Functional analysis of human MT and related visual cortical areas using magnetic resonance imaging. *Journal of Neuroscience* 15.4: 3215–3230.

Tootell, R. B. H., Hadjikhani, N. K., Vanduffel, W., Liu, A. K., Mendola, J. D., Sereno, M. I., and Dale, A. M. 1998. Functional analysis of primary visual cortex (V1) in humans. *Proceedings of the National Academy of Sciences U.S.A.* 95: 811–817.

Treisman, A. 1991. Search, similarity and the integration of features between and within dimensions. *Journal of Experimental Psychology: Human Perception and Performance* 27: 652–676.

Tsao, D. Y., Freiwald, W. A., Tootell, R. B., and Livingstone, M. S. 2006. A cortical region consisting entirely of face-selective cells. *Science* 311: 670–674.

Tune, L., Brandt, J., Frost, J. J., Harris, G., et al. 1991. Physostigmine in Alzheimer's disease: Effects on cognitive functioning, cerebral glucose metabolism analyzed by positron emission tomography and cerebral blood flow analyzed by single phonon emission tomography. *Acta Psychiatrica Scandinavica* 366S: 61–65.

Turkeltaub, P. E., Eden, G. F., Jones, K. M., and Zeffiro, T. A. 2002. Meta-analysis of the functional neuroanatomy of single-word reading: Method and validation. *NeuroImage* 16: 765–780.

Uttal, W. R. 2000. *The War Between Mentalism and Behaviorism.* Mahwah, NJ: Lawrence Erlbaum Associates.

Uttal, W. R. 2001. *The New Phrenology: The Limits of Localizing Cognitive Processes in the Brain.* Cambridge, MA: MIT Press.

Vaidya, C. J., Austin, G., Kirkorian, G., Ridlehuber, H. W., Desmond, J. E., Glover, G. H., and Gabrieli, J. D. E. 1999. Selective effects of methylphenidate in attention deficit hyperactivity disorder: A functional magnetic resonance study. *Proceedings of the National Academy of Sciences U.S.A.* 95: 14494–14499.

Vaidya, C. J., Bunge, S. A., Dudukovic, N. M., Zalecki, C. A., Elliott, G. R., and Gabrieli, J. D. E. 2005. Altered Neural Substrates of Cognitive Control in Childhood ADHD: Evidence from Functional Magnetic Resonance Imaging. *American Journal of Psychiatry* 162: 1605–1613.

van Essen, D. C., and Gallant, J. L. 1994. Neural mechanisms of form and motion processing in the primate visual system. *Neuron* 13: 1–10.

Van Orden, G. C., and Paap, K. R. 1997. Functional neuroimages fail to discover pieces of mind in parts of the brain. *Philosophy of Science* 64: S85–S94.

van Turennout, M., Ellmore, T., and Martin, A. 2000. Long-lasting cortical plasticity in the object naming system. *Nature Neuroscience* 3: 1329–1334.

Verhaeghen, P., and Basak, C. 2005. Ageing and switching of the focus of attention in working memory: Results from a modified N-back task. *Quarterly Journal of Experimental Psychology A* 58: 134–154.

Vern, B. A., LaGuardia, J., Leheta, B. I., Schuette, W. H., and Juel, V. C. 1997a. Correlation of increases in cortical blood volume and cytochrome aa3 oxidation with enhanced electrographic activity and eye movement bursts during REM sleep in cats. *Annals of Neurology* 42: 458.

Vern, B. A., Leheta, B. J., Juel, V. C., LaGuardia, J., Graupe, P., and Schuette, W. H. 1998. Slow oscillations of cytochrome oxidase redox state and blood volume in unanesthetized cat and rabbit cortex: Interhemispheric synchrony. *Advances in Experimental Medicine and Biology* 454: 561–570.

Vern, B. A., Leheta, B. J., Juel, V. C., LaGuardia, J., Graupe, P., and Scuette, W. H. 1997b. Interhemispheric synchrony of slow oscillations of cortical blood volume and cytochrome aa_3 redox state in unanesthetized rabbits. *Brain Research* 775: 233–239.

Vern, B. A., Schuette, W. H., Juel, V. C., and Radulovacki, M. 1987. A simplified method for monitoring the cytochrome aa3 redox state in bilateral cortical areas of unanesthetized cats. *Brain Research* 415: 188–193.

Vern, B. A., Schuette, W. H., Leheta, B., Radulovacki, M., and Juel, V. 1988. Low frequency oscillation of cortical oxidative metabolism in waking and sleep. *Cerebral Blood Flow & Metabolism* 8: 215–226.

Vuilleumier, P., Henson, R. N., Driver, J., and Dolan, R. J. 2002. Multiple levels of visual object constancy revealed by event-related fMRI of repetition priming. *Nature Neuroscience* 5: 491–499.

Vul, E., Harris, C., Winkielman, P., and Pashler, H. 2009. Puzzlingly high correlations in fMRI studies of emotion, personality, and social cognition. *Perspectives on Psychological Science.*

Wager, T. D., Keller, M. C., Lacey, S. C., and Jonides, J. 2005. Increased sensitivity in neuroimaging analyses using robust regression. *NeuroImage* 26.1: 99–113.

Wager, T. D., and Smith, E. E. 2003. Neuroimaging studies of working memory: a meta-analysis. *Cognitive, Affective, and Behavioral Neuroscience* 3: 255–274.

Wagner, A. D., Schacter, D. L., Rotte, M., Koutstaal, W., Maril, A., Dale, A. M., et al. 1998. Building memories: Remembering and forgetting of verbal experiences as predicted by brain activity [see comments]. *Science* 281: 1188–1191.

Wallis, G., and Bulthoff, H. 1999. Learning to recognize objects. *Trends in Cognitive Sciences* 3: 22–31.

Walton, K. 1984. Transparent pictures: On the nature of photographic realism. *Critical Inquiry* 11: 246–276.

Wandell, B. A. 1999. Computational neuroimaging of human visual cortex. *Annual Review of Neuroscience* 22: 145–173.

Warnking, J. Dojat, M., Guérin-Dugué, A., Delon-Martin, C., Olympieff, S., Richard, N., Chéhikian, A., and Segebarth, C. 2002. fMRI retinotopic mapping—Step by step. *NeuroImage* 17: 1665–1683.

Wei, X., Yoo, S. S., Dickey, C. C., Zou, K. H., Guttmann, C. R. G., and Panych, L. P. 2004. Functional MRI of auditory verbal working memory: Long-term reproducibility analysis. *NeuroImage* 21.3: 1000–1008.

Weisberg, D. S., Keil, F. C., Goodstein, J., Rawson, E., and Gray, J. R. 2008. The seductive allure of neuroscience explanations. *Journal of Cognitive Neuroscience* 20.3: 470–477.

Weisskoff, R. M., Baker, J., Belliveau, J., Davis, T. L., Kwong, K. K., Cohen, M. S., and Rosen, B. R. 1993. Poser spectrum analysis of functionally-weighted MR data: What's in the noise? *Proceedings of the SMRM, 12th Annual Meeting* (p. 7). New York.

White, T., O'Leary, D., Magnotta, V., Arndt, S., Flaum, M., and Andreasen, N. C. 2001. Anatomic and functional variability: The effects of filter size in group fMRI data analysis. *NeuroImage* 13.4: 577–588.

Williams, M. A., Baker, C. I., Op de Beeck, H. P., Shim, W. M., Dang, S., Triantafyllou, C., and Kanwisher, N. G. 2008. Feedback of visual object information to foveal retinotopic cortex. *Nature Neuroscience* 11: 1439–1445.

Williams, M. A., Dang, S., and Kanwisher, N. G. 2007. Only some spatial patterns of fMRI response are read out in task performance. *Nature Neuroscience* 10: 685–686.

Wimsatt, W. C. 2007. *Re-engineering Philosophy for Limited Beings: Piecewise Approximations to Reality*. Cambridge, MA: Harvard University Press.

Winston, J. S., O'Doherty, J., Kilner, J. M., Perrett, D. I., and Dolan, R. J. 2007. Brain systems for assessing facial attractiveness. *Neuropsychologia* 45.1: 195–206.

Winterer, G., Hariri, A. R., Goldman, D., and Weinberger, D. R. 2005. Neuroimaging and human genetics. Genes, Cognition and Psychosis Program, National Institute of Mental Health National Institutes of Health, Bethesda, Maryland. *International Review of Neurobiology* 67: 325–383.

Wohlschlager, A. M., Specht, K., Lie, C., Mohlberg, H., Wohlschlager, A., Bente, K., et al. 2005. Linking retinotopic fMRI mapping and anatomical probability maps of human occipital areas V1 and V2. *NeuroImage* 26.1: 73–82.

Wollheim, R. 1987. *Painting as an Art*. Princeton, NJ: Princeton University Press.

Wong, E. C., Boskamp, E., and Hyde, J. S. 1992. A volume optimized quadrature elliptical endcap birdcage brain coil. *Proceedings of the ISMRM, 11th Annual Meeting* (p. 401). Berlin.

Wong, E. C., and Hyde, J. S. 1997. The design of surface gradient coil for MRI. *Proceedings of the SMRM, 10th Annual Meeting* (p. 346). New York.

Wong-Riley, W., Antuono, P., Ho, K. C., Egan, R., Hevner, R., Liebl, W., et al. 1997. Cytochrome oxidase in Alzheimer's disease: biochemical, histochemical and immunohistochemical analyses of the visual and other systems. *Vision Research* 37: 3593–3608.

Woolrich, M. 2008. Robust group analysis using outlier inference. *NeuroImage* 41.2: 286–301.

Worsley, K. J., Liao, C. H., Aston, J., Petre, V., Duncan, G. H., Morales, F., and Evans, A. C. 2002. A general statistical analysis for f[MRI] data. *NeuroImage* 15.1: 1–15.

Worsley, K. J., Marrett, S., Neelin, P., Vandal, A. C., Friston, K. J., and Evans, A. C. 1996. A unified statistical approach or determining significant signals in images of cerebral activation. *Human Brain Mapping* 4: 58–73.

Xiong, J., Parsons, L. M., Gao, J. H., and Fox, P. T. 1999. Interregional connectivity to primary motor cortex revealed using MRI resting state images. *Human Brain Mapping* 8.2–3: 151–156.

Xiong, J., Parson, L. M., Pu, Y., Gao, J. H., and Fox, P. T. 1998. Improved inter-regional connectivity mapping by use of covariance analysis within rest condition. *Proceedings of the 6th ISMRM* (p. 1480). Sydney, Australia.

Xu, Y. 2005. Revisiting the role of the fusiform face area in visual expertise. *Cerebral Cortex* 15.8: 1234–1242.

Yacoub, E., Shmuel, A., Logothetis, N., and Ugurbil, K. 2007. Robust detection of ocular dominance columns in humans using Hahn Spin Echo BOLD functional MRI at 7 Tesla. *NeuroImage* 37: 1161–1177.

Yoo, S. S., Hu, P. T., Gujar, N., Jolesz, F. A., and Walker, M. P. 2007. A deficit in the ability to form new human memories without sleep. *Nature Neuroscience* 10.3: 385–392.

Yovel, G., and Kanwisher, N. 2004. Face perception: Domain specific, not process specific. *Neuron* 44.5: 747–748.

Yule, G. U. 1971. *The Statistical Papers of George Udny Yule*. Santa Ana, CA: Griffin Publishers.

Zhang, J. 2006. Causal Discovery in Causally Insufficient Systems. PhD Thesis, Carnegie Mellon University, Pittsburgh, PA.

Zilles, K., Palomero-Gallagher, N., and Schleicher, A. 2004. Transmitter receptors and functional anatomy of the cerebral cortex. *Journal of Anatomy* 205.6: 417–432.

Zonta, M., Angulo, M. C., Gobbo, S., Rosengarten, B., Hossmann, K. A., Pozzan, T., and Carmignoto, G. 2003. Neuron-to-astrocyte signaling is central to the dynamic control of brain microcirculation. *Nature Neuroscience* 6: 43–50.

Contributors

William Bechtel   Department of Philosophy, University of California, San Diego, La Jolla, California

Bharat Biswal   Department of Radiology, University of Medicine and Dentistry of New Jersey, Newark, New Jersey

Matthew Brett   MRC Cognition and Brain Sciences Unit, Cambridge University, Cambridge, United Kingdom

Martin Bunzl   Department of Philosophy, Rutgers University, Newark, New Jersey

Max Coltheart   Macquarie Centre for Cognitive Science, Macquarie University, Sydney, Australia

Karl J. Friston   Wellcome Trust Centre for Neuroimaging, University College London, London, United Kingdom

Joy J. Geng   Institute of Cognitive Neuroscience, University College London, London, United Kingdom

Clark Glymour   Department of Philosophy, Carnegie Mellon University, Pittsburg, Pennsylvania

Kalanit Grill-Spector   Department of Psychology and Neuroscience Institute, Stanford University, Sanford, California

Stephen José Hanson   Department of Psychology, Rutgers University, Newark, New Jersey

Trevor Harley   School of Psychology, University of Dundee, Dundee, United Kingdom

Gilbert Harman   Department of Philosophy, Princeton University, Princeton, New Jersey

James V. Haxby   Department of Psychology, Dartmouth College, Hanover, New Hampshire

Rik N. Henson Department of Neuroscience, University of Cambridge, Cambridge, United Kingdom

Nancy Kanwisher McGovern Institute for Brain Research, Massachusetts Institute of Technology, Cambridge, Massachusetts

Colin Klein Philosophy Department, University of Illinois at Chicago, Chicago, Illinois

Richard Loosemore Surfing Samurai Robots, Inc., Genoa, New York

Sébastien Meriaux Neurospin, I2BM, CEA, Gif-sur-Yvette, France

Christopher Mole Department of Philosophy at the University of British Columbia, British Columbia, Canada

Jeanette A. Mumford Department of Psychology, University of California, Los Angeles, Los Angeles, California

Russell A. Poldrack Department of Psychology, University of California, Los Angeles, Los Angeles, California

Jean-Baptiste Poline Neurospin, I2BM, CEA, Gif-sur-Yvette, France

Richard C. Richardson Department of Philosophy, University of Cincinnati, Cincinnati, Ohio

Alexis Roche Neurospin, I2BM, CEA, Gif-sur-Yvette, France and ETHZ, Zurich, Switzerland

Adina L. Roskies Department of Philosophy, Dartmouth College, Hanover, New Hampshire

Pia Rotshtein School of Psychology, University of Birmingham, Birmingham, United Kingdom

Rebecca Saxe Saxelab, Massachusetts Institute of Technology, Cambridge, Massachusetts

Philipp Sterzer Department of Psychiatry, Charité Campus Mitte, Berlin, Germany

Bertrand Thirion Institut National de Recherche en Informatique en Automatique, Neurospin, Gif-sur-Yvette, France

Edward Vul Department of Brain and Cognitive Sciences, Massachusetts Institute of Technology, Cambridge, Massachusetts

Index